Endocrinology of the Heart

Editors: W. Kaufmann and G. Wambach

With 122 Figures and 36 Tables

Springer-Verlag
Berlin Heidelberg New York
London Paris Tokyo Hong Kong

Prof. Dr. W. Kaufmann
Prof. Dr. G. Wambach
Medizinische Klinik II und Poliklinik der Universität
Ostmerheimer Straße 200
D-5000 Köln 91

ISBN-13:978-3-540-51409-1 e-ISBN-13:978-3-642-83858-3
DOI: 10.1007/978-3-642-83858-3

Library of Congress Cataloging-in-Publication Data
Endocrinology of the heart / editors, W. Kaufmann and G. Wambach.
p. cm.
Articles chiefly in English; 2 articles in German.
Includes bibliographical references.
ISBN-13:978-3-540-51409-1 (U.S.)
1. Atrial natriuretic peptides–Physiological effect. 2. Heart–Physiology. 3. Heart–Pathophysiology. 4. Endocrine glands–Diseases–Complications and sequelae. I. Kaufmann, Werner, 1924- II. Wambch, G.
[DNLM: 1. Heart–physiology. 2. Heart Diseases–physiopathology. 3. Natriuretic Peptides, Atrial. WG 202 E56]
QP572.A82E53 1989
616.1'7–dc20
DNLM/DLC
for Library of Congress 89-21677
CIP

2127/3335-543210

Table of Contents

ANP in Healthy Volunteers

ANP and Cardiac Diseases

Thyroid Hormones and the Heart

Sympathetic Activity and the Heart

The Heart in Various Endocrine Systems

Author's Addresses

Prof. Dr. Klaus Addicks
Anatomisches Institut
Joseph-Stelzmann-Str. 9
D-5000 Köln 41

Prof. Dr. Peter H. Althoff
Klinikum der Joh.-W.-Goethe-Universität
Zentrum der Inneren Medizin
Theodor-Stern-Kai
D-6000 Frankfurt a.M. 70

Dr. R. H. A. Becker
Hoechst AG
Department of Cardiology
H 821
D-6230 Frankfurt/Main

Dr. Michael Böhm
Ludwig-Maximilian-Universität
Klinikum Großhadern
Med. Klinik, Forschungslab. B
Marchioninistr. 15
D-8000 München 70

Dr. G. Brabant
Medizinische Hochschule Hannover
Abt. für Klin. Endokrinologie
Konstanty-Gutschow-Straße 8
D-3000 Hannover 61

Dr. Paul Brugger
Abt. f. Gesundheitsvorsorge der PVARB
Faberstr. 29
A-5021 Salzburg

Dr. Neil Butkow
University of the Witwatersrand
Medical School
7 York Road
SA-2193 Johannesburg

Dr. Fritz Casper
Universit.-Frauenklinik
Langenbeckstr. 1
D-6500 Mainz

Prof. Dr. Herbert Dahlheim
Dept. of Physiology
University of Munich
Pettenkofer Str. 12
D-8000 München 2

Dr. Manfred Dahm
Universitätskliniken Mainz
Langenbeckstr. 1
D-6500 Mainz

Dr. Stefan Degenhardt
Med. Univ.-Klinik II
Josef-Stelzmann-Str. 9
D-5000 Köln 41

Prof. Dr. Franz Dienstl
University of Innsbruck
Clinic for Internal Medicine
Anichstr. 35
A-6020 Innsbruck

Dr. Cornelius J. Doorenbos
University Hospital
Dept. of Nephrology, C3-P
Rijnsburger Weg 10
NL-2333 AA Leiden

Dr. Leonidas Duntas
Univ. Klinik
Abt. Innere Medizin I
Steinhövelstr. 9
D-7900 Ulm

Dr. Hans Dusleag
Med. Universitätsklinik
Auenbruggerplatz 15
A-8036 Graz

Dr. Klaus Ehlenz
Abt. f. Endokrinologie und
Stoffwechsel der Med. Klinik
Baldinger Str.
D-3550 Marburg

Dr. W. G. Forssmann
Anatomisches Institut der Universität
III. Lehrstuhl
Im Neuenheimer Feld 307
D-6900 Heidelberg

Dr. D. Franzen
Med. Universitätsklinik III
Josef-Stelzmann-Str. 9
D-5000 Köln 41

Dr. M. Gagelmann
Anatomisches Institut der Universität
III. Lehrstuhl
Im Neuenheimer Feld 307
D-6900 Heidelberg

Prof. Dr. D. Ganten
Deutsches Institut zur Bekämpfung
des Hohen Blutdrucks
Im Neuenheimer Feld 366
D-6900 Heidelberg

Prof. Dr. J. Genest
Institut de Recherches Cliniques
de Montréal
110 Quest
Avenue des Pins
Montréal, Qué. H2W 1R7, Canada

Dr. R. Griebenow
Medizinische
Universitätsklinik II
und Poliklinik
Ostmerheimer Str. 200
D-5000 Köln 91

Dr. Peter Gross
Universität Heidelberg
Med. Universitätsklinik
Bergheimer Str. 56 A
D-6900 Heidelberg

Dr. L. Heinemann
Universität Düsseldorf
Abt. Ernährung u. Stoffwechsel
Moorenstr. 5
D-4000 Düsseldorf

Prof. Dr. H.-J. Hirche
Institut für Physiologie
Robert-Koch-Str. 39
D-5000 Köln 41

Dr. C. Hirth
Bayer AG
Institut für Pharmakologie
Postfach 10 17 09
D-5600 Wuppertal 1

Prof. Dr. J. Holtz
Institut für Angewandte Physiologie
und Balneologie
Hermann-Herder-Straße 7
D-7800 Freiburg

Prof. Dr. T. Inagami
Department of Biochemistry
Vanderbilt University
Nashville, Tennessee 37232, USA

Dr. Detlev Jäger
Abt. f. Kardiologie und Angiologie
„Bergmannsheil“
Gilsingstr. 14
D-4630 Bochum

Prof. Dr. Eckart Jungmann
Abt. f. Endokrinologie
Zentrum f. Innere Medizin
Universitäts-Klinikum
Theod.-Stern-Kai 7
D-6000 Frankfurt a/M 70

Dr. Georg Kahaly
II Med. Univ. Klinik Endokrinologie
Bau 303
Langenbeckstr. 1
D-6500 Mainz 1

Dr. M. Kentsch
Hövelnstr. 5
D-2400 Lübeck

Dr. Klaus Kienast
Med. Universitätsklinik
Abt. f. Endokrinologie
Hufelandstr. 55
D-4300 Essen

Prof. Dr. F. Kokot
Dept. Nephrology
Silesian School of Medicine
Ul. Francuska 20
PL-40027 Katovice, Poland

Prof. Dr. H. Kramer
Med.-Univ. Poliklinik
Wilhelmstraße 35–37
D-5300 Bonn1

Prof. Dr. M. Lehmann
Klinikum der Albert-Ludwigs-Universität
Abt. Sport- und Leistungsmedizin
Hugstetterstraße 55
D-7800 Freiburg

Dr. T. T. van Loenhout
Canisius-Wilh. Hospital
Dept. Cardiology
NL-Nijmegen

Dr. A. Machraoui
Kardiolog. Abt. "Bergmannsheil"
Gilsingstr. 14
D-4630 Bochum 1

Prof. Dr. Franco Mantero
Via Ospedale Civile, 105
I-Padova

Dr. Bernhard Manz
Abt. f. Exp. Endokrinologie
Univ.-Klinik
Johann-Gutenberg-Universität
Langenbachstr. 1
D-6500 Mainz

Dr. Peter Meyer
German Army Hospital Ulm
Oberer Eselsberg 40
D-7900 Ulm

Dr. N. Natcheff
Dept. of Physiologie
Medical Academy of Sofia
G.-Sofijski-Str. 1
BU-1431 Sofia

Dr. Stefan Niesert
Frauenklinik der Medizinischen
Hochschule Hannover
Oststadtkrankenhaus
Podbielskistr. 380
D-3000 Hannover 51

Prof. Dr. W. Oelkers
Med. Klinik-Endokrinologie
Klinikum Steglitz, FU Berlin
Hindenburgdamm 30
D-1000 Berlin 45

Dr. Wolf Osterode
Medizinische Universitätsklinik
Lazarettgasse 14
A-1090 Wien

Dr. Barbara Pietsch
Med. Universitätsklinik
Auenbruggerplatz 15
A-8036 Graz

Dr. Hans Georg Predel
Med. Universitäts-Poliklinik
Wilhelmstr. 35–37
D-5300 Bonn

Prof. Dr. D. J. Ramsay
Department of Physiology
University of San Francisco
San Francisco, CA 94 143-0400, USA

Prof. Dr. W. Rascher
Universitätsklinikum Essen
Klinik und Poliklinik für Kinder- und Jugendmedizin
Hufelandstraße 55
D-4300 Essen 1

Prof. Dr. G. Riegger
Universität Würzburg
Joseph-Schneider-Straße 2
D-8700 Würzburg

Dr. Alexander von Ruecker
Institut für Klin. Biochemie
Universität Bonn
Sigmund-Freud-Str. 25
D-5300 Bonn 1

Dr. Scherberich
Zentrum für Innere Medizin
Universität Frankfurt
Abt. Endokrinologie
Theodor-Stern-Kai 7
D-6000 Frankfurt

Dr. Wolfgang Schnizer
Inst. f. Med. Balneologie und Klimatologie
Universität München
Marchioninistr. 17
D-8000 München 70

Dr. S. Shaw
Medizinische Poliklinik
Inselspital Bern
CH-3010 Bern

Prof. Dr. H. Sonnenberg
Department of Physiology
University of Toronto
Toronto, Canada M5S 1A8

Dr. Gerhard Stark
Med. Universitätsklinik
Auenbruggerplatz 15
A-8036 Graz

Dr. Hans-Jürgen Talartschik
Medizinische Klinik
Abt. Nephrologie
Robert-Koch-Str. 40
D-3400 Göttingen

Dr. Ilkka Tikkanen
Minerva Inst. f. Med. Research
P.O. Box 819
SF-00101 Helsinki

Prof. Dr. G. Wambach
Medizinische Klinik II und Poliklinik
der Universität
Ostmerheimer Straße 200
D-5000 Köln 91

Dr. Siegfried Wieshammer
Universitätsklinik Ulm
Steinhövelstr. 9
D-7900 Ulm

Prof. Dr. H. G. Zimmer
Physiologisches Institut
Universität München
Pettenkoferstraße 12
D-8000 München 2

Introduction

The significance and substance of this symposium is based upon highly impressive development: In 1955 Otto H. Gauer and James P. Henry were able to demonstrate that volume increments of the left atrium of the heart led to increased renal sodium and water excretion, a phenomenon which was considered to indicate the existence of volume regulation. Since Paintal found increased electrical activity in afferent vagus fibres from these stretched left atrium, the diuretic response was attributed to inhibitory effects on ADH secretion coming about via the integrating action of the hypophysis. Never at this time in the late 50's, neither Gauer himself nor his associates (myself included) at the Kerckhoff Institute in Bad Nauheim, Germany, nor any scientist arguing about the results of Gauer, with Gauer, came up with the idea that the hormone being produced by the heart itself might be involved in the regulatory process. It must be assumed, that the specific granules in close vicinity of the artrial muscle fibers described by Kisch, also in 1955, were either not known to or neglected by physiologists and clinicians. Eventually, the break came 25 years later in 1980 when De Bold and Sonnenberg, who is present today, and coworkers and associates, injected extracts of rat atria into rats and observed the significant diuresis and natriuresis. Since it was evident to them that the granules behaved like a depository of a hormone, it was consequently concluded that the heart pump does operate as an endocrine gland as well. The publication of De Bold, Sonnenberg and others was followed by competitive and stimulating research activities in many countries of the world. The atrial natriuretic peptide was quickly isolated, it's amino acid sequence was determined and it's mechanism of action could be characterized. Up to now there is conclusive evidence that besides its natriuretic and diuretic action, ANP leads to vasodilatation and inhibits renin and aldosterone secretion. Yet, additional facts on the production side of natriuretic peptide and the mechanism of action have come to light. At the cellular level the atrial peptide seems to activate the enzyme guanylate cyclase, and, hence, stimulates GMP which is strongly considered to be the second messenger of ANP activity. A large body of information on the significance of ANP has been accumulated in recent years, so that a new concept of pressure and volume regulation could be established. It is evident that the antagonistic relationship between the renin-angiotensin aldosterone system and the atrial peptide must considered to be essential parameters in the context. In view of the many results published in recent years and the data about to be presented today and tomorrow, a systematization is just mandatory. We are going to start with a session on the morphology of the myoendocrine cell and the biochemistry and physiology of cardiac hormones. A session on the pathophysiological findings and the clinical relevance as in congestive heart failure, arterial hypertension, renal insufficiency and liver cirrhosis will follow. Furthermore, the heart as target organ of different endocrine factors, such as thyroid hormones, catecholamines, renin-angiotensin, growth hormone and endogenous opiodes will be presented at the meeting. In order to get an idea of the essence of the excellent research work performed in our field of interest, two poster sessions are going to take place during the conference. The symposium will be closed with a round table discussion in which the role of ANP in the regulation of fluid volume and blood pressure should be characterized in order to bridge the gap between the initial concept of Gauer and Henry and the facts known today.

The proceedings of the stimulating symposium are now in your hands. We like to take the opportunity to thank the Bayer Company for the sponsoring of the symposium. In addition, we want to express our gratitude to Boehringer Mannheim for making this publication possible.

Cologne, October 1988

W. Kaufmann
G. Wambach

Atrial Natriuretic Peptide: Morphology and Physiology

Morphology of the Myoendocrine Cardiac Cell and Extra-Auricular Systems Producing Cardiac Hormones*

W. G. Forssmann, S. Feller, M. Meyer, and P. Schulz-Knappe

Department of Anatomy and Cell Biology, University of Heidelberg, Heidelberg, FRG

Summary. This presentation is a review on cardiac hormones with special reference to the morphology of cardiac myoendocrine cells and extra-auricular CDD-producing systems. The fact that the heart is an endocrine organ and the center of a multiple endocrine, paracrine, and neuronal system was elaborated during the last decade. First, an attempt is made to summarize the essential historical aspects concerning the recent discoveries, then the myoendocrine cell of the heart atria, including its secretion cycle, is described. Among the numerous extra-auricular cell systems which synthesize and/or store cardiac polypeptides are (1) the cardiac conductive system, (2) the nervous system, (3) the adrenal medulla, and (4) the kidney, which are presented as new organs related to these regulatory polypeptides. Also some phylogenetic aspects are accounted for. From actual data it is evident that cardiac polypeptides are a family of differentially processed and expressed regulatory substances forming a multilocal and multifunctional system which is involved in many functions of the body, particularly in the regulation of the cardiovascular organs and of bodyfluid and electrolyte homeostasis.

Key words: Myoendocrine Cells – Endocrine Heart – Cardiodilatin – Atrial Natriuretic Polypeptide – Urodilatin - Morphology – Brain – Adrenal Medulla – Kidney

* Dedicated to Professor Viktor Mutt at the occasion of his 65th anniversary.

Introduction

For centuries, cardiovascular research has been focussed on William Harvey's discovery that the heart is a mechanical pump [72] and the dynamic center of blood circulation. Furthermore Marcello Malpighi's description of the capillary circulation contributed highly to the basic concepts of the cardiovascular system [106]. A revolutionary discovery of our century is that the heart is also an endocrine organ (Fig. 1). In 1956, electron microscopy facilitated Bruno Kisch's finding of new organellas in the heart atria [93–95], and functional data by Gauer and Henry enhanced the assumption that diuresis is stimulated by atrial dilatation [66, 75]. These two crucial observations have been thoroughly substantiated since then, because according to many studies, it is evident that the heart produces polypeptide hormones and, therefore, also has a function as an endocrine organ [18, 31, 45–47, 50, 51, 97, 98, 120, 167].

First indications of an involvement of granulated atrial myoendocrine cells in the regulation of water-electrolyte balance, depending on the status of total body fluid, were published in 1976 by Marie et al. [107]. In 1981, DeBold et al. [32] showed that acid atrial extracts stimulate diuresis as well as sodiuresis. A vasorelaxant effect of cardiac atrial extracts was subsequently described by Deth et al. in 1982 [35] and in 1983 by Currie et al. [27], our group [53], and others [69]. Hence two different biological tests were provided to perform the chromatographic isolation of various bioactive substances from cardiac atria of the rat, porcine and human species. A variety of names such

1956	**Bruno Kisch**	**Discovery of atrial granules**
1956	**Gauer, Henry**	**Discovery of cardiorenal reflex**
1964	**Jamieson, Palade**	**Secretory nature of specific granules**
1976	**Marie, Guillemot, Hatt**	**Fluid-electrolyte balance and granule index**
1981	**DeBold**	**Diuretic effect of atrial extracts**
1982 **1983**	**Deth** **Forssmann, Currie**	**Vasorelaxant effect of atrial extracts**
1983	**Flynn, DeBold**	**Isolation of Cardionatrin**
1983	**Forssmann et al.**	**Isolation of Cardiodilatin**
1984	**Matsuo, Kangawa**	**Isolation of human ANP**
1984	**Greenberg et al.**	**Characterization of human CDD/ANP gene**
1986	**Forssmann et al.**	**Isolation of human circulating CDD**
1988	**Matsuo, Sudoh**	**Isolation of BNP (Brain Natriuretic Polypeptide)**
1988	**Schulz-Knappe, Forssmann**	**Isolation of human Urodilatin**

Fig. 1. Historical events leading to the recent concept that the heart is an endocrine organ and the discoveries dealing with different polypeptides of the CDD/ANP family related to extracardiac synthesis and storage sites (see references [27, 32, 35, 44, 53, 66, 70, 75, 84, 88, 93, 107, 141, 151])

as cardiodilatin (CDD [48, 53]), cardionatrin [42], atrial natriuretic factor (ANF [18, 69]), atrial natriuretic polypeptide (ANP [88]), atriopeptin [28], auriculin [7], etc. were given to these polypeptides. In 1984, the human gene structure of cardiac hormones was published by Seidman et al. [143] and Greenberg et al. [70] who elaborated the expression of the entire molecule of this polypeptide-hormone family. In 1988, two closely related peptide hormones were found. The one (= BNP, brain natriuretic polypeptide) isolated from porcine brain by Matsuo's group [151, 152] is probably the product of a related but different gene; the other one CDD-95-126, named urodilatin, was isolated from human urine by our group [141] and may be derived from the prohormone coded by the cardiodilatin gene. The amino acid sequences of these peptides reveal different CDD/ANP-producing potencies, depending upon from which organ they originate e.g. brain, heart or kidney (see below).

Morphology of the Endocrine Heart

The morphological features of the endocrine heart may be analyzed on three scales of magnification (Fig. 15): (1) macroscopical distribution of the myoendocrine cells, (2) immunohistochemical localization of cardiac hormones within the myoendocrine cells, and (3) intracellular localization of cardiac hormones under normal, experimental and pathological conditions of the endocrine heart. Numerous morphological studies were published in the 1960ies and 1970ies [10, 11, 16, 17, 20, 22, 29, 30, 34, 40, 62, 81, 84, 108, 112, 131, 157, 160] showing the differences between atrial and ventricular myocytes and substantiating the presence of a specific function of the atrial appendages long before the cardiac polypeptide hormones were characterized via physiological and biochemical means.

Routine methods of immunohistochemistry, i.e. peroxidase-antiperoxidase (PAP) and fluorescein-isothiocyanat (FITC) methods were used to study the distribution of CDD-IR cells [8, 19, 23, 24, 41, 48, 52, 68, 71, 73, 79, 86, 87, 105, 111, 113, 127, 132, 133, 134, 156, 161, 163, 164, 178] within the entire heart (Figs. 2 and 3). Recently, we could also develop an antibody against BNP which readily stains atrial myoendocrine cells (Figs. 10 and 11). In mammalian species, a compact endocrine organ within the thin-walled, trabecular parts of the atria is distinguished, which corresponds to the most distensible parts of the atria – the atrial appendages. A diffuse distribution of endocrine cells in the heart, which are mainly related to the conductive system (see also below) is characteristic (Fig. 3). Light microscopy of myoendocrine cells also indicates the specific immunoreaction of antibodies directed against CDD at the subcellular level: the perinuclear regions exhibit small spots representing an endocrine secretory apparatus. These areas are called *perinuclear Golgi complexes*. Nevertheless, in the remaining parts of the large myoendocrine cells, i.e. in the *telenuclear* zone, the same cytoplasmic organellas may be found; we call them either *interfibrillar* or *subsarcolemmal Golgi complexes*. In electronmicroscopical pictures, these dictiosomes exhibit accumulations of rough endoplasmic reticulum, Golgi cisternae, and secretory granules (Fig. 12 to 14). Proof for the intragranular localisation of CDD-specific immunoreactivity is given by the immunogold method (Figs. 14 and 16). Also BNP can be demonstrated by use of this method, but since it is stored in much lower concentrations in the atrial specific granules than CDD we observe only a faint staining by routine methods, which can, however, be enhanced by adequate dilution and incubation time in the immunohistochemical process (Fig. 17). From comparative biochemical and immunohistochemical studies it is evident that the storage form of cardiac hormones is CDD-1-126: the bulk of extractable CDD in the atria is present in this large prohormonal form [24, 48, 60, 89, 145, 158], and all antibodies raised from synthetic segments of epitopes belonging to CDD-1-126 may be used for identical staining of the granules of the myoendocrine cells [24]. Furthermore, a cleaving enzyme which converts CDD-1-126 into the circulating CDD-99-126 form is located either in the matrix of the secretory granules, in the cell membrane of the myoendocrine cell, or in the endothelium of the efferent vasculature, because the release via exocytosis is accompanied by an immediate generation of CDD-99-126, which is the circulating bioactive form of the molecule. Recent results strongly support the assumption that the processing enzyme is located in the secretory granules [60, 82, 171] and activated simultaneously with the event of exocytosis.

As far as the gene expression of CDD within the atrial endocrine tissue is concerned we may summarize: the CDD gene is located on the human chromosome I. [116, 176]. Several examples of restriction fragment length polymorphismus (RFLPs) are known [56–58, 124, 125]. It consists of three exons which contain the information for the CDD preprohormone. Thus, the knowledge at the DNA and mRNA level concerning cardiac hormones was rapidly and consistently completed by numerous groups [3, 43, 56, 57, 58, 63, 64, 65, 70, 71, 92, 104, 116, 118, 121, 123, 124, 125, 128, 143, 144, 149, 168, 173, 176, 179]. As mentioned above the posttranslational processing has not yet entirely been clarified. However, some details are known about the enzymatic degradation of circulating CDD, namely that a specific renal endopeptidase cleaves CDD between positions Cys^{105} and Phe^{106}, where the cysteine-phenylalanine bond is located, thus altering the ring structure of the molecule and terminating its biological activity [61, 129, 174].

Secretion Cycle of the Myoendocrine Cell

The basis for the understanding of the secretory cycle of cardiac hormones has been studied extensively, models have been provided to understand the stimulus for synthesis and secretion [2, 4, 5, 9, 13, 26, 37, 44, 73, 87, 94, 100, 102, 110, 148, 155, 158, 178], processing [14, 15, 60, 71, 80, 82, 123, 139, 144, 154, 171, 175], receptor binding [12], as well as circulation and degradation [25, 36, 44, 61, 78, 90, 103, 117, 119, 129, 135, 142, 147, 150, 159, 166, 167, 175] of CDD/ANP; approaches to these problems were made by use various methods. Also recently, mor-

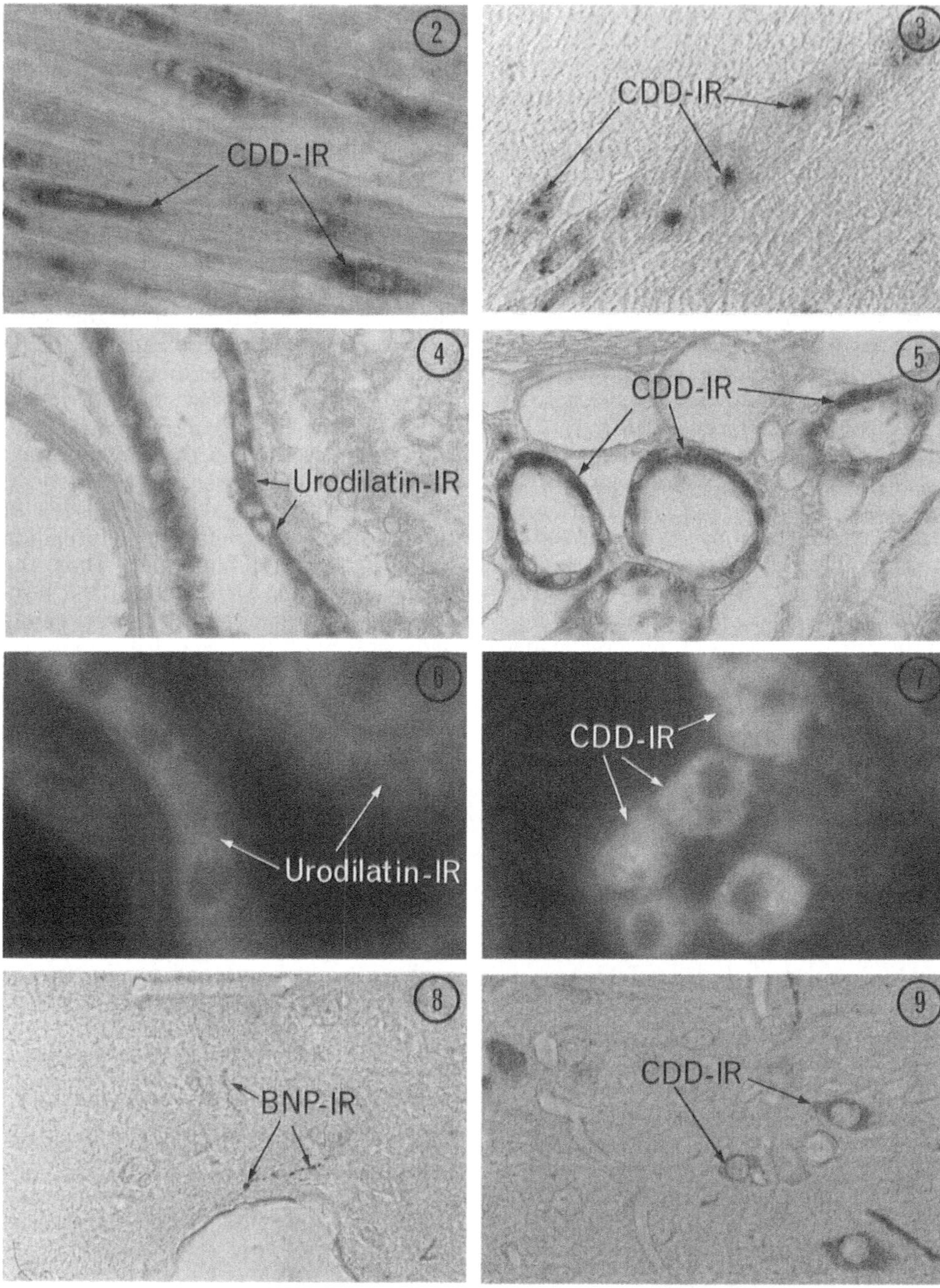

Fig. 2. Myoendocrine cells of the porcine left atrial appendage showing the immunoreactive cardiodilatin (CDD-IR) using an antibody directed against the C-terminus (CDD-99-126) of the atrial prohormone. The perinuclear region of atrial myoendocrine cells are stained showing the specific labeling by the peroxidase-antiperoxidase (PAP)- method. × 512

Fig. 3. Ventricular conductive cells of the porcine heart showing the immunoreaction for cardiodilatin (CDD-IR) using an antibody directed against the N-terminus (CDD-1-7) of the atrial prohormone. The

Golgi regions of these cells belonging to the intraseptal branches of the left bundle are specifically stained by the peroxidase-antiperoxidase (PAP)-method whereas the ventricular myocardiocytes exhibit no CDD-IR. × 512

Fig. 4. Porcine kidney tubular cells of the distal segment showing an immunoreaction for urodilatin using an antibody directed against the N-terminal epitope of urodilatin (= CDD-95-101). This antiserum does not stain the myoendocrine cells containing the atrial prohormone. The nuclei of the distal tubular cells are not stained and the specific labeling by the peroxidase-antiperoxidase (PAP)-method is seen diffusely in the tubular cells. × 512

Fig. 5. The same kidney tubular cells as in Figure 4 exhibit also an immunoreaction for circulating cardiodilatin (CDD-99-126) using an antibody directed against the epitopes of the ring-structured part of the molecule between the positions Cys^{101} and Cys^{119} of cardiodilatin. Antisera of this characteristic do stain the myoendocrine cells containing the atrial prohormone. Again the nuclei of the distal tubular cells are not immunoreactive and the specific staining by the peroxidase-antiperoxidase (PAP)-method is documented in the tubular cells. × 512

Fig. 6. Porcine kidney tubular cells stained by the fluoresceine-isothiocyanate (FITC)-method showing an immunoreaction for urodilatin (CDD-95-101) as in Figure 4. Note that the nuclei of the distal tubular cells are again not stained indicating the specific localisation of urodilatin-IR in the cytoplasm of the distal tubular cells. × 512

Fig. 7. Adrenal medullary cells stained by the fluoresceine-isothiocyanate (FITC)-method showing an immunoreaction for cardiodilatin (CDD-99-126) as in Figure 2. Note the fine granular distribution of the CDD-IR in the cytoplasm of this population of adrenal medullary cells and that the nuclei are not stained by the FITC-reaction. The specific localisation of a precursor molecule of the CDD-family is also substantiated by the fact that N-terminally directed antisera (e.g. CDD-8-24) have been shown to produce an identical staining in the adrenal medulla. × 1024

Fig. 8. Detection of BNP-IR (brain natriuretic polypeptide) varicosities in the monkey brain (Tupaia belangeri) found in the periventricular nucleus of the hypothalamus. The nerves are stained by an antibody raised against synthetic porcine BNP-26. × 512

Fig. 9. Detection of CDD-IR (cardiodilatin-immunoreaction) in perikarya and varicosities of the monkey brain (Tupaia belangeri) found in the dorsal area of the hypothalamus. The perikarya and nerve fibers are stained by an antibody raised against synthetic human/porcine CDD-99-126 (= alpha ANP) (modified from [55]). × 256

phological studies concerning myoendocrine cells were presented [26, 33, 49, 76, 136, 137, 153]. The highly accelerated activation of the secretory apparatus of myoendocrine cells following acute changes in body-fluid balance and its effects on atrial wall tension are well studied [100, 102, 136]. We carried out investigations in which (1) volume reduction was achieved by producing acute hemorrhage of about 20% of blood volume in rats and (2) volume load was increased by infusion of small quantities of plasma-expanding saline. A marked involution of the Golgi apparatus is seen after acute hemorrhage; progranules, a sign of secretory activity, completely diminished. By contrast, after volume overload the secretory apparatus exhibits extremely enhanced stimulation: the Golgi cisternae contain more progranules and they can easily be stained by the immunogold method. Furthermore, an increased stainability by the immunogold reaction against CDD is observed in the Golgi complex and in the endoplasmic reticulum. This is not observed in inhibited or basal secretion of myoendocrine cells [49, 136, 162]. The increased activity of myoendocrine cells also allows the observation of exocytotic events [49, 153] which are virtually not found in control animals. The combined use of HPLC and RIA in these experiments demonstrates that during stimulated and inhibited reactions only one molecular form exists in the plasma, eluting at the same position as the synthetic CDD-99-126. The elevated plasma-concen-

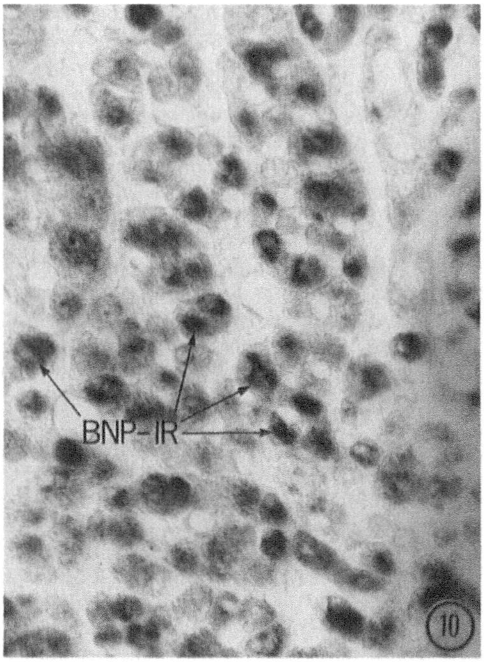

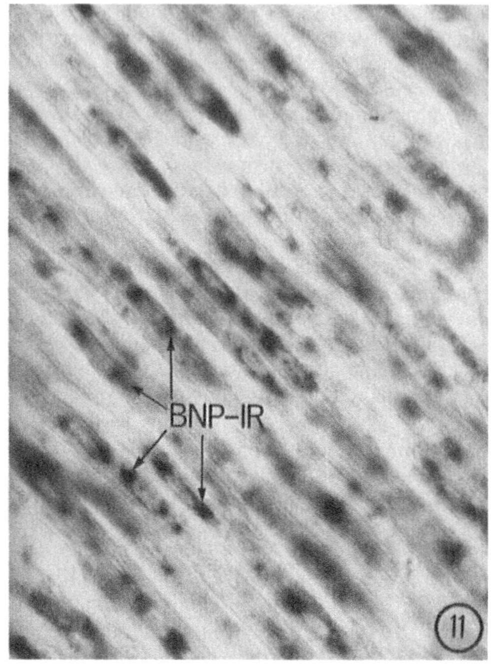

Fig. 10. Myoendocrine cells of the porcine left atrial appendage showing the immunoreaction for brain natriuretic polypeptide (BNP-IR) using an antibody directed against BNP-26. The perinuclear region of atrial myoendocrine cells exhibit strong staining in this transverse section through atrial myoendocrine cells showing the specific immunoreaction by the peroxidase-antiperoxidase (PAP)-method. × 600

Fig. 11. Myoendocrine cells of the porcine left atrial appendage as in Figure 10, however in longitudinal section, show the immunoreaction for brain natriuretic polypeptide (BNP-IR) using an antibody directed against BNP-26. The perinuclear region of atrial myoendocrine cells contain the specific labeling by the peroxidase-antiperoxidase (PAP)-method. × 600

tration after volume load and the reduced concentration after hemorrhage can easily be documented by use of this technique. Hence, from the above quoted studies on the secretory cycle and processing of cardiac hormones we conclude that the finding of CDD-1-126 as the storage form and CDD-99-126 as the circulating form of heart hormones account for the general concept of the events happening in the myoendocrine cell during the secretory cycle.

Extra-Auricular Localisation of Cardiodilatin in the Heart

The secretory granules, first described by Kisch in 1956 [93], are mainly encountered in a specific part of a population of atrial myocytes, as elaborated by Jamieson and Palade 1964 [84]. They were also shown to occur in other sites of cardiac tissue, namely in the bundle of HIS, by Bompiani, Hatt and Rouiller in 1959 [16]. However, until recently, there was no evidence for ventricular conductive fibers to contain secretory granules, except for some results by Mochet et al. 1974 [115], who obtained results indicating an active protein synthesis in the ventricular conductive tissue of rat. Immunohistochemical results were published [8, 23, 132, 133, 134, 172] showing that ventricular immuno-reactive CDD-fibers do exist which was later confirmed by use of further techniques [64, 73, 172]. In normal hearts of mammalian species these fibers are confined to the conductive system (Figs. 3 and 18) as documented in several recent publications [8, 67, 163, 164]. It was reported that an endocrine function occurs in ventricular myocardial fibers in phylogenesis as well as in pathological states, namely in cardiomyopathia. In Figure 3, staining of porcine conductive cells of the ventricular septum by the peroxidase-antiperoxidase method is illustrated. After thorough examination of the Purkinje fibers of the ventricular excitatory system, a secretory apparatus analogous to that in the myoendocrine cells, which is responsible for the production of peptides, was detected. Sections through the conductive cells in the bundle of HIS illustrate a well-developed ergastoplasma and Golgi apparatus, including some secretory granules. An attempt was made to prove the occurrence of CDD in the ventricle by biological, immunocytochemical, and biochemical-radioimmunological means. The results may be summarized as follows: after the application of septal peptide extracts to an RP-column, epitope-specific immunhistochemistry (Fig. 18), mRNA hybridization and determination of vasorelaxant bioactivity in septal tissue, the combination of HPLC and RIA confirmed that the conductive fibers contain a site for the synthesis of CDD. However, from the quantity of septal CDD we conclude that the atria constitute the major site in the body for the production of CDD, which is responsible for the maintenance of plasma concentration.

The Adrenal Medulla as a Cardiodilatin-Producing Site

Although it has been established that CDD systems are encountered in several organs (see Fig. 2), e.g. in the nervous system [54, 55, 59, 65, 83, 85, 91, 121, 126, 132, 140, 146, 155, 165, 177], pituitary gland [111], lung [6, 161], kidney [38, 39, 40, 111], adrenal gland [38, 83, 111, 114, 130], various vessels [6, 63, 101, 149, 161] and gastrointestinal tract [21, 170], only results concerning the adrenal glands and the kidney will be emphasized in the following discussion.

It is well-known that adrenal medullary cells produce a number of neuropeptides, such as VIP, SP, NT, OP, CGRP and NPY [77, 96]. Recently, we investigated several questions arising from the occurrence of CDD in the adrenal gland: (1) Is CDD synthesized in the adrenal gland? (2) Which cells of the adrenals produce CDD, and (3) what is the functional impact of CDD in the adrenal gland? [114]. The site of CDD immunoreaction in the adrenal was determined by antibodies against CDD-99-126 and CDD-8-24 (Figs. 7 and 19). Electron microscopical immunocytochemistry demonstrates that the CDD-IR is located in the secretory granules of a certain population of chromaffine adrenal medullary cells (Fig. 19). The existence of N- and C-terminal CDD prohormone-IR is evident from immunohistochemistry, and the potency of synthesis can be shown by a highly sensitive mRNA-blot hybridization technique [114]. The existence of CDD in the adrenal medulla is also confirmed by extraction of the corresponding peptide [130]. The occurrence of CDD in these cells raises the question about its functional significance. As CDD-specific receptors have been detected in the adrenal medulla [74] a local, paracrine function of CDD in the adrenal gland may be postulated.

The Kidney and Cardiodilatin: An Intrarenal Paracrine System

It has been suggested that cardiac hormones may be excreted in human urine, as radioimmunoassayable amounts can be detected in samples taken from normal and diseased individuals [138]. However, our investigation did not give evidence for a correlation between plasma and urine secretion in most patients [109, 138]. The isolation of human *urodilatin* from 1,000 l of human urine was carried out by Schulz-Knappe et al. in 1988 and revealed that urine and blood CDD-IR are different by nature [141]. In fact, the N-terminus of urodilatin is an extension of CDD-99-126 by four amino acids (see Fig. 21).This suggests that urodilatin may be a renal peptide processed from a precursor molecule in a different manner than the CDD prohormone in the heart. We used antibodies directed against N- and C-terminal epitopes of CDD-1-126 (see Fig. 5), which showed a specific staining of renal distal tubules [38, 39, 41]. Furthermore, mRNA isolation followed by a dot blot

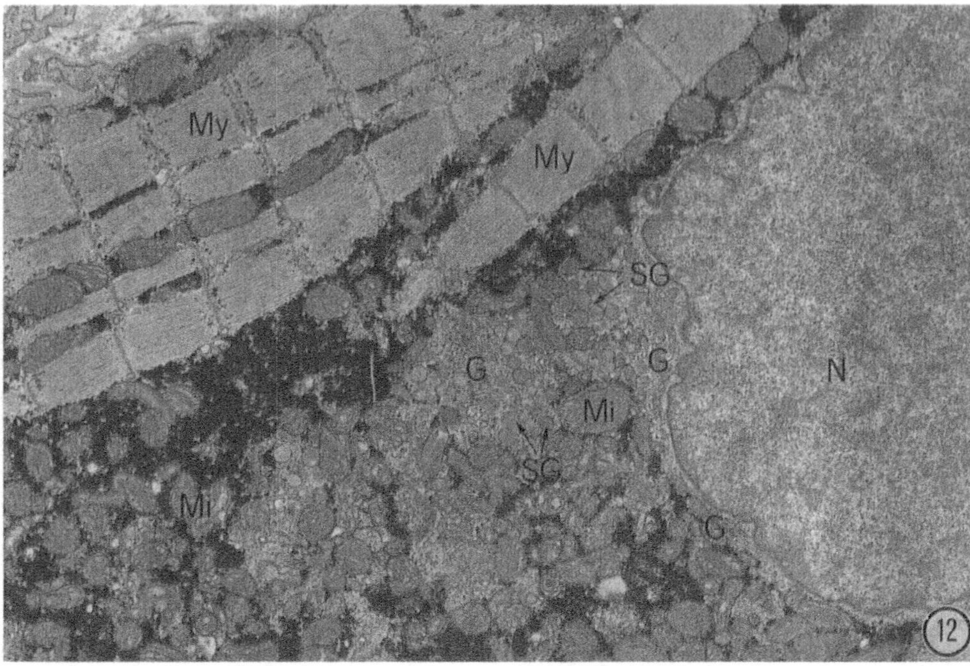

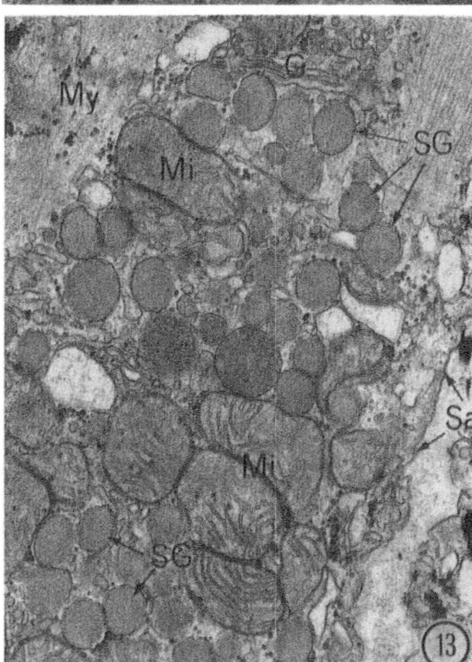

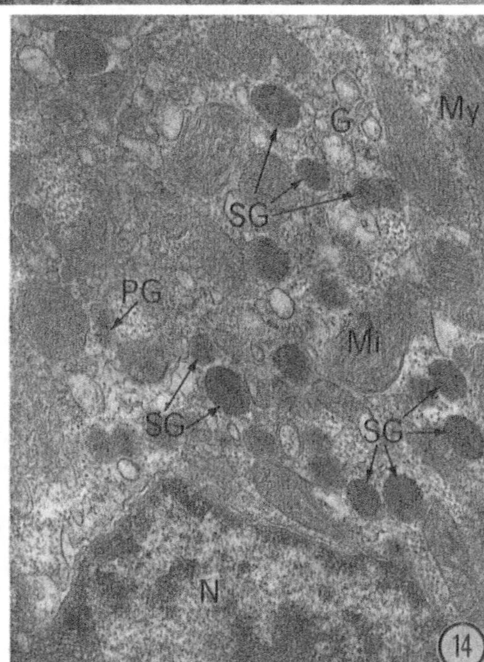

Fig. 12. Electron microscopy of an atrial myoendocrine cell of the human heart showing the endocrine activity of this type of myocardial cells in the Golgi region. Note the perinuclear region corresponds to the stained area in Figure 2 at the light microscopical level. Golgi apparatus (G) surrounded by the secretory granules (SG), progranules, cell nucleus (N), mitochondria (Mi), myofibrils (My). × 10 000

Fig. 13. Electron microscopy of an atrial myoendocrine cell of the human heart showing the telenuclear arrangement of the secretory machine. The Golgi region is located in the subsarcolemmal (or, as not shown, in the interfibrillar) space. Golgi apparatus (G) surrounded by the secretory granules (SG), progranules (PG), sarcolemma (Sa), mitochondria (Mi), myofibrils (My). × 28 350

Fig. 14. Electron microscopical immunocytochemistry of an atrial myoendocrine cell of the human heart showing the CDD-IR in the secretory granules around the Golgi region. The specific granules are specifically stained for CDD-IR using an antibody directed against CDD-99-126. The Golgi apparatus (G) is surrounded by labeled secretory granules (SG) and progranules (PG). Note also glycogen plaques (Gly), mitochondria (Mi), myofibrils (My), and the cell nucleus (N). × 23 800

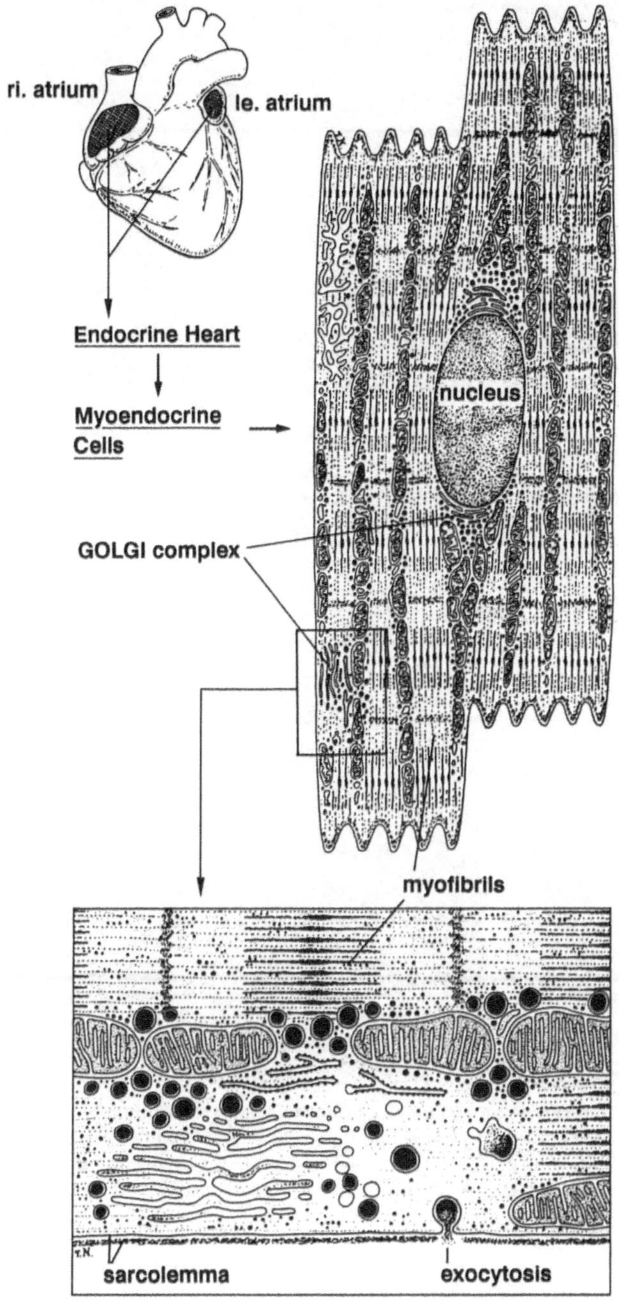

Fig. 15. Schematic drawing of the endocrine heart at the different scales of morphology: a) localisation of the compact endocrine organ in the atrial appedanges, b) myoendocrine cell as the functional unit of the endocrine heart, and c) the endocrine subcellular secretory apparatus including the rough endoplasmic reticulum, the Golgi complex, secretory granules, and showing the event of exocytosis

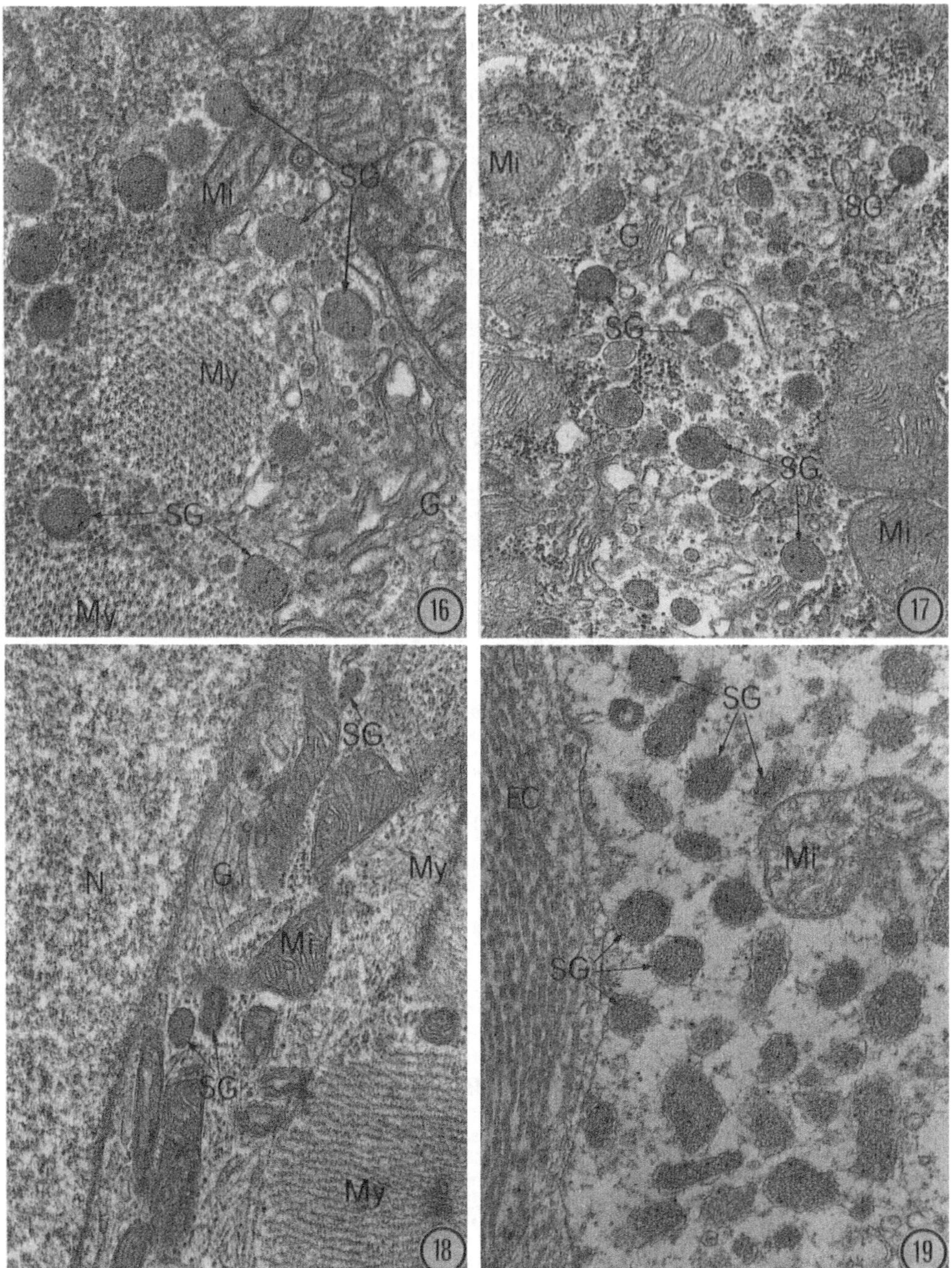

Fig. 16. Ultrastructural immunocytochemistry of an atrial myoendocrine cell of the human heart as in Figure 13 showing the CDD-IR of secretory granules. The specific granules also exhibit CDD-IR after using an antibody directed against CDD-8-24 is applied. The Golgi region (G) contains immunogold-labeled specific secretory granules (SG). Note further mitochondria (Mi) and myofibrils (My). × 38150

Fig. 17. BNP-IR-26 is also found using electron microscopical immunocytochemistry in atrial myoendocrine cells. Around the Golgi region secretory granules (SG) are found which are slightly stained by BNP-specific antibodies such as in Figures 8, 10, and 11. Note further mitochondria (Mi). × 35425

Fig. 18. Electron microscopy of a conductive ventricular cell of the porcine heart showing the comparable discrete secretory machine of CDD-production as in the atrial myoendocrine cell. This Golgi region is located in the areas stained for CDD-IR as seen in Figure 3. The Golgi apparatus (G) is surrounded by few secretory granules (SG), mitochondria (Mi), myofibrils (My), and the cell nucleus (N). × 25425

Fig. 19. Electron microscopy of a porcine adrenal medullary cell exhibiting CDD-production as in the atrial myoendocrine cell. The secretory granules (SG), mitochondria (Mi), extra-cellular space (EC). × 35970

showed that kidney tissue possesses a CDD-producing capacity [39]. Recent studies using an antibody directed against the amino acids 95–101 of the CDD prohormone, which is the free N-terminus of urodilatin, resulted in a good staining of the kidney tubules (Figs. 4 and 6), but no reaction was found in the heart atrium. CDD-immunoreactive material is synthesized and secreted by a human embryonic kidney cell line [39]. This supports the hypothesis that urodilatin is another polypeptide which may be produced in median segments (distal tubules) of the nephron, is luminally secreted and exerts a paracrine effect on more distally located receptors in the collecting duct, thus causing a strong diuresis. This postulated function, however, has yet to be proven by physiological methods. Some effects of CDD-95-126 are given by Gagelmann et al. [60].

The Nervous System and Cardiodilatin: Neuropeptides of the CDD-Family

The occurrence of CDD-IR in the PNS and CNS of different species is now well accepted. The presence of this peptide was discovered by immunocytochemistry in the atrial nerve endings and the corresponding subesophageal ganglion of the avertebrate Helix pomatia, where it forms a neurosecretory neuro-cardiac axis [121]. Later, the presence of CDD was confirmed in the nervous system of many mammalian species using radioimmunological, biochemical analytical [65, 165], and immunocytochemical [55, 91, 146; 177] techniques (Fig. 9). Recently, Matsuo's group isolated BNP (brain natriuretic polypeptide) from porcine brain (see Sudoh et al., 1988 [151, 152], a peptide related to the CDD family. Staining by an antibody against CDD-99-126 or BNP may cross-react; hence, the localization of brain polypeptide of the different forms of molecules has still to be investigated in order to make conclusive statements about BNP and CDD systems in the mammalian brain. Differential staining of neuronal structures may be obtained by the application of CDD-99-126 or BNP–26 antibodies (Figs. 8 and 9). In any case CDD-like peptides are found in many regions of the central and peripheral nerous systems. Of great interest is the possible functional implication of brain-born CDD-like peptides. To a significant extent they are located in hypothalamic areas which are somehow related to fluid uptake regulation and cardiovascular regulation. Thus they may interact in functional systems of similar physiological regulations by peripheral and control interactions.

Conclusions

This study shows that polypeptide hormones, first discovered in the heart, are also produced in many other organs (Fig. 20). This polypeptide family seems to have numerous functions as hormonal, neurosecretory and neuronal signal transmitters. Several molecular forms of bioactive post-translational expression products of the CDD gene are now well-known, e.g. circulating CDD (= alpha ANP), urodilatin and shorter molecules generated in the brain. Certainly, also brain natriuretic peptide

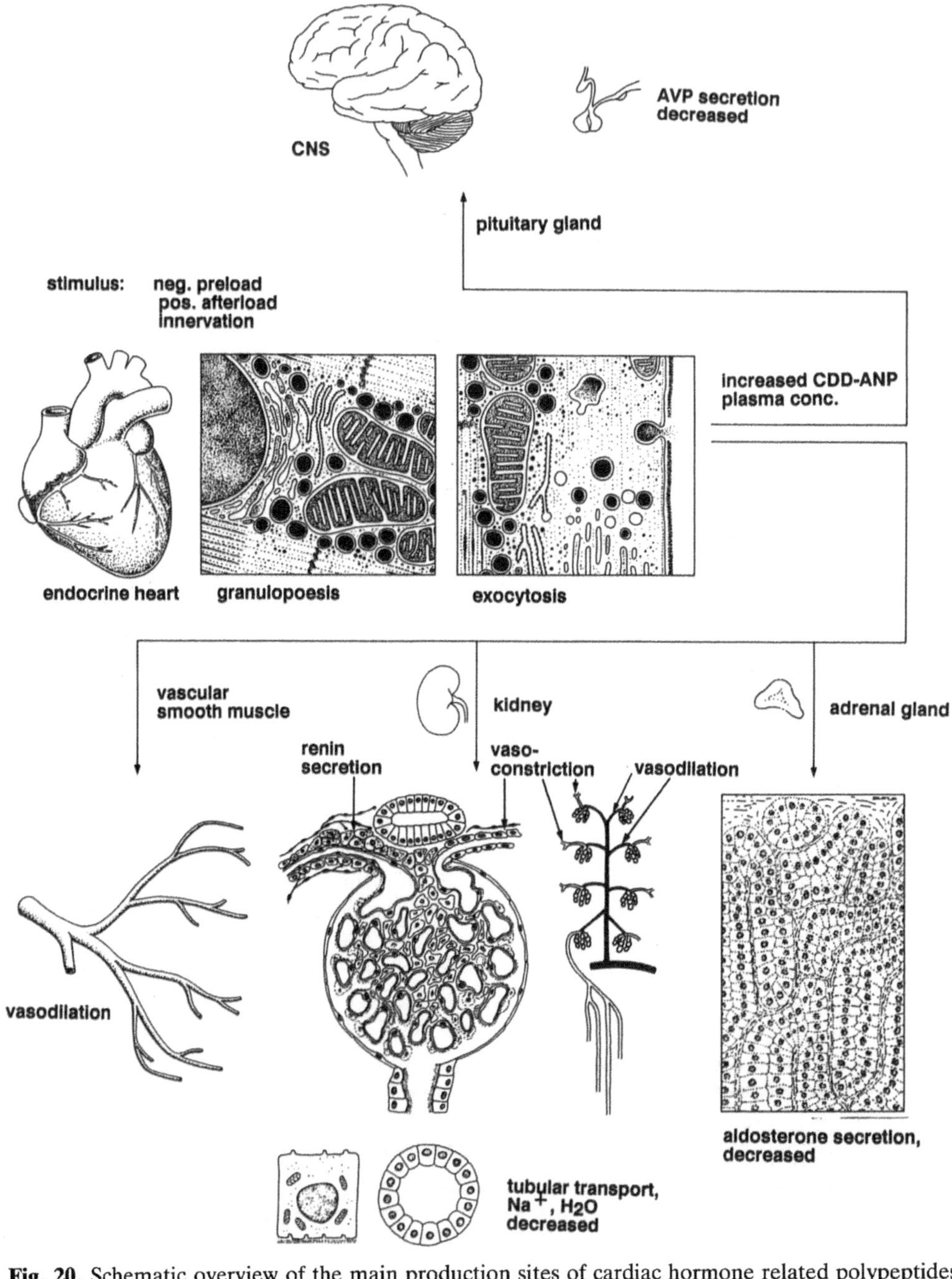

Fig. 20. Schematic overview of the main production sites of cardiac hormone related polypeptides. Further organs containing cardiac hormone-related polypeptides are mentioned in Figure 21

Tissue	Analyzing Methods RIA	IH	IC	mRNA
HEARD				
atria	+++	+++	+++	+++ (0.5-2%)
ventricle	+	+	+	+ (0.01%)
septum	+	+	+	+
VESSELS				
aortic arch	+		+	+
vena pulmonalis	+	+		
vena cava	+	+		
lung	+	+		+
CNS				+ (0.001%)
thalamus	+	+		
hypothalamus	+	+		+ (0.00025%)
bulbus olfactorius	+	+		
hypophysis	+	+		
brain stem	+	+		+ (0.001%)
(different regions)				+ (0.005-0.001%)
cerebral cortex	+	+		+
spinal cord	+	+		
PNS				
autonomic ganglia	+	+	+	
sensory ganglia	+	+	+	
ADRENAL MEDULLA	+	+	+	+
KIDNEY	+	+	+	+
PANCREAS	+	+*		
SALIVARY GLANDS	+	+	+	
THYMUS	+	+		**
STOMACH	+			**
DUODENUM	+			

* internalization from blood
** high-molecular-weight polypeptide detected, mRNA not yet investigated

Fig. 21. Table summarzing the findings of heart hormone related productions sites. Note the proof of storage or synthesis of cardiac polypeptides in extra-auricular sites is established by radioimmunoassay (RIA), immunohistochemistry (IH), immunocytochemistry (IC), as well as by in situ hybridisation and/or mRNA extraction (mRNA). (references see text, for mRNA values see [65], for thymus see [169])

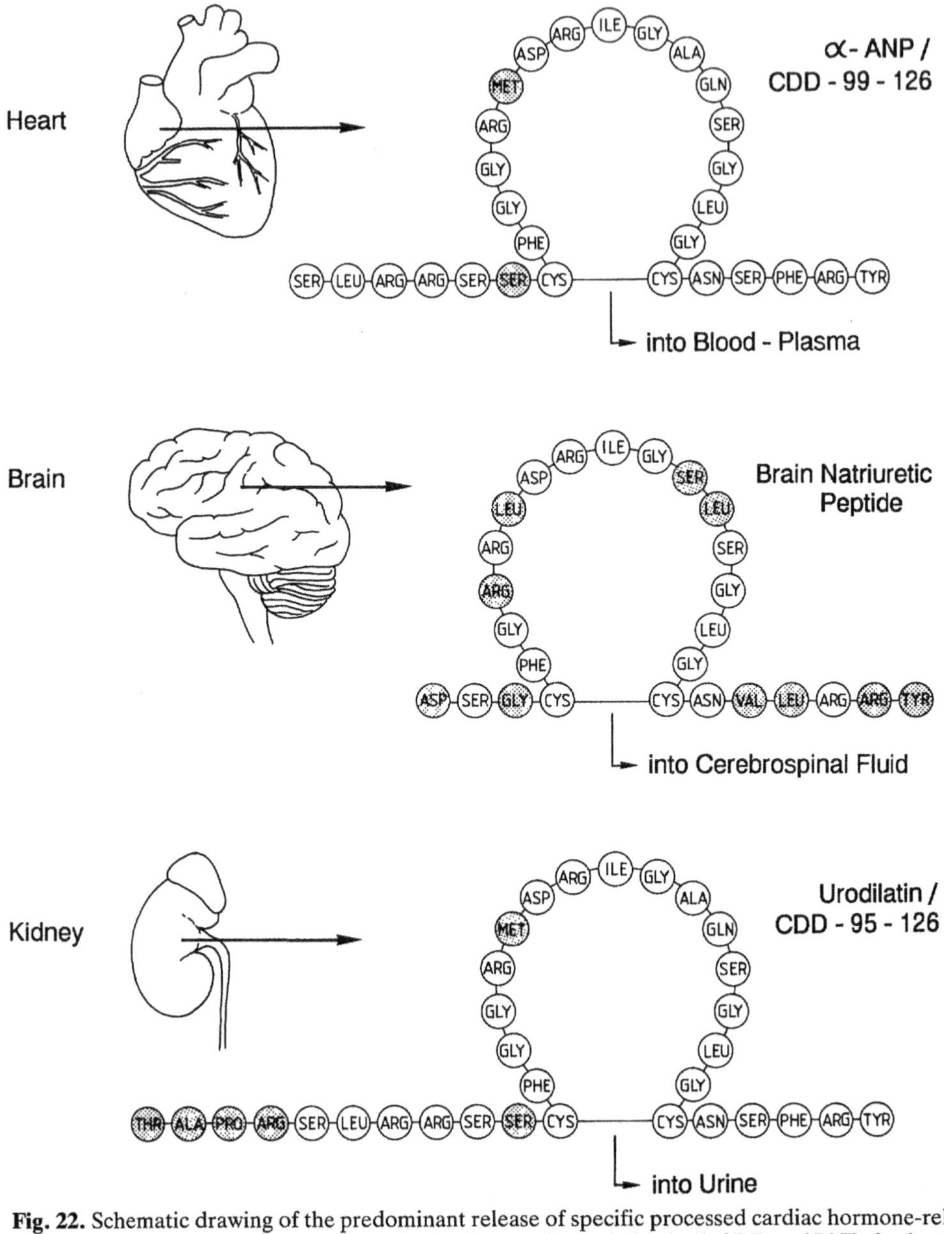

Fig. 22. Schematic drawing of the predominant release of specific processed cardiac hormone-related polypeptides into body fluids. Cerebrospinal fluid contains probably both CDD and BNP, further BNP is also detectable in low amounts in the blood plasma

(BNP), which is probably derived from a different gene, belongs to this polypeptide family which is functionally involved in the regulation of many target organs or cell systems. As many sites of the body have been found to contain specific receptors for the peptide released from the endocrine heart or extra-cardiac CDD-producing sites, these cardiac polypeptides are probably involved manyfold in the regulation of body functions (Fig. 22), of which the majority is still unknown, especially during phylogenesis during which the CDD-peptides may play a changing role (Fig. 23). Their

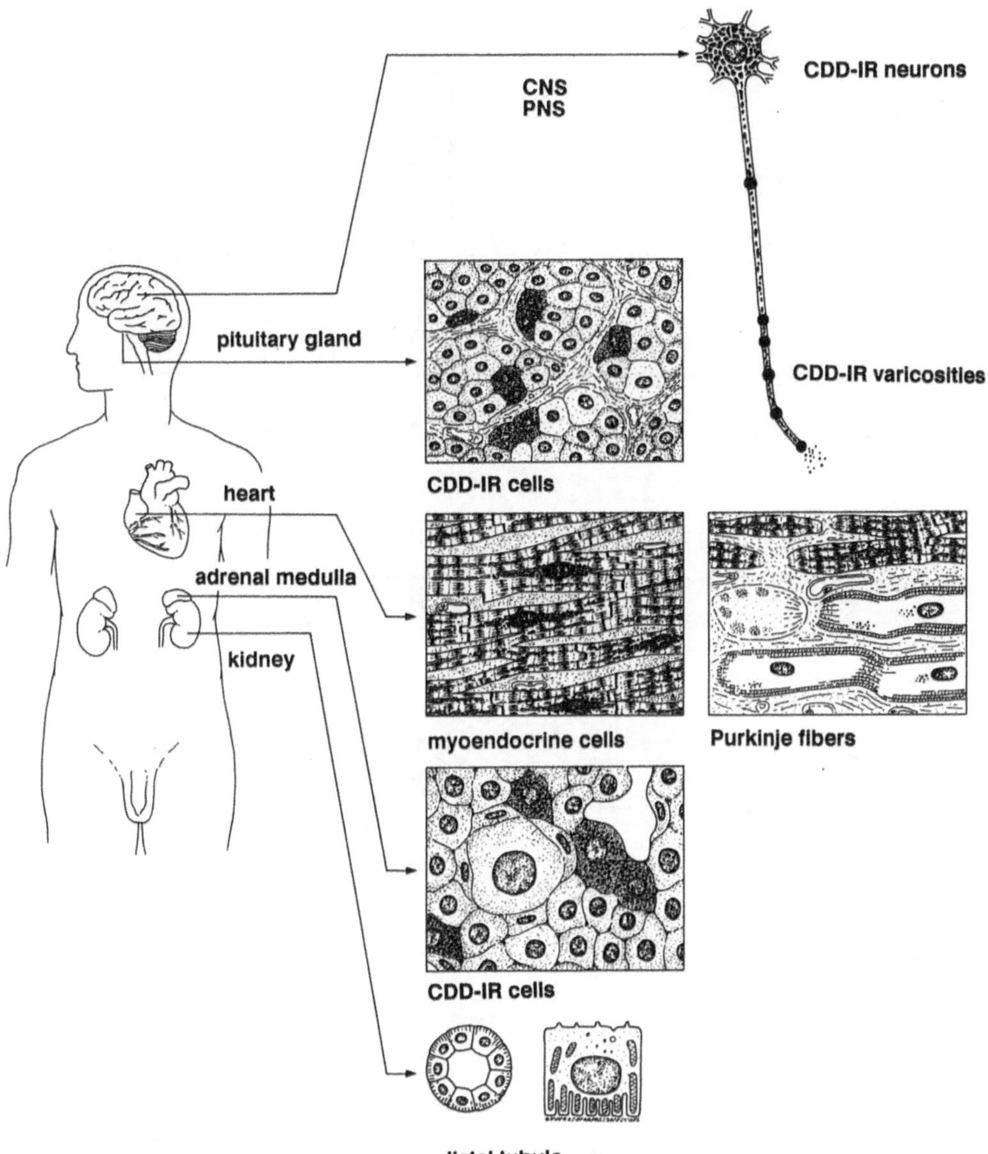

Fig. 23. Important target organs exhibiting receptors for cardiac hormone-related polypeptides and the physiological effet in these organs. Further comment see text

predominant physiological role, however, may be their involvement in the establishment of body fluid homeostasis, blood volume, and blood pressure. As far as we know today, major target organs for CDD/ANP are (Fig. 22): (1) the pituitary gland, where vasopressin secretion is inhibited, (2) vascular smooth muscle cells of various vessels, which are influenced in their luminal width (3) renal tubular and collecting duct cells of which sodium and water reabsorption is decreased, (4) the granulated cells of the juxtaglomerular apparatus from which renin secretion is reduced and (5) the zona glomeru-

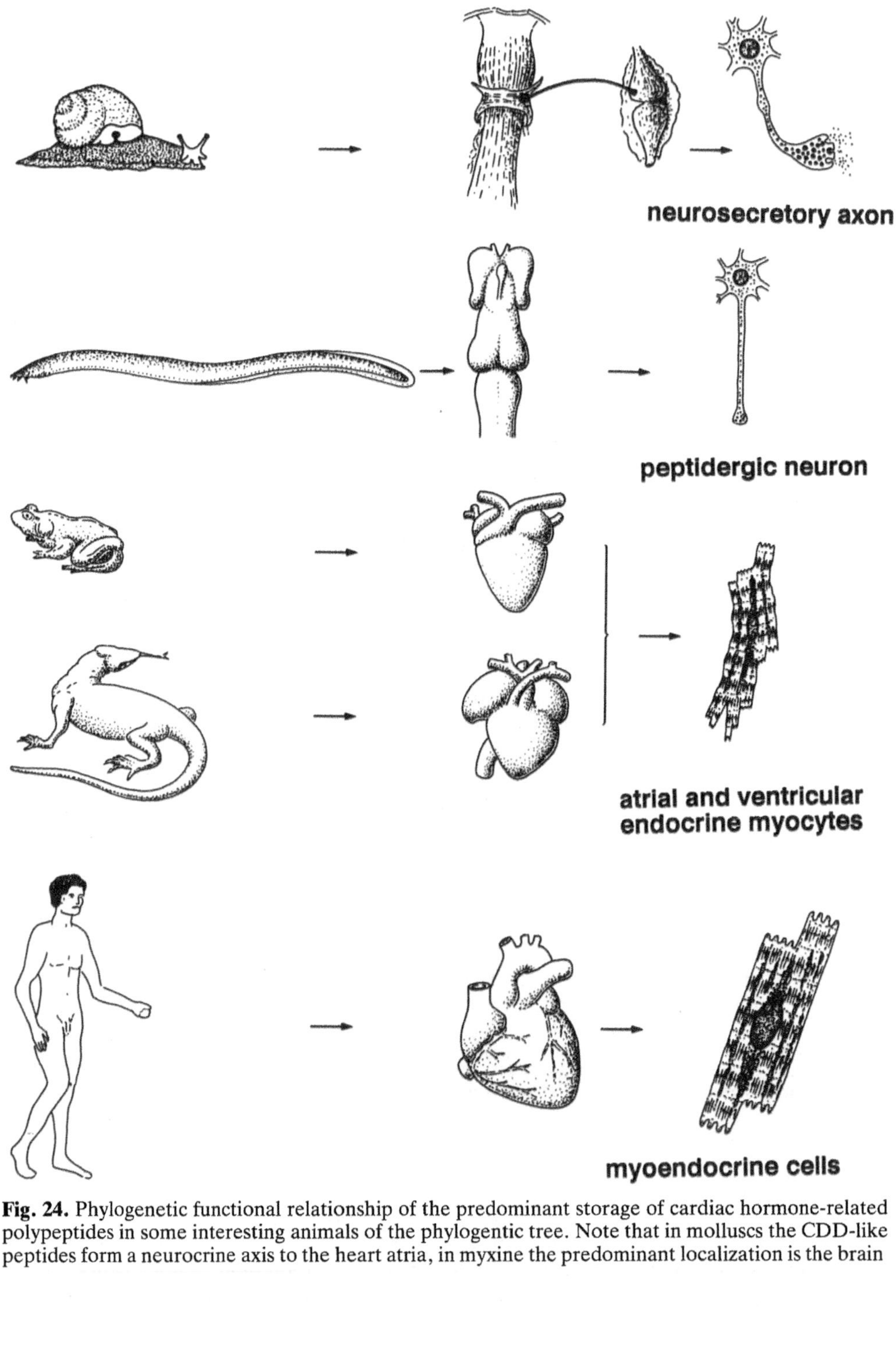

Fig. 24. Phylogenetic functional relationship of the predominant storage of cardiac hormone-related polypeptides in some interesting animals of the phylogentic tree. Note that in molluscs the CDD-like peptides form a neurocrine axis to the heart atria, in myxine the predominant localization is the brain

losa of the adrenal cortex, where aldosterone production is decreased. One major effect exerted by these cardiac hormones may be to decrease blood volume and blood pressure via the reduction of the peripheral resistence and the excretion of urine. These parameters are considered to be of fundamental clinical importance.

We are indebted for technical help and for preparing the manuscript to B. Brühl, B. Herbold, G. Sürig, E. and R. Botz, R. Nonnemacher, I. Stenull, and J. Sis. The program on cardiac endocrinology was supported by the German Research Foundation (SFB 320, grant A 3) and a grant of Bissendorf Peptide GmbH (BRAUN-COP88)

References

1. Ackermann DM, Edwards BS, Wold LE, Burnette JC (1986) Atrial natriuretic peptide: localization in the human heart. JAMA 256:1048
2. Angoletti G, Rodella A, Ferrari R, Harris P (1987) Release of atrial natriuretic peptide-like immunoreactive material during stretching of the rat atrium in vitro. J Mol Cell Cardiol 19:217–220
3. Argentin S, Nemer M, Drouin J, Scott GK, Kennedy BP, Davies PL (1985) The gene for rat atrial natriuretic factor. J Biol Chem 260:4568–4571
4. Arjamaa O, Ruskoaho H, Tuominen M, Vakkuri O, Leppäluoto J (1988) The concentration of atrial natriuretic peptide (ANP) is decreased in plasma but not in atria in hypophysectomised rats. Life Sci 42:589–596
5. Arjamaa O, Vuolteenaho O (1985) Sodium ion stimulates the release of atrial natriuretic polypeptides (ANP) from rat atria. Biochem Biophys Res Commun 132:375–381
6. Asai J, Nakazato M, Toshimori H, Matsukura S, Kangawa K, Matsuo H (1987) Presence of atrial natriuretic polypeptide in the pulmonary vein and vena cava. Biochem Biophys Res Commun 146:1465–1470
7. Atlas SA, Kleinert HD, Camargo MJ, Januszewicz A, Sealey T (1984) Purification, sequencing and synthesis of natriuretic and vasoactive rat atrial peptide. Nature 309:717–719
8. Back H, Stumpf WE, Ando E, Nokihara K, Forssmann WG (1986) Immunocytochemical evidence for CDD/ANP-like peptides in strands of myoendocrine cells associated with the ventricular conduction system of the rat heart. Anat Embryol 175:223–226
9. Baertschi AJ, Hausmaninger C, Walsh RS, Mentzer RM Jr, Wyatt DA, Pence RA (1986) Hypoxia-induced release of atrial natriuretic factor (ANF) from the isolated rat and rabbit heart. Biochem Biophys Res Commun 140:427–433
10. Battig CG, Low FN (1961) The ultrastructure of human cardiac muscle and its associated tissue space. Am J Anat 108:349
11. Berger JM, Bencosme SA (1971) Fine structural cytochemistry of granules in atrial cardiocytes. J Mol Cell Cardiol 3:111–120
12. Bianchi C, Gutkowska J, Thibault G, Garcia R, Genest J, Cantin M (1985) Radioautographic localization of ^{125}I-atrial natriuretic factor (ANF) in rat tissues. Histochemistry 82:441–452
13. Bilder GE, Schofield TL, Blaine EH (1986) Release of atrial natriuretic factor. Effects of repetitive stretch and temperature. Am J Physiol 251:F817–F821
14. Bloch KD, Scott JA, Zisfein JB, Falon JT, Margolies MN, Seidman CE, Matsueda GR, Homcy CJ, Graham RM, Seidman JG (1985) Biosynthesis and secretion of proatrial natriuretic factor by cultured rat cardiocytes. Science 230:1168–1171
15. Bloch KD, Seidman JG, Naftilan JD, Fallon JT, Seidmann CE (1986) Neonatal atria and ventricles secrete atrial natriuretic factor via tissue-specific secretory pathways. Cell 47:695–702
16. Bompiani GD, Rouiller CH, Hatt PY (1959) Le tissu de conduction du coeur chez le rat. Étude au microscope électronique. I. Le tronc commun du faisceau de His et les cellules claires de l'oreillette droite. Arch Mal Coeur 52:1257–1274
17. Cantin M, Benchimol S, Castonguay Y, Berlinguet JC, Huet M (1975) Ultrastructural cytochemistry of atrial muscle cells. V. Characterization of specific granules in the human left atrium. J Ultrastr Res 52: 179–192
18. Cantin M, Genest J (1985) The heart and the atrial natriuretic factor. Endocr Rev 6:107–127
19. Cantin M, Gutkowska J, Thibault G, Milne RW, Ledoux S, MinLi S, Chapeau C (1984) Immunocytochemical localization of atrial natriuretic factor in the heart and salivary glands. Histochemistry 80:113–127
20. Cantin M, Timm-Kennedy M, El-Khatib E, Huet M, Yunge L (1979) Ultrastructural cytochemistry of atrial muscle cells. VI. Comparative study of specific granules in right and left atrium of various animal species. Anat Rec 193:55–96

21. Chabot JG, Morel G, Kopelman H, Belles-Isles M, Heisler S (1987) Atrial natriuretic factor and exocrine pancreas: autoradiographic localization of binding sites and ultrastructural evidence for internalization of endogeneous ANF. Pancreas 2:404–413
22. Chang WWL, Bencosme SA (1969) Quantitative electron microscopic analysis of the specific granule population of rat atrium. Can J Physiol Pharmacol 47:483–485
23. Chapeau C, Gutkowska J, Schiller PW, Milne RW, Thibault G, Garcia R, Genest J, Cantin M (1985) Localization of immunoreactive synthetic atrial natriuretic factor (ANF) in the heart of various animal species. J Histochem Cytochem 33:541–550
24. Christmann MP, Nokihara K, Feller S, Forssmann WG (1988) Demonstration of the storage form of cardiac hormones by the use of segment-specific antibodies against cardiodilatin (CDD). Acta Histochemica (in press)
25. Condra CL, Leidy EA, Bunting P, Colton CD, Nutt RF, Rosenblatt M, Jacobs JW (1988) Clearance and early hydrolysis of atrial natriuretic factor in vivo. J Clin Invest 81:1348–1354
26. Cuevas P, Golitsin A, Gonzales AM, Forssmann WG (1987) Ultrastructural evidence of cardiodilatin in rat transplanted heart. Transplantation Proc 19:3789–3791
27. Currie MG, Geller DM, Cole BR, Boylan JG, YuSheng W, Holmberg SW, Needleman P (1983) Bioactive cardiac substances: potent vasorelaxant activity in mammalian atria. Science 221:71–73
28. Currie MG, Geller DM, Cole BR, Siegel NR, Fok KF, Adams SP, Eubanks SR, Gallupi GR, Needleman P (1984) Purification and sequence analysis of bioactive atrial peptides (atriopeptins). Science 223:67–69
29. DeBold AJ (1978) Morphometric assessment of granulation in rat atrial cardiocytes: effect of age. J Mol Cell Cardiol 10:717–724
30. DeBold AJ (1979) Heart atria granularity effects of changes in waterelectrolyte balance. Proc Soc Exp Biol Med 161:508–511
31. DeBold AJ (1985) Atrial natriuretic factor: A hormone produced by the heart. Science 230:767–770
32. DeBold AJ, Borenstein HB, Veress AT, Sonnenberg H (1981) A rapid and potent natriuretic response to intravenous injection of atrial extracts in rats. Life Sci 28:89–94
33. DeBold AJ, DeBold ML, Sarda IR (1986) Functional-morphological studies on in vitro cardionatrin release. J Hypertension 4 (Suppl):S3–S7
34. DeBold AJ, Raymond JJ, Bencosme SA (1978) Atrial specific granules of the rat heart light microscopic staining and histochemical reactions. J Histochem Cytochem 26:1094–1102
35. Deth RC, Wong K, Fukozawa S, Rocco R, Smart JL, Lynch CJ, Awad R (1982) Inhibition of rat aorta contractile response by natriuresis-inducing extract of rat atrium. Fed Proc 41:983
36. Devine E, Artman L, Budzik G, Bush E, Hollemann W (1986) Distribution and elimination of intravenously administered atrial natriuretic hormone (ANH) to normal and nephrectomized rats. Red Proc 45:1738
37. Dietz JR (1987) Control of atrial natriuretic factor release from a rat heart-lung preparation. Am J Phsiol 252:R498–R502
38. Feller S, Meyer M, Hock D, Forssmann WG (1988) Extraaurikuläre Lokalisation von Cardiodilatin. Acta Anat 132:80
39. Feller S, Schulz-Knappe P, Forssmann WG (1988) The kidney as a paracrine, urodilatin-producing organ. Circulation 78, [Suppl II]:429
40. Fenoglio JJ jr, Pham TD, Hordof A, Edie RN, Wit AL (1979) Right atrial ultrastructure in congenital heart disease. II. Atrial septal defect: effects of volume overload. Am J Cardiol 43:820–827
41. Flügge G, Inagami T, Fuchs E (1987) Atrial natriuretic peptide detected by immunocytochemistry in peripheral organs of Tupaia belangeri. Histochemistry 86: 479–483
42. Flynn TG, DeBold ML, DeBold AJ (1983) The amino acid sequence of an atrial peptide with potent diuretic and natriuretic properties. Biochem Biophys Res Commun 117:859–865
43. Flynn TG, Davies PL, Kennedy BP, DeBold ML, DeBold AJ (1985) Alignment of rat cardionatrin sequences with the preprocardionatrin sequence from complementary DNA. Science 228:323–235
44. Forssmann K, Hock D, Herbst F, Schulz-Knappe P, Talartschik J, Scheler F, Forssmann WG (1986) Isolation and structural analysis of the circulating human cardiodilatin (alpha ANP). Klin Wochenschr 64: 1276–1280
45. Forssmann WG (1986) Cardiac hormones. I. Review on the morphology, biochemistry, and molecular biology of the endocrine heart. Eur J Clin Invest 16:439–451
46. Forssmann WG (1987) Das Herz, ein endokrines Organ (Referat). Verh Anat Ges 81:97–108
47. Forssmann WG (1988) Morphological review: immunohistochemistry and ultrastructure of the endocrine heart. In: Forss-

mann WG, Scheuermann DW, Alt J (eds). Functional morphology of the endocrine heart. Steinkopff, Darmstadt, pp 13–42
48. Forssmann WG, Birr C, Carlquist M, Christmann M, Finke R, Henschen A, Hock D, Kirchheim H, Kreye V, Lottspeich F, Metz J, Mutt V, Reinecke M (1984) The auricular myocardiocytes of the heart constitute an endocrine organ. Characterization of a porcine cardiac peptide hormone, cardiodilatin-126. Cell Tissue Res 238: 425–430
49. Forssmann WG, Greenberg J, Schulz-Knappe P, Rippegather G (1989) Morphological changes induced by stimulation and inhibition of atrial myoendocrine cells. Eur J Clin Invest (in press)
50. Forssmann WG, Heidland A, Lang RE (eds) (1986) I. Workshop on cardiac hormones "Potential role in health and disease". Klin Wochenschr 64 [Suppl VI]: 1–117
51. Forssmann WG, Hock D (1988) Morphologie und Biochemie des endokrinen Herzens. In: Kreye VAW, Bussmann WD (Hrsg) ANP – Atriales natriuretisches Peptid und das kardiovaskuläre System. Steinkopff, Darmstadt, S 1–9
52. Forssmann WG, Hock D, Kirchheim F, Metz J, Mutt V, Reinecke M (1984) Cardiac hormones: morphological and functional aspects. Clin Exp Hypertension A6: 1873–1878
53. Forssmann WG, Hock D, Lottspeich F, Henschen A, Kreye V, Christmann M, Reinecke M, Metz J, Carlquist M, Mutt V (1983) The right auricle of the heart is an endocrine organ: Cardiodilatin as a peptide hormone candidate. Anat Embryol 168: 307–313
54. Forssmann WG, Lang RE, Aoki A, Reinecke M, Rippegather G, Hock D (1987) Cardiodilatin as a neuropeptide (Cardiac polypeptide hormones are also neuropeptides). Exp Brain Res 16:43–50
55. Forssmann WG, Mutt V (1985) Cardiodilatin-immunoreactive neurons in the hypothalamus of Tupaia. Anat Embryol 172:1–5
56. Frossard PM, Gonzalez PA, Greenberg B, Fiddes JC, Atlas SA (1986) Bgl II dimorphism at the human atrial natriuretic peptide (ANP) gene locus. Nucl Acid Res 14: 5121
57. Frossard PM, Coleman RT (1986) Human atrial natriuretic peptides (ANP) gene locus: Bgl I RFLP. Nucl Acid Res 14:9223
58. Frossard PM, Coleman RT, Morrison NA (1987) Human natriuretic peptides (ANP) gene locus: Bsm I RFLP. Nucl Acid Res 15:7656
59. Fujio N, Ohashi M, Nawata H, Kato K, Tateishi J, Matsuo H, Ibayashi H (1987) Unique distribution of natriuretic hormones in dog brain. Reg Pept 18:131–137
60. Gagelmann M, Feller S, Hock D, Schulz-Knappe P, Forssmann WG (1989) Biochemistry of the differential release, processing and degradation of cardiac and related peptide hormones. In: Kaufmann W, Wurmbach G (eds) Endocrinology of the heart. Springer, Berlin Heidelberg New York, pp 27–40
61. Gagelmann M, Hock D, Forssmann WG (1988) Urodilatin (CDD/ANP–95–126) is not biologically inactivated by a peptidase from dog kidney cortex membranes in contrast to atrial natriuretic peptide/cardiodilatin (alpha-hANP/CDD–99–126). FEBS Lett 223:249–254
62. Garcia R, Cantin M, Thibault G, Ong H, Genest J (1982) Relationship of specific granules to the natriuretic and diuretic activity of rat atria. Experientia (Basel) 38:1071–1073
63. Gardner DG, Deschepper CF, Baxter JD (1987) The gene for the atrial natriuretic factor is expressed in the aortic arch. J Hypertension 9:103–106
64. Gardner DG, Deschepper CF, Ganong WF, Hane S, Fiddes J, Baxter JD, Lewicki J (1986) Extra-atrial expression of the gene for atrial natriuretic factor. Proc Natl Acad Sci USA 83:6697–6701
65. Gardner DG, Vlasuk GP, Baxter JD, Fiddes JC, Lewicki JA (1987) Identification of atrial natriuretic factor gene transcripts in the central nervous system of the rat. Proc Natl Acad Sci USA 84:2175–2179
66. Gauer OH, Henry JP (1963) Circulatory basis of fluid volume control. Physiol Rev 43:423–481
67. Göbel J, Back H, Forssmann K, Daffner C, Stumpf WE, Forssmann WG (1988) Evidence for the existence of cardiac hormones in the conductive system of the mammalian heart. In: Forssmann WG, Scheuermann DW, Alt J (eds) Functional morphology of the endocrine heart. Steinkopff, Darmstadt, pp 43–49
68. Göbel J, Metz J, Forssmann WG (1986) Korrelation zwischen myoendokrinen Zellen und peptiderger Innervation im Herz. Verh Anat Ges 80:551–553
69. Grammer RT, Fukumi H, Inagami T, Misono KS (1983) Rat atrial natriuretic factor: purification and vasorelaxant activity. Biochem Biophys Res Commun 116: 696–703
70. Greenberg BD, Bencen GH, Seilhamer JJ, Lewicki JA, Fiddes JC (1984) Nucleotide

sequence of the gene encoding human atrial natriuretic factor precursor. Nature 312: 656-658
71. Hamid Q, Wharton J, Terenghi G, Hassall CJS, Aimi J, Taylor KM, Nakazato H, Dixon JE, Burnstock G, Polak JM (1987) Localization of atrial natriuretic peptide mRNA and immunoreactivity in the rat heart and human atrial appendage. Proc Natl Acad Sci USA 84:6760–6764
72. Harveii G (1625) De motu cordis et sanguinis en animalibus. Anatomica exercitatio. Lugduni Batavorum. Ex officina Ioannis Maire
73. Hassall CJS, Wharton J, Gulbenkian S, Anderson JV, Frater J, Bailey DJ, Merighi A, Bloom SR, Polak JM, Burnstock G (1988) Ventricular and atrial myocytes of newborn rats synthesize and secrete atrial natriuretic peptide in culture: light- and electron-microscopical localisation and chromatographic examination of stored and secreted molecular forms. Cell Tissue Res 251: 161–169
74. Heisler S, Morrier E (1988) Bovine adrenal medullary cells contain functional atrial natriuretic peptide receptors. Biochem Biophys Res Commun 150:781–787
75. Henry JP, Gauer OH, Reeves JL (1956) Evidence of the atrial location of receptors influencing urine flow. Circ Res 4:85–90
76. Herbst WM, Mall G, Weers J, Mattfeldt T, Lang RE, Forssmann WG (1988) Combined quantitative morphological and biochemical study on atrial granules (AG). In: Forssmann WG, Scheuermann DW, Alt J (eds) Functional morphology of the endocrine heart. Steinkopff, Darmstadt, pp 75–82
77. Heym C, Kummer W (1988) Regulatory peptides in paraganglia. Progr Histochem Cytochem 18:1–95
78. Hirata Y, Ishii M, Matsuoka H, Sugimoto T, Iizuka M, Uchida Y, Serizawa T, Sato H, Kohmoto O, Mochizuki T, Sugimoto T, Miyata A, Kangawa K, Matsuo H (1987) Plasma concentrations of alpha-human atrial natriuretic polypeptide and cyclic GMP in patients with heart disease. Am Heart J 113:1463–1469
79. Hock D, Fey E, Brühl B, Forssmann WG (1988) Das endokrine Herz beim Rind. Verh Anat Ges 82 (in press)
80. Hock D, Schriek U, Fey E, Forssmann WG, Mutt V (1987) Isolation of bovine cardiodilatin by fast protein liquid chromatography and reverse phase high-performance liquid chromatography. J Chromatogr 397:347–353
81. Huet M, Benchimol S, Castonguay Y, Cantin M (1974) Ultrastructural cytochemistry of atrial muscle cells. III. Reactivity of specific granules in man. Histochemistry 41:87–105
82. Imada T, Takayanagi R, Inagami T (1988) Purification of a specific peptidase in bovine atria for the processing of pro-atrial natriuretic factor. Biol Chem Hoppe-Seyler 369:113–120
83. Inagaki S, Kubota Y, Kito S, Kangawa K, Matsuo H (1986) Immunoreactive atrial natriuretic polypeptides in the adrenal medulla and sympathetic ganglia. Reg Pept 15:249–260
84. Jamieson JD, Palade GE (1964) Specific granules in atrial muscle cells. J Cell Biol 123:151–172
85. Jirikowski GF, Back H, Forssmann WG, Stumpf WE (1986) Coexistence of atrial natriuretic factor (ANF) and oxytocin in neurons of the rat hypothalamus. Neuropeptides 8:243–249
86. Jockusch H, Füchtbauer EM, Füchtbauer A, Leger JJ, Leger J, Maldonado CA, Forssmann WG (1986) Long-term expression of isomyosins and myoendocrine functions in ectopic grafts of atrial tissue. Proc Natl Acad Sci USA 83:7325–7329
87. Kaczmarczyk G, Forssmann WG, Noble MIM, Gaul E, Schnoy N (1987) Atrial granules in the dog heart after cardiac denervation. Cell Tissue Res 249:701–705
88. Kangawa K, Matsuo H (1984) Purification and complete amino acid sequence of alpha-human atrial natriuretic polypeptide (alpha-hANP). Biochem Biophys Res Commun 118:131–139
89. Kangawa K, Tawaragi Y, Oikawa S, Mizuno A, Sakuragawa Y, Nakazoto H, Fukuda A, Minamino N, Matsuo H (1984) Identification of rat gamma atrial natriuretic polypeptide and characterization of the cDNA encoding its precursor. Nature 312: 152–155
90. Katsube N, Schwartz D, Needleman P (1986) Atriopeptin turnover: quantitative relationship between in vivo changes in plasma levels and atrial content. J Pharmacol Exp Ther 239:474–479
91. Kawata M, Nakao K, Morii N, Kiso Y, Yamashita H, Imura H, Sano Y (1985) Atrial natriuretic polypeptide: topographical distribution in the rat brain by radioimmunoassay and immunohistochemistry. Neuroscience 16:521–546
92. Kennedy BP, Marsden JJ, Flynn TG, DeBold AJ, Davies PL (1984) Isolation and nucleotide sequence of a cloned cardionatrin cDNA. Biochem Biophys Res Commun 122:1076–1082

93. Kisch B (1956) Electron microscopy of the atrium of the heart. I. Guinea pig. Exp Med Surg 14:99–112
94. Kisch B (1959) Electron microscopic investigations of the heart of cattle. I. The atrium of the heart of cows. Exp Med Surg 17: 247–261
95. Kisch B (1963) A significant electron microscopic difference between the atria and the ventricles of the mammalian heart. Exp Med Surg 21:193–221
96. Kondo H (1985) Immunohistochemical analysis of the localization of neuropeptides in the adrenal gland. Arch Histol Jap 48:453–481
97. Kramer HJ (ed) (1987) Natriuretic hormones in hypertension. Official satellite symposium to the 11th meeting of the International Society of Hypertension, Heidelberg, September 7–9, 1986. Klin Wochenschr 65 [Suppl VIII]:1–161
98. Kreye VAW, Bussmann WD (Hrsg) (1987) ANP – Atriales natriuretisches Peptid und das kardiovaskuläre System. Steinkopff, Darmstadt
99. Lachance D, Garcia R, Gutkowska J, Cantin M, Thibault G (1986) Mechanisms of release of atrial natriuretic factor. I. Effect of several agonists and steroids on its release by atrial minces. Biochem Biophys Res Commun 135:1090–1098
100. Lang RE, Thölken H, Ganten D, Luft FC, Ruskoaho H, Unger Th (1985) Atrial natriuretic factor – a circulating hormone stimulated by volume loading. Nature 314:264–266
101. Larsen TH, Arjamaa O, Järvinen M, Saetersdal T (1987) Immunohistochemical localization of ANP in the pulmonary veins of the rat. Acta Histochem Cytochem 20:471–476
102. Ledsome JR, Wilson N, Courneya CA, Rankin AJ (1985) Release of atrial natriuretic peptide by atrial distension. Can J Physiol Pharmacol 63:739–742
103. Luft FC, Lang RE, Arnoff GR, Ruskoaho RH, Toth M, Ganten M, Sterzel RB, Unger T (1986) Atriopeptin III kinetics and pharmacodynamics in normal and anephric rats. J Pharmacol Exp Ther 236:416–418
104. Maki M, Takayanagi R, Misono KS, Pandey KN, Tibbetts C, Inagami T (1984) Structure of rat atrial natriuretic factor precursor deduced from cDNA sequence. Nature 309:722–724
105. Maldonado CA, Saggau W, Forssmann WG (1986) Cardiodilatin-immunoreactivity in specific atrial granules of human heart revealed by the immunogold stain. Anat Embryol 173:295–298
106. Malpighi M (1686) Opera omnia (Londra, 1686–87; Leida, 1987). Cited from: Belloni L (ed) Opere scelte di Marcello Malphighi. Tipografia Torinese S.p.A., Torino, pp 75–99
107. Marie JP, Guillemot H, Hatt PY (1976) Le degré de granulation des cardiocytes auriculaires. Étude planimétrique au cours de différents apports d'eau et de sodium chez le rat. Pathol Biol 24:549–554
108. Martinez-Palomo A, Bencosme SA (1966) Electron microscopic observations on myocardial specific granules and residual bodies in vertebrates. Anat Rec 154:473
109. Marumo F, Sakamoto H, Ando K, Ishigama T, Kawakami M (1986) A highly sensitive radioimmunoassay of atrial natriuretic peptide (ANP) in human plasma and urine. Biochem Biophys Res Commun 137: 231–236
110. Matsubara H, Nishikawa M, Umeda Y, Taniguchi T, Iwasaka T, Kurimoto T, Yamane Y, Inada M (1987) The role of atrial pressure in secreting atrial natriuretic polypeptides. Am Heart J 113:1457–1462
111. McKenzie JC, Tanaka I, Misono KS, Inagami T (1985) Immunocytochemical localization of atrial natriuretic factor in the kidney, adrenal medulla, pituitary, and atrium of rat. J Histochem Cytochem 33:828–832
112. McNutt NS, Fawcett DW (1969) The ultrastructure of the cat myocardium. II. Atrial muscle. J Cell Biol 42:46–67
113. Metz J, Mutt V, Forssmann WG (1984) Immunohistochemical localization of cardiodilatin in myoendocrine cells of the cardiac atria. Anat Embryol 170:123–127
114. Meyer M, Feller S, Gagelmann M, Hock D, Nokihara K, Forssmann WG (1988) Lokalisation von Cardiodilatin (CDD) im Nebennierenmark. Verh Anat Ges 82 (in press)
115. Mochet M, Moravec J, Guillemot H, Hatt PY (1975) The ultrastructure of rat conductive tissue; an electron microscopic study of the atrioventricular node and the bundle of His. J Mol Cell Cardiol 7:879–889
116. Mullins JJ, Zeng Q, Gross KW (1987) Mapping of the mouse atrial natriuretic factor gene. Evidence for tight linkage to the Fv-1 locus. Hypertension 9:518–521
117. Murthy KK, Thibault G, Garcia R, Gutkowska J, Genest J, Cantin M (1986) Degradation of atrial natriuretic factor in the rat. Biochem J 240:461–469
118. Nakayama K, Ohkubo H, Hirose T, Inayama S, Nakanishi S (1984) mRNA sequences for human cardiodilatin-atrial natrituretic factor precursor and regulation of precursor mRNA in rat atria. Nature 310: 699–701

119. Naruse M, Naruse K, Obana K, Kurimoto F, Sakurai H, Honda T, Higashida T, Demura H, Inagami T, Shizume K (1986) Immunoreactive alpha-human atrial natriuretic polypeptide in human plasma. Peptides 7:141–145
120. Needleman P (1986) Atriopeptin biochemical pharmacology. Fed Proc 45:2096–2100
121. Nehls M, Reinecke M, Lang RE, Forssmann WG (1985) Biochemical and immunological evidence for a cardiodilatin-like substance in the snail neurocardiac axis. Proc Natl Acad Sci USA 82:7762–7766
122. Nemer M, Chamberland M, Sirois D, Argentin S, Drouin J, Dixon RAF, Zivin RA, Condra JH (1984) Gene structure of human cardiac hormone precursor, pronatriodilatin. Nature 312:654–656
123. Nemer M, Lavigne JP, Drouin J, Thibault G, Gannon M, Antakly T (1986) Expression of atrial natriuretic factor in heart ventricular tissue. Peptides 7:1147–1152
124. Nemer M, Sirois D, Drouin J (1986) Xho I polymorphism at the human pronatriodilatin (hPND) gene locus. Nucl Acid Res 14:8696
125. Nemer M, Sirois D, Drouin J (1986) Taq I polymorphism at the 3' end of the human pronatriodilatin gene (hPND). Nucl Acid Res 14:8697
126. Netchitailo P, Feuilloley M, Pelletier G, Leboulenger F, Cantin M, Gutkowska J, Vaudry H (1987) Atrial natriuretic factor-like immunoreactivity in the central nervous system of the frog. Neuroscience 22:341–359
127. Nokihara K, Ando E, Forssmann WG (1987) Isolation of cardiodilatin from porcine atria using immunoaffinity chromatography and production of monoclonal antibody. In: Miyazawa T (ed) Peptide Chemistry 1986. Protein Research Foundation, Osaka, pp 7–10
128. Oikawa S, Imai M, Ueno A, Tanaka S, Noguchi T, Nakazato H, Kangawa K, Fukuda A, Matsuo H (1984) Cloning and sequence analysis of cDNA encoding a precursor for human atrial natriuretic polypeptide. Nature 309:724–726
129. Olins GM, Spear KL, Siegel NR, Zurcher-Neely HA (1987) Inactivation of atrial natriuretic factor by the renal brush border. Biochem Biophys Acta 901:97–100
130. Ong H, Lazure C, Nguyen TT, McNicoll N, Seidah N, Chrétien M, De Léan A (1987) Bovine adrenal chromaffin granules are a site of synthesis of atrial natriuretic factor. Biochem Biophys Res Commun 147:957–963
131. Poche R (1958) Submikroskopische Beiträge zur Pathologie der Herzmuskelzelle bei Phosphorvergiftung, Hypertrophie, Atrophie und Kaliummangel. Virchows Arch 331:165–248
132. Reinecke M, Betzler D, Forssmann WG (1987) Immunocytochemistry of cardiac polypeptide hormones (Cardiodilatin/atrial natriuretic polypeptide) in brain and hearts of Myxine glutinosa (Cyclostomata). Histochemistry 86:233–239
133. Reinecke M, Betzler D, Forssmann WG, Thorndyke M, Askensten U, Falkmer S (1987) Electronmicroscopical, immunohistochemical, immunocytochemical and biological evidence for the occurrence of cardiac hormones (ANP/CDD) in chondrichthyes. Histochemistry 87:531–538
134. Reinecke M, Nehls M, Forssmann WG (1985) Phylogenetic aspects of cardiac hormones as revealed by immunocytochemistry, electron microscopy, and bioassay. Peptides 6 [Suppl 3]:321–331
135. Riegger GAJ, Elsner D, Kromer EP, Daffner C, Forssmann WG, Muders F, Pascher EW, Kochsiek K (1988) Atrial natriuretic peptide in congestive heart failure in the dog. Circulation (in press)
136. Rippegather G, Maldonado CA, Schulz-Knappe P, Hock D, Lang RE, Forssmann WG (1987) Morphologie der myoendokrinen Zellen des Rattenherzens bei akuten Veränderungen des Blutvolumens. Verh Anat Ges 81:109–113
137. Rippegather G, Saggau W, Forssmann WG (1987) Pathomorphologie des endokrinen Herzens. In: Kreye VAW, Bussmann WD (Hrsg) ANP – Atriales natriuretisches Peptid und das kardiovasculäre System. Steinkopff, Darmstadt, pp 169–178
138. Rippegather G (1988) Pathomorphology of the endocrine heart. In: Forssmann WG, Scheuermann DW, Alt J (eds) Functional morphology of the endocrine heart. Steinkopff, Darmstadt, pp 145–152
139. Rittenhouse J, Moberly L, O'Donnell ME, Owen NE, Marcus F (1986) Phosphorylation of atrial natriuretic peptides by cyclic AMP-dependent protein kinase. J Biol Chem 261:7607–7610
140. Saper CB, Standaert DG, Currie MG, Schwartz D, Geller DM, Needleman P (1985) Atriopeptin-immunoreactive neurons in the brain: presence in cardiovascular regulatory areas. Science 227:1047–1049
141. Schulz-Knappe P, Forssmann K, Herbst F, Hock D, Pipkorn R, Forssmann WG (1988) Isolation and structural analysis of "urodulatin", a new peptide of the cardiodilatin-(ANP)-family, extracted from human urine. Klin Wochenschr 66:752–759

142. Schwartz D, Geller DM, Manning PT, Siegel NR, Fok KF, Smith CE, Needleman P (1985) Ser-Leu-Arg-Arg-Atriopeptin III: the major circulating forms of atrial peptide. Science 229:397–400
143. Seidman CE, Bloch KD, Klein KA, Smith JA, Seidman JG (1984) Nucleotide sequences of the human and mouse atrial natriuretic factor genes. Science 226: 1206–1209
144. Seidman CE, Bloch KD, Zisfein J, Smith JA, Haber E, Homcy C, Duby AD, Choi E, Graham RM, Seidman JG (1985) Molecular studies of the atrial natriuretic factor gene. Hypertension 7 [Suppl I]:31–34
145. Shields PP, Glembotski CC (1988) The post-translational processing of rat pro-atrial natriuretic factor by primary atrial myocyte cultures. J Biol Chem 263:8091–8098
146. Skofitsch G, Jacobowitz DM, Eskay RL, Zamir N (1985) Distribution of atrial natriuretic factor-like immunoreactive neurons in the rat brain. Neuroscience 16:917–948
147. Sonnenberg JL, Sakane Y, Jeng AY, Koehn JA, Ansell JA, Wennogle LP, Ghai RD (1988) Identification of protease 3.4.24.11 as the major atrial natriuretic factor degrading enzyme in the rat kidney. Peptides 9:173–180
148. Sonnenberg H, Veress AT (1984) Cellular mechanism of release of atrial natriuretic factor. Biochem Biophys Res Commun 124: 443–449
149. Springall DR, Bhatnagar M, Wharton J, Hamid Q, Gulbenkian S, Hedges M, Meleagros L, Bloom SR, Polak JM (1988) Expression of the atrial natriuretic peptide gene in the cardiac muscle of rat extrapulmonary and intrapulmonary veins. Thorax 43:44–52
150. Stephenson SL, Kenny AJ (1987) The hydrolysis of alpha-human atrial natriuretic peptide by pig kidney microvillar membranes is initiated by endopeptidase-24.11. Biochem J 243:183–187
151. Sudoh T, Kangawa K, Minamino N, Matsuo H (1988) A new natriuretic peptide in procine brain. Nature 332:78–81
152. Sudoh T, Minamino N, Kangawa K, Matsuo H (1988) Brain natriuretic peptide-32; N-terminal six amino acid extended form of brain natriuretic peptide identified in porcine brain. Biochem Biophys Res Commun 155:726–732
153. Sugawara M (1987) Ultrastructural evidence for exocytotic release of atrial natriuretic polypeptide in the rat atrial muscle with the use of the tannic acid method. Biomedical Res 8:9–17
154. Takayanagi R, Imada T, Inagami T (1987) Synthesis and presence of atrial natriuretic factor in rat ventricle. Biochem Biophys Res Commun 142:483–488
155. Tanaka I, Inagami T (1986) Release of immunoreactive atrial natriuretic factor from rat hypothalamus in vitro. Eur J Pharmacol 122:353–355
156. Tang J, Fei H, Xie CW, Suen MZ, Han JS, Webber RJ, Chang D, Chang JK (1984) Characterization and localization of atriopeptin in rat atrium. Peptides 5:1173–1177
157. Theron JJ, Biagio R, Meyer AC, Boekkoois (1978) Ultrastructural observations on the maturation and secretion of granules in atrial myocardium. J Mol Cell Cardiol 10: 567–572
158. Thibault G, Garcia R, Gutkowska J, Bilodeau J, Lazure C, Seidah NG, Chretien M, Genest J, Cantin M (1987) The propeptide Asn1-Tyr126 is the storage form of rat atrial natriuretic factor. Biochem J 241: 265–272
159. Thibault G, Garcia R, Gutkowska J, Lazure C, Seidah NG, Chretien M, Genest J, Cantin M (1986) Identification of the released form of atrial natriuretic factor by the perfused rat heart. Proc Soc Exp Biol Med 182:137–141
160. Tomisawa M (1969) Atrial specific granules in various mammals. Arch Histol Jap 30: 449–465
161. Toshimori H, Nakazato M, Toshimori K, Asai J, Matsukura S, Oura C, Matsuo H (1988) Distribution of atrial natriuretic polypeptide-(ANP)-containing cells in the rat heart and pulmonary vein. Cell Tissue Res 251:541–546
162. Toshimori H, Toshimori K, Oura C, Matsuo H (1987) Immunohistochemical study of atrial natriuretic polypeptides in the embryonic, fetal and neonatal rat heart. Cell Tissue Res 248:627–633
163. Toshimori H, Toshimori K, Oura C, Matsuo H (1987) Immunohistochemistry and immunocytochemistry of atrial natriuretic polypeptide in porcine heart. Histochemistry 86:595–601
164. Toshimori H, Toshimori K, Oura C, Matsuo H, Matsukura S (1988) Immunohistochemical identification of Purkinje fibers and transitional cells in a terminal portion of the impulse-conducting system of porcine heart. Cell Tissue Res 253:47–53
165. Ueda S, Sudoh T, Fukuda K, Kangawa K, Minamino N, Matsuo H (1987) Identification of alpha atrial natriuretic peptide 4–28 (and 5–28) in porcine brain. Biochem Biophys Res Commun 149:1055–1062
166. Vanneste Y, Michel A, Dimaline R, Naj-

dovski T, Deschodt-Lanckman M (1988) Hydrolysis of alpha-human atrial natriuretic peptide in vitro by human kidney membranes and purified endoprotease-24-11. Biochem J 254:531–537

167. Weidmann P, Saxenhofer H, Ferrier C, Shaw SG (1988) Atrial natriuretic peptide in man. In: Forssmann WG, Scheuermann DW, Alt J (eds) Functional morphology of the endocrine heart. Steinkopff, Darmstadt, pp 161–186
168. Vlasuk GP, Miller J, Bencen GH, Lewicki JA (1986) Structure and analysis of the bovine atrial natriuretic peptide precursor gene. Biochem Biophys Res Commun 136: 396–403
169. Vollmar AM, Schulz R (1988) Evidence for the presence of ANP-precursor material in the rat thymus. Biochem Biophys Res Commun 155:700–708
170. Vuolteenaho O, Arjamaa O, Vakkuri O, Maksniemi T, Nikkilä L, Kangas J, Puurunen J, Ruskoaho H, Leppäluoto J (1988) Atrial natriuretic peptide (ANP) in rat gastrointestinal tract. FEBS Lett 233:79–82
171. Wypij DM, Harris RB (1988) Atrial granules contain an amino-terminal processing enzyme of atrial natriuretic factor. J Biol Chem 263:7079–7086
172. Yamada H, Saito Y, Mukoyama M, Nakao K, Yasue H, Ban T, Imura H, Sano Y (1988) Immunohistochemical localization of atrial natriuretic polypeptide (ANP) in human atrial and ventricular myocardiocytes. Histochemistry 89:411–413
173. Yamanaka M, Greenberg B, Johnson L, Seilhammer J, Brewer M, Friedemann T, Miller J, Atlas S, Laragh J, Lewicki J, Fiddes J (1984) Cloning and sequence analysis of the cDNA for the rat atrial natriuretic factor precursor. Nature 309:719–722
174. Yandle TG, Crozier I, Nicholls G, Espiner E, Carne A, Brennan S (1987) Amino acid sequence of atrial natriuretic peptides in human coronary sinus plasma. Biochem Biophys Res Commun 146:832–839
175. Yandle TG, Richards AM, Nicholls MG, Cueno R, Espiner EA, Livesey JH (1986) Metabolic clearance rate and plasma half live of alpha-human atrial natriuretic peptide in man. Life Sci 38:1827–1833
176. Yang-Feng TL, Floyd-Smith G, Nemer M, Drouin J, Francke U (1985) The pronatriodilatin gene is located on the distal short arm of human chromosome 1 and on mouse chromosome 4. Am J Hum Genet 37: 1117–1128
177. Zamir N, Skofitsch G, Eskay RL, Jacobowitz DM (1985) Distribution of immunoreactive atrial natriuretic peptides in the central nervous system of the rat. Brain Res 365:105–111
178. Zisfein JB, Sylvestre D, Homcy CJ, Graham RM (1987) Analysis of atrial natriuretic factor biosynthesis and secretion in adult and neonatal rat atrial cardiocytes. Life Sci 41:1953–1959
179. Zivin R, Chondra JH, Dixon RAF, Seidah NG, Chrétien M, Nemer M, Chamberland M, Drouin J (1984) Molecular cloning and characterization of DNA sequences encoding rat and human atrial natriuretic factors. Proc Natl Acad Sci USA 81:6325–6329

Biochemistry of the Differential Release, Processing and Degradation of Cardiac and Related Peptide Hormones*

M. Gagelmann, S. Feller, D. Hock, P. Schulz-Knappe, and W. G. Forssmann

Institute of Anatomy and Cell Biology III, University of Heidelberg, FRG

Summary. Investigations during the last few years supported the existence of two major forms of cardiac peptides. In the heart, a prohormone of 126 amino acid residues (CDD-1-126) is stored, while CDD-99-126/ANP (= αANP) is the circulating form in the blood plasma. By use of a similar isolation procedure, as used for the isolation of circulating CDD-99-126/ANP, a biological active peptide, strongly related to CDD-99-126/ANP, was purified from urine, indicating excretion from the kidneys. Sequence analysis shows that the main form of urinary cardiodilatin is a 32 amino acid residue containing molecule (urodilatin-95-126) similar to CDD-99-126/ANP except N-terminal extension by four amino acid residues. The prolongation first of all indicates that urodilatin is not derived from a plasma form and obtained by filtration and renal clearance. Secondly, it demonstrates that urodilatin undergoes a different posttranslational process during excretion than CDD-99-126/ANP. Both, synthetic human cardiodilatin (CDD-99-126)/atrial natriuretic peptide (ANP) and urodilatin (95-126) are phosphorylated by the catalytic subunit of cAMP-dependent protein kinase at a serine residue in position 104. Phosphorylated peptides exhibit decreased relaxing potency compared to unphosphorylated peptides. CDD-99-126/ANP is rapidly removed from the circulation by clearance and proteolytic degradation. Inactivation of CDD-99-126/ANP in the kidneys occurs by an endoprotease-24.11 present in the cortical membranes. Due to the enzymatic reaction a major cleavage occurs within the ring structure between Cys^{105} and Phe^{106}. In contrast, N-terminal extension by four amino acid residues (Thr-Ala-Pro-Arg) and cAMP-dependent phosphorylation of CDD-99-126/ANP inhibit proteolysis by kidney cortical membranes.

Key words: Cardiodilatin (CDD-99-126) – Atrial natriuretic peptide – Urodilatin (CDD-95-126) – cAMP-dependent phosphorylation – Bioactivity – Relaxation – Degradating activity – Protease 3.4.24.11 – Kidney cortical membranes

Introduction

Specific granules of mammalian heart atria [35, 42] have been suggested to contain a natriuretic and diuretic substance [7] which was characterized as a polypeptide [13, 16]. In these secretory granules, the polypeptide is stored in a large molecular form (Fig. 1) as a prohormone of 126 amino acids [17, 18, 19]. The latest experiments with purified bovine granule preparations strongly indicate that the prohormone and a processing protease are co-stored in the granules with the protease probably being localized in the granular membranes [34, 80]. The processing protease specifically cleaves the prohormone between arginine and serine in position 98 and 99 [34, 80] thereby releasing the circulating peptide (CDD-99-126/ANP; αANP). As the protease is inactive at pH 6.5 and below [80] and the storage granules are acidic [71] processing of the prohormone into the circulating peptide probably takes place during exocytosis of the granules. Isolated perfused hearts release the circulating atrial peptide that comprises the amino acid residues Ser^{99} to Tyr^{126} [70, 76]. The circulating bioactive peptide in the blood plasma contains 28 residues of the C-terminus of the prohormone (Fig. 1) with a disulfide bridge between the cysteine residues in position 106 and 121 [15, 19, 67].

* Dedicated to Viktor Mutt (Stockholm) to his 65th anniversary

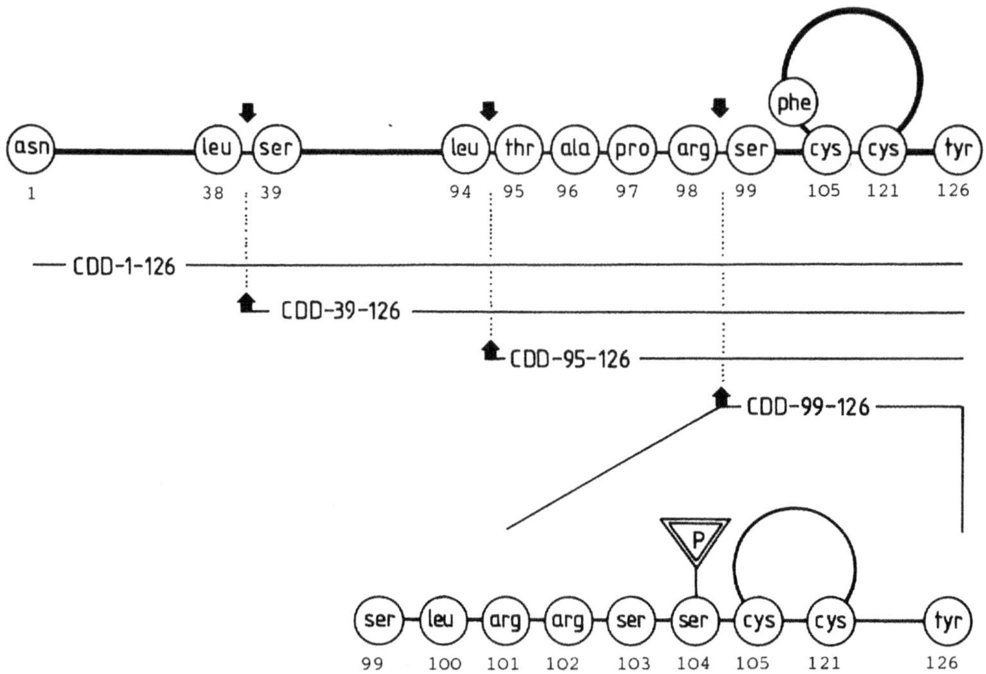

Fig. 1. Schematic illustration of the prohormone (CDD-1-126), shorter prohormone (CDD-39-126), urodilatin (CDD-95-126) and cardiodilatin (CDD-99-126)/atrial natriuretic peptide (ANP) showing parts of the amino acid sequence. In the lower part of the figure, the position of the cAMP-dependent phosphylated serine residue in position 104 is given

The peptide exhibits potent natriuretic, diuretic and vasorelaxant activity. The largest fraction of peptides extracted from large scale extractions of the polypeptides from porcine myoendocrine cells of the atrial tissue by the method of Mutt [51], which involves heating is the prohormone [17]. In addition, as a side fraction, CDD-39-126 consisting of 88 amino acids (Fig. 1) may be extracted [31]. The CDD-39-126 is biologically active, as the final 28 amino acids correspond to human alpha ANP. Several groups have published a large number of cardiac peptide hormones from rat, human and porcine atria (for rev. see ref. [18]). The great variety of fragments may be due to proteolytic degradation during the isolation procedure as also suggested by Flynn et al. [13]. Heat treatment, however, enables purification of the natural cleavage products.

Cardiac hormones are known to occur in other organs, as revealed by mRNA hybridization [27], polypeptide extraction [62] and immunological studies [12, 20, 48]. By use of the same isolation procedure as for the isolation of circulating CDD/ANP from human blood [15], a peptide of 32 amino acids was isolated from human urine [66]. The amino acid sequence is similar to the CDD-99-126/ANP, except that the molecule is N-terminally extended by the tetrapeptide Thr^{95}-Ala^{96}-Pro^{97}-Arg^{98} (Fig. 1) indicating different processing compared to CDD-99-126/ANP in the heart.

Two brain natriuretic peptides of 26 [74] and 32 [75] amino acid residues with a remarkable sequence homology but distinct to CDD-99-126/ANP were isolated from porcine brain. Both peptides elicit a similar pharmacological spectrum as CDD-99-126/ANP [74, 75].

The cardiac peptides exhibit a common amino acid sequence, Arg^{101}-Arg^{102}-Ser^{103}-Ser^{104} (Fig. 1). The sequence Arg-Arg-X-Ser is a recognition sequence for the catalytic subunit of cAMP-dependent protein kinase [4] which phosphorylates the serine in position 104 [2, 24, 59, 63]. In vitro phosphorylation of a synthetic CDD/ANP analog (CDD/ANP-101-126) enhances the Na/K/Cl co-transport in cultured vascular smooth muscle cells [63]. Phosphorylated synthetic CDD-99-126 is less potent than unphosphorylated peptide in respect to vasorelaxant activity [24, 59] and receptor binding properties [59]. As urodilatin exhibits a large homology to CDD-99-126/ANP with respect to the amino acid sequence, similar pharmacological effects are expected for phosphorylated urodilatin.

Exogenously administered CDD-99-126/ANP exhibits a short half-life time [6, 8, 37, 50, 82, 83]. From human coronary sinus blood, a circulating form (CDD-106-126) of CDD/ANP, was detected by amino acid sequence analysis indicating a single cleavage within the ring structure between Cys^{105} and Phe^{106}. The proteolytic product is biological inactive, as will be demonstrated below, and amounts to 20–30% of the total CDD/ANP content [84]. The kidney is considered to be the important site for the clearance and subsequent degradation of circulating CDD/ANP [45]. Incubation of synthetic CDD/ANP with preparations of kidney cortical membranes demonstrate a specific proteolytic activity in the membranes, which catalyzes the same cleavage between Cys^{105} and Phe^{106} [25, 43, 60, 61, 73, 77] as also found in the blood [84]. The cleavage site is specific for endoprotease-24.11 [73, 77], and it was recently shown that endoprotease-24.11 activity is the predominant ANP-degradating activity in the kidney [72]. Immunohistochemical studies support that urodilatin most probably originates from distal tubule cells of the kidneys [10, 12], from where it is secreted into the lumen. Therefore, one should expect that urodilatin exerts an effect in the kidney and thus should be inert against proteolysis by endoprotease-24.11.

The close location of the cAMP-dependent phosphorylation site (Ser^{104}) and the bond (Cys^{105}-Phe^{106}) in the ring sensitive to endoprotease-24.11 cleavage rises the question whether cAMP-dependent phosphorylation may influence the endoproteolytic cleavage of CDD-99-126/ANP by the protease.

Materials and Methods

The catalytic subunit of cAMP-dependent protein kinase (EC 2.7.1.37) was isolated from bovine cardiac muscle [41]. Synthetic cardiodilatin/ANP (CDD-99-126) and urodilatin (95-126) were from Bissendorf Biochemicals (Hannover, FRG). Bovine cardiac cardiodilatin-39-126 was prepared as described [31]. Trifluoroacetic acid (TFA) and acetonitrile were from Applied Biosystems. All other reagents were of the highest grade available and obtained from local suppliers.

Preparation of phosphorylated peptides was as described [25]. The catalytic subunit of cAMP-dependent protein kinase was added in a concentration that ensures complete phosphorylation within 40 min. The reaction was stopped by freezing with liquid nitrogen. Purification of phosphorylated peptide by reverse phase high performance liquid chromatography (RP-HPLC) was as described [25]. Phosphorylated and unphosphorylated peptides elute as single peaks.

Purification of phosphorylated peptide by cation exchange HPLC. The phosphorylated peptide separated by RP-HPLC was submitted to a cation exchanger column (4 × 50 mm) using a HPLC device from LKB equipped with two pumps, a 2152 Controller, a 2151 Variable Wavelength Monitor, and a Rheodyne Injector (1 ml loop). The column was developed with a linear gradient of NaCl in 10 mM Na_2HPO_4 (pH 5) at a flow rate of 0.7 ml/min (absorbance 230 nm). All steps were performed at room temperature. The starting concentration was 100 mM NaCl. The phosphorylated peptide elutes at lower salt concentration compared to the unphosphorylated material [26]. The peak was collected, lyophilized and stored at −70°C. Contaminating salt was removed by another RP-HPLC as described above.

Bioactivity tests were done with aortic smooth muscle strips from New Zealand rabbits as reported [24].

Preparation of membranes from dog kidney cortex and proteolysis basically followed the procedure described by Koehn et al. [43] except for some modifications [25].

Results and Discussion

I. Localization and Structure of the CDD/ANP Gene

In 1984, shortly after publication of the first amino acid sequences for atrial natriuretic peptides, several groups sequenced cDNA's coding the human and rat preprohormone [30, 36, 38, 46, 52, 53, 57, 68, 81, 86]. Up to the present, sequences of cardiodilatin/atrial natriuretic peptide, cDNA's and genes of several mammals are known [1, 14, 30, 32, 36, 46, 49, 52, 53, 57, 58, 68, 69, 78, 81, 86]. The gene is located on the short arm of human chromosome 1, as demonstrated by in situ hybridization [85]. Studies indicate that it is located near the Friend virus susceptibility locus Fv-1 [55]. The Fig. 2 summarizes the informations available on the localization and structure of human CDD/ANP gene, mRNA, and posttranslational processing products.

Transcription of the various mammalian CDD/ANP genes and processing of the primary transcripts results in mRNAs of approximately 950 bases. The mRNAs code a signal peptide of 23 to 25 amino acid residues, followed by a 126 amino acid residue prohormone which, in some species, is elongated by 2 C-terminal arginines. This prolongated reading frame is due to a single nucleotide change. The arginines are probably removed early after synthesis, as they are absent in all of the prohormones sequenced so far from artrial and adrenal tissue. The 3′ end of the mRNA contains one or two polyadenylation signal sequences. In all CDD/ANP genes known today, the mRNA coding region is interrupted by two introns, thus generating 3 exons. Exon 1 codes for the signal peptide and 20 N-terminal amino acids of the prohormone, exon 2 for the rest of the prohormone, except 1 to 3 C-terminal amino acid residues, which are contained in exon 3. Intron 2 covers 2 Alu sequences, further a putative binding site for the glucocorticoid receptor complex.

Two CAAT-boxes (sequences thought to regulate the transcription frequency) and a region with homology to part of the SV 40 enhancer sequence are located in the non transcribed 5′flank of the CDD/ANP gene. Experiments with transgenic mice have documented that this region ensures tissue specific gene expression [11, 21, 22, 23, 54, 55]. Comparison of the sequence of mammalian CDD/ANP genes shows a high degree of homology, up to over 90% for the nucleotides coding the circulating 28 amino acid residue hormone, but also in the noncoding regions. The mentioned 5′flank reaches e.g. 79% homology between human and mouse gene, a conservativity which may be due to its relevance for specific expression of the gene. Restriction fragment length polymorphisms (RFLP's) are known for the restriction enzymes Taq I, Xho I, Bsm I, Bgl I and II [29], but no hints exist for a correlation of a certain allelic type to inheritable diseases.

II. Posttranslational Processing

Influence of cAMP-Dependent Phosphorylation on the Biological Activity

Phosphorylation is critical to the regulation of many cellular processes including differentiation and proliferation. Several peptide hormones are phosphorylated by isolated protein kinases. Phosphorylation of peptid hormones has been shown for prolactin [56], for peptide derived from proopiomelanocortin [9] and for the α subunit of human chorionic gonadotropin [65]. Rittenhouse et al. [63] reported that cAMP-dependent protein kinase phosphorylates synthetic peptides related to CDD/ANP in vitro. They found that phosphorylated ANP-peptides are more potent than unphosphorylated forms in stimulating Na/K/Cl co-transport in cultured vascular smooth muscle cells, whereas Olins et al. [59] and Gagelmann et al. [24] reported that phosphorylated CDD/ANP exhibits decreased vasorelaxant potency on living muscle strips. With primary cultures of neonatal rat cardiocytes being used, the sites of cAMP-dependent phosphorylation were identified as Ser^{39} and Ser^{50} in the prohormone, while no phosphorylation of Ser^{104} could be detected [2]. Recently, however, Rittenhouse et al. [64] demonstrated that in situ in atria the prohormone is phosphorylated at the cAMP-dependent site. Despite the overall extent of Ser^{104} phosphorylation was low by a cAMP-dependent pathway. So far it has

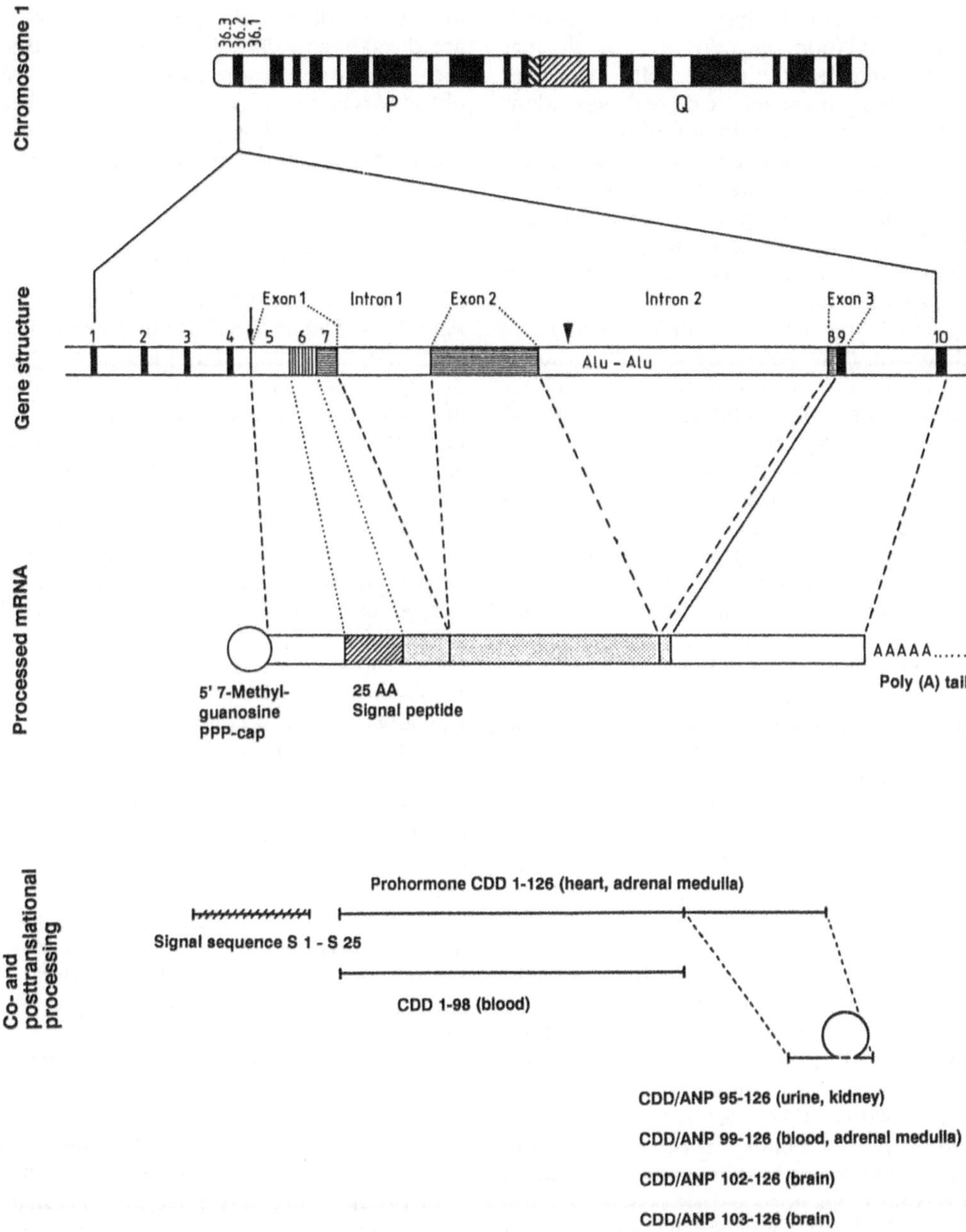

Fig. 2. Human cardiodilatin (CDD-99-126)/atrial natriuretic peptide (ANP) gene. Localization, gene structure, mRNA and natural peptides (1, region with homology to part of the SV 40 enhancer sequence; 2, putative CAAT-box 1; 3, putative CAAT-box 2; 4, TATA-box; 5, Transcribed, non coding 5'-area; 6, signal sequence coding area; 7, 8, short prohormone coding regions; 9, stop codon (opal); 10, signal sequence for polyadenylation; Alu-Alu, 2 Alu-sequences (tandem); Arrow head, putative binding site for glucocorticoid receptor complex

been considered that cAMP-dependent phosphorylation only occurs in distinct compartments within the cells. Most recently [44], however, a cAMP-dependent ecto-protein kinase in addition ot other ecto-protein kinase activities was for the first time found on the cell surface of HeLa cells. These data suggest that cells are capable to modify extracellular proteins and peptides of the immediate environment by phosphorylation.

Atrial natriuretic peptide (ANP)/cardiodilatin (CDD-99-126) as well as the N-terminal deleted prohormone (CDD-39-126) are phosphorylated in the presence of ATP and catalytic subunit of cAMP-dependent protein kinase. The phosphorylated site was characterized as the serine in position 104 [26, 59, 63]. On precontracted rabbit aorta muscle strips, phosphorylated CDD-99-126/ANP (4.5×10^{-10} M final concentration) exhibits only little or no effect, while aorta strips considerably relax at this concentration with unphosphorylated peptide [26]. During stepwise incubation with unphosphorylated, phosphorylated and again unphosphorylated CDD-99-126 relaxation, only occurs in presence of unphosphorylated peptide. Administration of the peptide in the reversed sequence (start with phosphorylated CDD-99-126) demonstrates a similar result: relaxation is only achieved with unphosphorylated peptide [26].

The time course of cAMP-dependent phosphorylation of urodilatin (95-126) by the catalytic subunit is similar as with CDD-99-126/ANP showing complete phosphorylation under our conditions [26]. As observed with CDD-99-126/ANP, the biological activity of phosphorylated urodilatin compared to unphosphorylated peptide on precontracted aorta strips is strongly depressed. Both, phosphorlylated and unphosphorylated urodilatin (1.22, 0.64, 0.18 nM, final concentration) exhibit a dose-dependent relaxing activity showing a stronger relaxing effect at higher concentrations. Again, administration of phosphorylated urodilatin in the same concentrations caused a less pronounced relaxation in all cases [26]. Receptor binding studies by Olins et al. [59] demonstrated that the decreased relaxant potency and the decreased receptor binding of phosphorylated peptide are directly correlated. This indicates that the decreased vasorelaxant potency of phosphorylated CDD-99-126/ANP and urodilatin are probably due to a decreased receptor binding to living vascular muscle.

Proteolytic Degradation of CDD-99-126/ANP and Urodilatin

The biological half-time of CDD-99-126/ANP in vivo is short, as it is rapidly removed from the circulation. The half-life rates of disappearance of exogenous CDD/ANP after injection is approximately 15 to 30 sec. in rat [8, 37] and 2.5 to 3.1 min in man [82, 83]. A proteolytic product of CDD-99-126/ANP was detected showing a single specific cleavage in the ring between Cys and Phe in position 105 and 106 (Fig. 3). The proteolytic product was isolated from human coronary sinus blood in a yield of 20 to 30% of the total CDD/ANP [84]. Several fragments (Fig. 3) are generated early after injection of CDD-99-126/ANP [25, 60] in vitro is age between Cys and Phe. This finding indicates that the proteolysis contributes to the clearance of CDD/ANP from the circulation. Similar specific proteolysis [25, 43, 60, 61, 72, 73, 77] causing inactivation of the CDD-99-126/ANP [25, 60] in vitro is catalyzed in the presence of a preparation of kidney membranes (Fig. 4, right panel). The proteolytic activity was identified as endoprotease-24.11 (EC 3.4.24.11), which is the major ANP-degradating activity in the kidney [72]. The endoprotease-24.11 is a widespread enzyme in the plasma membranes of many tissues [3, 28, 47] and cleaves exclusively peptide bonds on the N-terminal side of hydrophobic amino acid residues [40], although some divergency has been observed in this respect [77]. As can be seen from Fig. 3, purified endoprotease-24.11 cleaves the peptide bond between Cys and Phe in position 105 and 106 among others. During 20 min incubation of synthetic CDD-99-126/ANP with a preparation of kidney cortical membranes, a single major product is generated, which elutes prior to the intact CDD-99-126/ANP during separation by RP-HPLC (Fig. 4, right panel). The proteolytic product was identified by amino acid sequence analysis showing a single

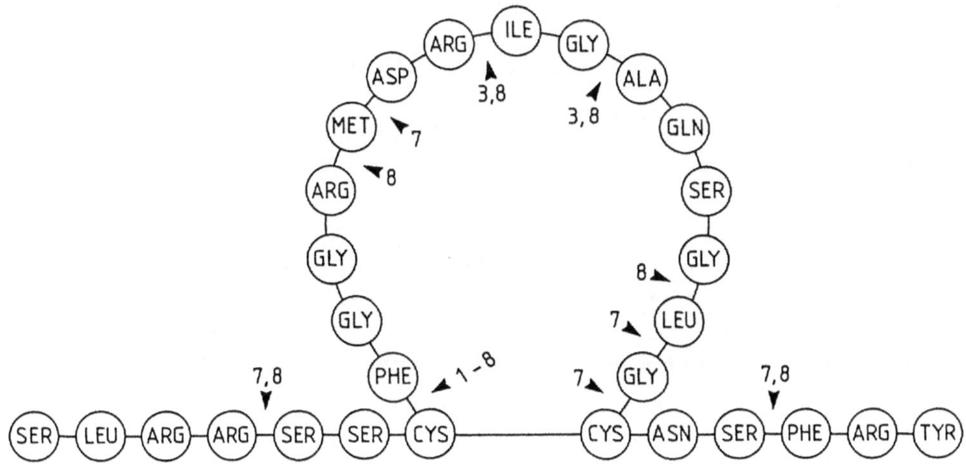

α - ANP / CDD - 99 - 126

HYDROLYSIS OF ATRIAL NATRIURETIC PEPTIDE/CARDIODILATIN BY:

1 ►	Kidney brush-border membranes	**Olins et al.** (1987)
2 ►	Kidney cortex membranes	**Koehn et al.** (1987)
3 ►	Kidney microvillar membranes and purified endoprotease-24.11	**Stephenson and Kenny** (1987)
4 ►	*In vivo* in human coronary sinus blood	**Yandle et al.** (1987)
5 ►	Purified endoprotease-24.11	**Sonnenberg et al.** (1988)
6 ►	Kidney cortex membranes	**Gagelmann et al.** (1988)
7 ►	*In vivo* in rat blood	**Condra et al.** (1988)
8 ►	Human kidney membranes and purified endoprotease-24.11	**Vanneste et al.** (1988)

Fig. 3. Cleavages reported to occur in synthetic CDD-99-126/ANP after treatment with kidney membranes and purified endoprotease-24.11 in vitro and in vivo after injection of the peptide into the circulation as well as after release from the heart. The numbers in the schematic drawing (upper) indicate the cleavage sites under the appropriate conditions by the different groups given below on the left in the lower panel

cleavage of the peptide between Cys and Phe. Prolonged incubation (40 min) almost completely removed the intact peptide [25]. The proteolytic activity is destroyed upon boiling of the membranes [25] or by preincubation with the protease inhibitor phosphoramidon [72, 73, 79].

The urodilatin isolated from human urine [66] exhibits a similar amino acid sequence as CDD-99-126/ANP except the already described N-terminal extension by four amino acid residues (Fig. 1). The same N-terminal amino acid residues are present in the prohormone (Fig. 1). Thus, if urodilatin is re-

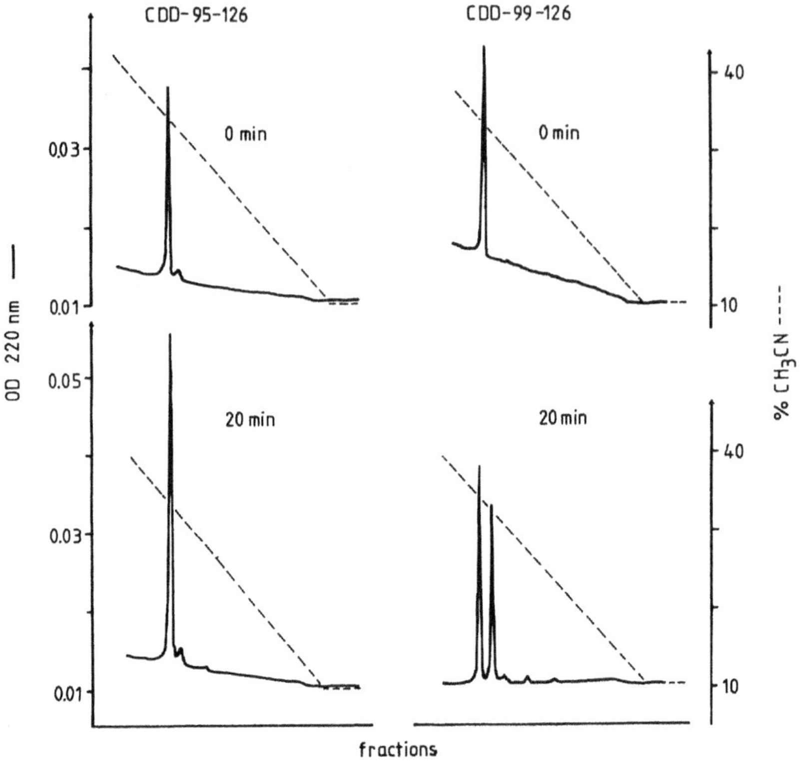

Fig. 4. Proteolysis of urodilatin (CDD-95-126; left panel) and CDD-99-126/ANP (right panel) by a membrane protease preparation from dog kidney cortex. In both cases 15 μg peptide were incubated with 12 μg membrane protein at the same conditions. After 0 (upper) and 20 min (lower) incubation, an aliquot corresponding to 5 μg peptide was removed from the reaction vessel and separated by RP-HPLC (Aquapore 4.6 × 400, RP-300, C8 from ABI). The column was developed with a linear acetonitrile (CH_3CN) gradient with 0.1% trifluoroacetic acid (dotted line). The absorbance was recorded at 220 nm (continuous line)

leased from a kidney prohormone, this proteolytic step must necessarily be mediated by another processing protease than in the heart granules. In the heart, specific cleavage of the prohormone occurs between Arg and Ser in position 98 and 99, whereas in the case of urodilatin, cleavage should occur between Leu and Thr in position 94 and 95 (Fig. 1). As mentioned before, urodilatin most probably is secreted from cells of the distal tubule region [10, 12]. It would, however, be difficult to understand how urodilatin could exert any biological effect in the kidney, if it is rapidly destroyed. Therefore, it is tempting to speculate that urodilatin may be inert against endoprotease-24.11 which is probably due to N-terminal prolongation. Incubation of urodilatin for 20 min with the kidney cortical membranes (Fig. 4, left panel) under the same conditions as in case of CDD-99-126/ANP demonstrates that urodilatin is stable against endoprotease-24.11. Prolonged incubation (40 min) of urodilatin with the membrane preparation leads to a certain decrease of the intact peptide. Only minor proteolysis, however, is observed without further increase of proteolytic product. This is not surprising, since crude membrane preparations are used; thus, one has to expect a variety of proteolytic activities [39]. The finding indicates that the presence of the tetra-peptide (Thr-Ala-Pro-Arg) prevents proteolysis and thus rapid metabolization by the kidney, while CDD-99-126/ANP undergoes hydrolysis and inactivation. In order to investigate whether N-terminal extension of the cardiac peptide is the important factor in one exper-

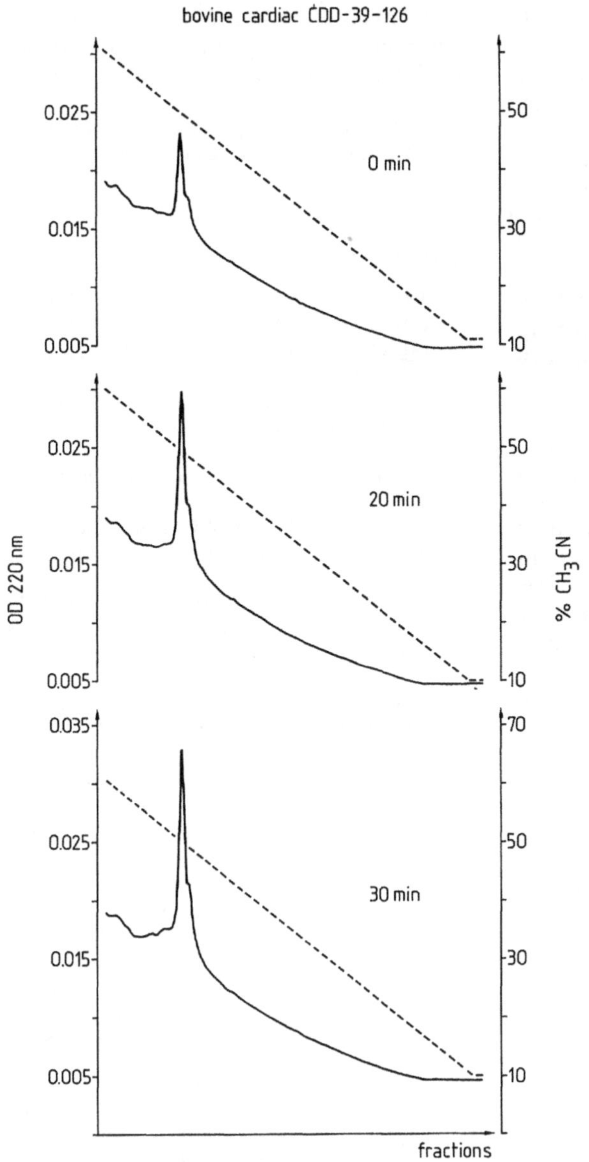

Fig. 5. Incubation of bovine cardiac CDD-39-126 with kidney cortical membranes for 0, 20 and 30 min. For the incubation 30 μg CDD-39-126 and 12 μg membrane preparation were used. The conditions for separation are identical to the conditions described in the legend to Fig. 4, except that an aliquot corresponding to 10 μg was used in case of 20 and 30 min incubation

iment (Fig. 5), the shorter form of the prohormone (CDD-39-126) was used as a substrate for the membrane preparation. As can be seen from Fig. 5, CDD-39-126 elutes from the RP-column at a higher acetonitrile concentration than CDD-99-126/ANP or urodilatin. Again, as observed before in case of urodilatin CDD-39-126, is not proteolytically destroyed by the membranes.

Influence of cAMP-dependent phosphorylation on proteolytic degradation of CDD-99-126/ANP by endoprotease-24.11

The close location of the cAMP-dependent phosphorylation site (Ser^{104}) and the cleaved peptide bond (Cys^{105}-Phe^{106}) raised the question whether or not phosphorylation at the cAMP-dependent site influences degradation by endoprotease-24.11. In order to answer this question, phosphorylated peptide was purified from contaminating unphosphorylated material. As the phosphoryl group transferred from ATP into the peptide contributes to the charge of the molecule, separation of the phosphorylated material from the unphosphorylated peptide by ion exchanger HPLC is enabled. At pH 5, the unphosphorylated CDD-99-126 elutes from the cation exchange column as a single peak at a salt concentration of approximately 230 mM NaCl. The phosphorylated CDD-99-126, however, binds more weakly to the cation exchanger and elutes at a lower salt concentration of 150 mM NaCl [26]. The salt from the cation exchanger step was removed by RP-HPLC. Endoprotease-24.11 activity was ensured by control incubation of CDD-99-126/ANP with the kidney membrane preparation. The phosphorylated CDD-99-126/ANP, however, incubated with the same membrane preparation containing the proteolytic activity under the same conditions as the control, shows only minor proteolysis [33].

Conclusion

The findings suggest that the N-terminal extension of urodilatin by at least four amino acid residues compared to CDD-99-126/ANP prevents proteolytic attack by endoprotease-24.11, which contributes to the major ANP-degradating activity in the kidney. Since urodilatin is excreted from the kidney, and since the kidney may be considered as the target tissue for peptide action, it appears logical that the secreted peptide has a design which prevents biological inactivation. The physiological roles of phosphorylation of CDD/ANP and related peptides remain to be further defined. Cyclic-AMP-dependent phosphorylation is unlikely to be involved in the process of storage or secretion. Cyclic-AMP-dependent phosphorylation or phosphorylation at the same site by another protein kinase may, however, be an important factor in the control of the biological activity of circulating CDD/ANP and urodilatin, as both phosphorylated peptides exhibit decreased vasorelaxant potency on vascular smooth muscle. Phosphorylation of CDD-99-126/ANP has a similar effect as the N-terminal prolongation in respect to proteolytic degradation by kidney cortical membranes.

Acknowledgements: Supported by Braunschweig Biotechnology Co., BRAUNKOP 88.

References

1. Argentin S, Nemer M, Drouin J, Scott GK, Kennedy BP, Davies PL (1985) The gene for rat atrial natriuretic factor. J Biol Chem 260:4568–4571
2. Bloch KD, Jones SW, Preibisch G, Seipke G, Seidman CE, Seidman JG (1987) Proatrial natriuretic factor is phosphorylated by rat cardiocytes in culture. J Biol Chem 262: 9956–9961
3. Bowes MA, Kenny AJ (1986) Endopeptidase-24.11 in pig lymph nodes. Biochem J 236:801–810
4. Carlson GM, Bechtel PJ, Graves DJ (1979) Chemical and regulatory properties of phosphorylase kinase and cyclic AMP-dependent protein kinase. Adv Enzymol 50:41–115
5. Condra CL, Leidy EA, Bunting P, Colton CD, Nutt RF, Rosenblatt M, Jacobs JW (1988) Clearance and early hydrolysis of atrial natriuretic factor in vivo. J Clin Invest 81:1348–1354
6. Crozier IG, Nicholls MG, Ikram H, Espiner EA, Gomez HJ, Warner NJ (1986) Heamodynamic effects of atrial peptide infusion in heart failure. Lancet II:1242–1245
7. DeBold AJ, Borenstein HB, Veress AT, Sonnenberg H (1981) A rapid and potent natriuretic response to intravenous injection of atrial extracts in rats. Life Sci 28:89–94
8. Devine E, Artman L, Budzik G, Bush E, Holleman W (1986) Distribution and elimination of intravenously administered atrial natriuretic hormone (ANH) to normal and nephrectomized rats. Fed Proc 45:1738
9. Eipper BA, Mains RE (1982) Phosphorylation of pro-adrenocorticotropin/endorphin-derived peptides. J Biol Chem 257: 4907–4915
10. Feller S, Meyer M, Hock D, Forssmann WG (1988) Extraaurikuläre Lokalisation von Cardiodilatin. Acta Anat 132:80
11. Field LJ (1988) Atrial natriuretic factor-SV 40 T antigen transgenes produce tumors and cardiac arrhythmias in mice. Science 239: 1029–1033
12. Flügge G, Inagami T, Fuchs E (1987) Atrial natriuretic peptide detected by immunocytochemistry in peripheral organs of Tupaia belangeri. Histochemistry 86:479–483

13. Flynn TG, DeBold ML, DeBold AJ (1983) The amino acid sequence of an atrial peptide with potent diuretic and natriuretic properties. Biochem Biophys Res Commun 117: 859–865
14. Flynn TG, Davies PL, Kennedy BP, DeBold ML, DeBold AJ (1985) Alignment of rat cardionatrin sequences with the preprocardionatrin sequence from complementary DNA. Science 228:323–325
15. Forssmann K, Hock D, Herbst F, Schulz-Knappe P, Talartschik J, Scheler F, Forssmann WG (1986) Isolation and structural analysis of the circulating human cardiodilatin (alpha ANP). Klin Wochenschr 64: 1276–1280
16. Forssmann WG, Hock D, Lottspeich F, Henschen A, Kreye V, Christmann M, Reinecke M, Metz J, Carlquist M, Mutt V (1983) The right auricle of the heart is an endocrine organ. Cardiodilatin as a peptide hormone candidate. Anat Embryol 168: 307–313
17. Forssmann WG, Birr C, Carlquist M, Christmann M, Finke R, Henschen A, Hock D, Kirchheim H, Kreye V, Lottspeich F, Metz J, Mutt V, Reinecke M (1984) The auricular myocardiocytes of the heart constitute an endocrine organ. Characterization of a porcine cardiac peptide hormone, cardiodilatin-126. Cell Tissue Res 238:425–430
18. Forssmann WG (1986) Cardiac hormones. I. Review on the morphology, biochemistry, and molecular biology of the endocrine heart. Eur J Clin Invest 16:439–451
19. Forssmann WG, Hock D, Mutt V (1986) Cardiac hormones: morphology and biochemistry. Klin Wochenschr 64 [Suppl VI]:4–12
20. Forssmann WG, Lang RE, Aoki A, Reinecke M, Rippegather G, Hock D (1987) Cardiodilatin as a neuropeptide (cardiac polypeptide hormones are also neuropeptides). Exp Brain Res 16:43–50
21. Frossard PM, Gonzalez PA, Greenberg B, Fiddes JC, Atlas SA (1986) BglII dimorphism at the human atrial natriuretic peptide (ANP) gene locus. Nucl Acids Res 14:5121
22. Frossard PM, Coleman RT (1986) Human atrial natriuretic peptides (ANP) gene locus: BglI RFLP. Nucl Acids Res 14:9223
23. Frossard PM, Coleman RT, Morrison NA (1987) Human natriuretic peptides (ANP) gene locus: BsmI RFLP. Nucl Acids Res 15: 7656
24. Gagelmann M, Hock D, Forssmann WG (1987) Relaxation of smooth muscle by cardiodilatin/atrial natriuretic peptide is inhibited by cAMP-dependent phosphorylation. FEBS Letters 225:251–254
25. Gagelmann M, Hock D, Forssmann WG (1988) Urodilatin (CDD/ANP-95-126) is not biologically inactivated by a peptidase from dog kidney cortex membranes in contrast to atrial natriuretic peptide/cardiodilatin (alpha hANP/CDD-99-126). FEBS Letters 233: 249–254
26. Gagelmann M, Hock D, Herbst F, Schulz-Knappe P, Forssmann WG (1989) Effect of cAMP-dependent phosphorylation on the bioactivity of cardiodilatin/atrial natriuretic factor and related peptides. Peptides [Suppl] (in press)
27. Gardner DG, Vlasuk GP, Baxter JD, Fiddes JC, Lewicki JA (1987) Identification of atrial natriuretic factor gene transcripts in the central nervous system of the rat. Proc Natl Acad Sci USA 84:2175–2179
28. Gee NS, Bowes MA, Buck P, Kenny AJ (1985) An immunoradiometric assay for endopeptidase-24.11 shows it to be a widely distributed enzyme in pig tissues. Biochem J 228:119–126
29. Graham RM, Bloch KD, Delaney VB, Bourke E, Seidman JG (1986) Bartter's syndrome and the atrial natriuretic factor gene. Hypertension 8:549–551
30. Greenberg BD, Bencen GH, Seilhamer JJ, Lewicki JA, Fiddes JC (1984) Nucleotide sequence of the gene encoding human atrial natriuretic factor precursor. Nature 312: 656–658
31. Hock D, Schriek U, Fey E, Forssmann WG, Mutt V (1987) Isolation of bovine cardiodilatin by fast protein liquid chromatography and reversed phase high-performance liquid chromatography. J Chromatogr 397:347–353
32. Hock D, Mayer W, Back H, Schriek U, Herbst F, Forssmann WG (1986) Isolation and characterization of bovine cardiodilatin (CDD). Biol Chem Hoppe-Seyler [Suppl] 367:267
33. Hock D, Gagelmann M, Dörner T, Forssmann WG (1989) Cyclic 3′,5′ monophosphate-dependent phosphorylation of cardiodilatin/atrial natriuretic peptide: reduced proteolysis by kidney cortex protease. (Submitted)
34. Imada T, Takayanagi R, Inagami T (1988) Purification of a specific peptidase in bovine atria for the processing of proatrial natriuretic factor. Biol Chem Hoppe-Seyler 369: 113–120
35. Jamieson JD, Palade GE (1964) Specific granules in atrial muscle cells. J Cell Biol 23:151–172
36. Kangawa K, Tawaragi Y, Oikawa S, Mizuno A, Sakuragawa Y, Nakazato H, Fukuda A, Minamino N, Matsuo H (1984) Identification of rat gamma atrial natriuretic polypeptide

and characterization of the cDNA encoding its precursor. Nature 312:152–155

37. Katsube N, Schwartz D, Needleman P (1986) Atriopeptin turnover: quantitative relationship between in vivo changes in plasma levels and atrial content. J Pharmacol Exp Ther 239:474–479
38. Kennedy BP, Marsden JJ, Flynn TG, DeBold AJ, Davies PL (1984) Isolation and nucleotide sequence of a cloned cardionatrin cDNA. Biochem Biophys Res Commun 122: 1076–1082
39. Kenny AJ, Maroux S (1982) Topology of microvillar membrane hydrolases of kidney and intestine. Physiol Rev 62:91–128
40. Kerr MA, Kenny AJ (1974) The purification and specificity of a neutral endopeptidase from rabbit kidney brush border. Biochem J 137:477–488
41. Kinzel V, Hotz A, König N, Gagelmann M, Pyerin W, Reed J, Kübler D, Hofmann F, Obst C, Gensheimer HP, Goldblatt D, Shaltiel S (1987) Chromatographic separation of two heterogeneous forms of the catalytic subunit of cyclic AMP-dependent protein kinase holoenzyme type I and type II from striated muscle of different mammalian species. Arch Biochem Biophys 253:341–349
42. Kisch B (1956) Electron microscopy of the atrium of the heart. I. Guinea pig. Exp Med Surg 14:99–112
43. Koehn JA, Norman JA, Jones BN, LeSueur L, Sakane Y, Ghai RD (1987) Degradation of atrial natriuretic factor by kidney cortex membranes. J Biol Chem 262: 11 623–11 627
44. Kübler D, Pyerin W, Bill O, Hotz A, Sonka J, Kinzel V (1988) Phosphorylation of kemptide by intact cells in a cAMP-dependent reaction: evidence for another ecto-protein kinase activity. Biol Chem Hoppe-Seyler 396:858
45. Luft FC, Lang RE, Arnoff GR, Ruskoaho RH, Toth M, Ganten M, Sterzel RB, Unger T (1986) Atriopeptin III kinetics and pharmacodynamics in normal and anephric rats. J Pharmacol Exp Ther 236:416–418
46. Maki M, Takayanagi R, Misono KS, Pandey KN, Tibbetts C, Inagami T (1984) Structure of rat atrial natriuretic factor precursor deduced from cDNA sequence. Nature 309: 722–724
47. Matsas R, Fulcher IS, Kenny AJ, Turner AJ (1983) Substance P and [Leu]enkephalin are hydrolyzed by an enzyme in pig caudate synaptic membranes that is identical with the endopeptidase of kidney microvilli. Proc Natl Acad Sci USA 80:3111–3115
48. McKenzie JC, Tanaka I, Misono KS, Inagami T (1985) Immunocytochemical localization of atrial natriuretic factor in the kidney, adrenal medulla, pituitary, and atrium of rat. J Histochem Cytochem 33:828–832
49. Mullins JJ, Zeng Q, Gross KW (1987) Mapping of the mouse atrial natriuretic factor gene. Evidence for tight linkage to the Fv-1 locus. Hypertension 9:518–521
50. Murthy KK, Thibault G, Garcia R, Gutkowska J, Genest J, Cantin M (1986) Degradation of atrial natriuretic factor in the rat. Biochem J 240:461–469
51. Mutt V (1959) Preparation of highly purified secretin. Arkiv Kemi 15:69–74
52. Nakayama K, Ohkubo H, Hirose T, Inayama S, Nakanishi S (1984) mRNA-sequence for human cardiodilatin-atrial natriuretic factor precursor and regulation of precursor mRNA in rat atria. Nature 310:699–701
53. Nemer M, Chamberland M, Sirois D, Argentin S, Drouin J, Dixon RAF, Zivin RA, Condra JH (1984) Gene structure of human cardiac hormone precursor, pronatriodilatin. Nature 312:654–656
54. Nemer M, Sirois D, Drouin J (1986) Xho I polymorphism at the human pronatriodilatin (hPND) gene locus. Nucl Acids Res 14:8696
55. Nemer M, Sirois D, Drouin J (1986) Taq I polymorphism at the 3′ end of the human pronatriodilatin gene (hPND). Nucl Acids Res 14:8697
56. Oetting WS, Tuazon PT, Traugh JA, Walker AM (1986) Phosphorylation of prolactin. J Biol Chem 261:1649–1652
57. Oikawa S, Imai M, Ueno A, Tanaka S, Noguchi T, Nakazato H, Kangawa K, Fukuda A, Matsuo H (1984) Cloning and sequence analysis of cDNA encoding a precursor for human atrial natriuretic polypeptide. Nature 309:724–726
58. Oikawa S, Imai M, Inuzuka C, Tawaragi Y, Nakazato H, Matsuo H (1985) Structure of dog and rabbit precursors of atrial natriuretic polypeptides deduced from nucleotide sequence of cloned cDNA. Biochem Biophys Res Commun 132:892–899
59. Olins GM, Mehta PP, Blehm DJ, Patton DR, Zupec ME, Whipple DE, Tjoeng FS, Adams SP, Olins PO, Gierse JK (1987) Phosphorylation of high- and low-molecular-mass atrial natriuretic peptide analogs by cyclic AMP-dependent protein kinase. FEBS Letters 224:325–330
60. Olins GM, Spear KL, Siegel NR, Zurcher-Neely HA (1987) Inactivation of atrial natriuretic factor by the renal brush border. Biochim Biophys Acta 901:97–100
61. Olins GM, Spear KL, Siegel NR, Reinhard EJ, Zurcher-Neely HA (1987) Atrial peptide inactivation by rabbit-kidney brush border membranes. Eur J Biochem 170:341–434

62. Ong H, Lazure C, Nguyen TT, McNicoll N, Seidah N, Chretien M, DeLean A (1987) Bovine adrenal chromaffin granules are a site of synthesis of atrial natriuretic factor. Biochem Biophys Res Commun 147: 957–963
63. Rittenhouse J, Moberly L, O'Donnell ME, Owen NE, Marcus F (1986) Phosphorylation of atrial natriuretic peptides by cyclic AMP-dependent protein kinase. J Biol Chem 261: 7607–7610
64. Rittenhouse J, Moberly L, Ahmed H, Marcus F (1988) Phosphorylation in situ of atrial natriuretic peptide prohormone at the cyclic AMP-dependent site. J Biol Chem 263: 3778–3783
65. Saccuzzo JE, Krzesicki RF, Perini F, Ruddon RW (1986) Phosphorylation of the secreted, free α subunit of human chorionic gonadotropin. Proc Natl Acad Sci USA 83: 9493–9496
66. Schulz-Knappe P, Forssmann K, Herbst F, Hock D, Pipkorn R, Forssmann WG (1988) Isolation and structural analysis of „urodilatin", a new peptide of the cardiodilatin-(ANP)-family, extracted from human urine. Klin Wochenschr 66:752–759
67. Schwartz D, Geller DM, Manning PT, Siegel NR, Fok KF, Smith CE, Needleman P (1985) Ser-Leu-Arg-Arg-Atriopeptin III: the major circulating forms of atrial peptide. Science 229:397–400
68. Seidman CE, Bloch KD, Klein KA, Smith JA, Seidman JG (1984) Nucleotide sequences of the human and mouse atrial natriuretic factor genes. Science 226:1206–1209
69. Seidman CE, Bloch KD, Zisfein J, Smith JA, Haber E, Homcy C, Duby AD, Choi E, Graham RM, Seidman JG (1985) Molecular studies of the atrial natriuretic factor gene. Hypertension [Suppl I] 7:31–34
70. Shields PP, Glembotski CC (1988) The post-translational processing of rat pro-artrial natriuretic factor by primary artrial myocyte cultures. J Biol Chem 263:8091–8098
71. Somlyo AV, Broderick R, Shuman H, Buhle EL, Somlyo AP (1988) Atrial-specific granules in situ have high calcium content, are acidic, and maintain anion gradients. Proc Natl Acad Sci USA 85:6222–6226
72. Sonnenberg JL, Sakane Y, Jeng AY, Koehn JA, Ansell JA, Wennogle LP, Ghai RD (1988) Identification of protease 3.4.24.11 as the major atrial natriuretic factor degrading enzyme in the rat kidney. Peptides 9: 173–180
73. Stephenson SL, Kenny AJ (1987) The hydrolysis of α-human atrial natriuretic peptide by pig kidney microvillar membranes is initiated by endopeptidase-24.11. Biochem J 243: 183–187
74. Sudoh T, Kangawa K, Minamino N, Matsuo (1988) A new natriuretic peptide in porcine brain. Nature 332:78–81
75. Sudoh T, Minamino N, Kangawa K, Matsuo H (1988) Brain natriuretic peptide-32: N-terminal six amino acid extended form of brain natriuretic peptide identified in porcine brain. Biochem Biophys Res Commun 155: 726–732
76. Thibault G, Garcia R, Gutkowska J, Lazure C, Seidah NG, Chrétien M, Genest J, Cantin M (1986) Identification of the released form of atrial natriuretic factor by the perfused rat heart. Proc Soc Exp Biol Med 182:137–141
77. Vanneste Y, Michel A, Dimaline R, Najdovski T, Deschodt-Lanckman M (1988) Hydrolysis of α-human atrial natriuretic peptide in vitro by human kidney membranes and purified endoprotease-24.11. Biochem J 254:531–537
78. Vlasuk GP, Miller J, Bencen GH, Lewicki JA (1986) Structure and analysis of the bovine atrial natriuretic peptide precursor gene. Biochem Biophys Res Commun 136:396–403
79. Vogt-Schaden M, Gagelmann M, Hock D, Herbst F, Forssmann WG (1989) Degradation of porcine brain natriuretic peptide (pBNP-26) by endoprotease–24.11 from kidney cortical membranes. Biochem Biophys Res Commun (in press)
80. Wypij DM, Harris RB (1988) Atrial granules contain an amino-terminal processing enzyme of atrial natriuretic factor. J Biol Chem 263:7079–7086
81. Yamanaka M, Greenberg B, Johnson L, Seilhamer J, Brewer M, Friedemann T, Miller J, Atlas S, Laragh J, Lewicki J, Fiddes J (1984) Cloning and sequence analysis of the cDNA for the rat atrial natriuretic factor precursor. Nature 309:719–722
82. Yandle TG, Crozier I, Espiner EA, Ikram H, Nicholls MG (1985) Production, plasma levels, and clearance of atrial natriuretic peptide in man. Hypertension 7:838
83. Yandle TG, Richards AM, Nicholls MG, Cuneo R, Espiner EA, Livesey JH (1986) Metabolic clearance rate and plasma half live of alpha-human atrial natriuretic peptide in man. Life Sci 38:1827–1833
84. Yandle T, Crozier I, Nicholls G, Espiner E, Carne A, Brennan S (1987) Amino acid sequence of atrial natriuretic peptides in human coronary sinus plasma. Biochem Biophys Res Commun 146:832–839
85. Yang-Feng TL, Floyd-Smith G, Nemer M, Drouin J, Francke U (1985) The pronatriodilatin gene is located on the distal short

arm of human chromosome 1 and on mouse chromosome 4. Am J Hum Genet 37: 1117–1128

86. Zivin RA, Chondra JH, Dixon RAF, Seidah NG, Chrétien M, Nemer M, Chamberland M, Drouin J (1984) Molecular cloning and characterization of DNA sequences encoding rat and human atrial natriuretic factors. Proc Natl Acad Sci 81:6325–6329

Intrarenal Mechanisms of Action of Atrial Natriuretic Factor

H. Sonnenberg

Department of Physiology, University of Toronto, Toronto, Canada

Summary. It is evident that atrial natriuretic factor (ANF), a peptide produced and stored in modified myocytes of cardiac atria, represents a hormone system involved in regulation of renal salt excretion. On intravenous injection ANF produces a large but short-lasting natriuresis. ANF causes significant alteration in intrarenal hemodynamics, raising glomerular filtration rate as well as medullary blood flow. These effects may be responsible for the observed increase in salt delivery to the medullary collecting duct system. In addition, specific inhibition of salt reabsorption along the duct itself has been documented. Although ANF has been shown to block an amiloride-sensitive sodium channel in this nephron segment, it is debatable whether this effect contributes to the natriuresis in vivo. The mechanism(s) of ANF-induced inhibition of medullary duct transport thus remain(s) to be determined.

Key words: Atrial natriuretic factor – Collecting duct transport – Microcatheterization – Microperfusion.

The effects of atrial natriuretic factor (ANF) on tubular sodium transport along the nephron have received much attention. Although the glomerulus, as well as proximal and distal tubules have been proposed as sites of action of the hormone, recent work has confirmed original micropuncture studies [2, 12] indicating that reduction of reabsorption in the medullary collecting duct system is a major feature of ANF natriuresis (for review see [11]). However, the mechanism of transport inhibition at this site has been controversial. Given the known effects of ANF on GFR and medullary blood flow it has been proposed that the increase in filtered sodium, combined with reduction in reabsorption in Henle's loop consequent to washout of the medullary solute gradient, would result in a large increase in the tubular load of sodium delivered to the medullary collecting duct. If transport capacity in this final segment is limited, a "spillover" into the urine could account for the natriuretic response to ANF [4, 16].

As seen in Fig. 1, however, the crucial requirement for this hypothesis is not met: Using the in vivo microcatheterization technique we have shown that fractional salt reabsorption in the duct remains constant at about 80% for deliveries up to 10% of filtered load [5]. It is evident, therefore, that this enormous duct transport capacity is more than adequate to compensate for the two- to threefold increase in delivery seen with ANF administration [12, 14]. Indeed, as also shown in Fig. 1, at any given level of delivery intravenous infusion of ANF [14], as well as increase of endogenous levels of the hormone by extracellular fluid volume expansion [17], are both associated with specific inhibition of sodium reabsorption along the collecting duct.

Although these data suggest direct interaction of ANF with cellular transport mechanisms for sodium, in vitro perfusion of tubular segments isolated from the medullary duct failed to show ANF-induced inhibition of net sodium reabsorption [8]. In addition, the traditional analogues of mammalian duct epithelium, isolated frog skin and toad bladder, also do not respond to the hormone by altering sodium transport. However, recently there have appeared studies from three different laboratories, within a few months of each other, indicating that ANF indeed had significant in vitro effects on renal cells. Using cultures of the renal tubular cell line LLC-PK_1, Goligorsky et al. [6] found that ANF reducded short-circuit current across confluent mono-

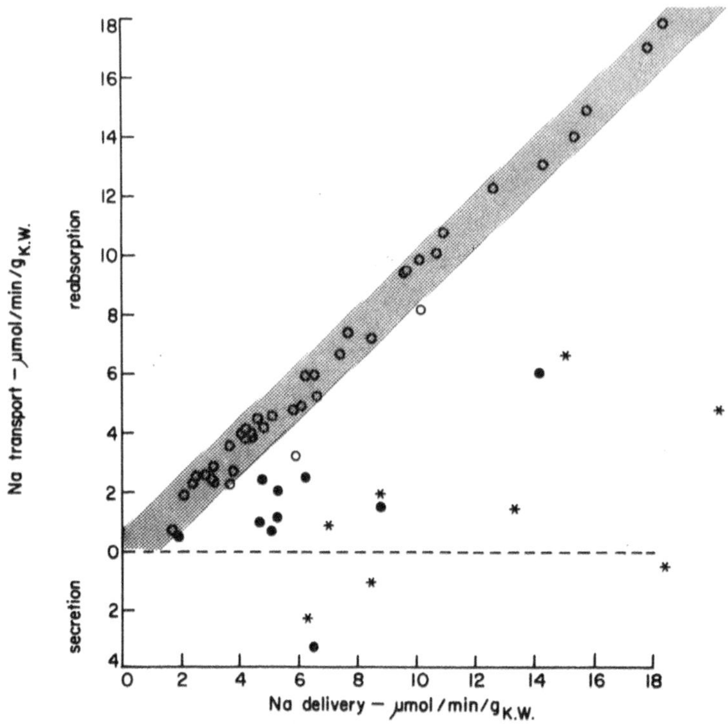

Fig. 1. Relationship of tubular delivery of sodium to the medullary collecting duct and reabsorption along the duct. Open circles represent individual control rats in which delivery was varied by experimental manipulations. Filled circles show data from rats infused with ANF; stars show data from animals during Ringer's infusion. (Data from ref's [5, 14, 17])

layers, an effect that was mimicked by c̄GMP. Cantiello and Ausiello [3] found that exposure of these cells to ANF increased c̄GMP production, and that either agent inhibited ^{22}Na uptake through a conductive pathway. Finally, Zeidel et al. used fresh suspensions of inner medullary collecting duct cells to show inhibition of ouabain-sensitive oxygen uptake which was not additive with amiloride [19], and was identical so that found with c̄GMP [20]. These results suggested that inhibition of sodium reabsorption in the collecting duct system by ANF was due to blockade of amiloride-sensitive sodium channels.

Although amiloride is not usually considered as affecting medullary duct function, inhibition of sodium reabsorption at this site is indeed in feature of the drug [15]. We therefore developed a modification of the microcatheterization technique which allows determination of unidirectional sodium efflux from duct lumen in vivo in the absence or presence of transport antagonists. The method may be described briefly as follows: Fine polyethylene catheters (OD ~ 20μ, length ~ 6 mm) are mounted on glass capillary tubes. The capillary is connected to a microperfusion pump [13], and the catheter inserted into a duct opening as usual [5, 14]. Perfusate contains ^{22}Na as well as ^{3}H-inulin. The pump is set to deliver 30 nl/min, and simultaneously urine is collected. Functioning of the perfusion system is monitored by measuring the urinary recovery of perfused inulin. A reduction of the sodium-to-inulin ratio in the collected urine then represents Na efflux out of the perfused collecting duct. In each rat, the catheter is advanced as far as possible into a duct opening at the tip of the exposed papilla, and a 5 min perfusion is begun. The catheter is then retracted by about 1 mm, a 5 min flushing period is allowed, followed by another 5 min collection at this new depth. In this way the whole extent of the

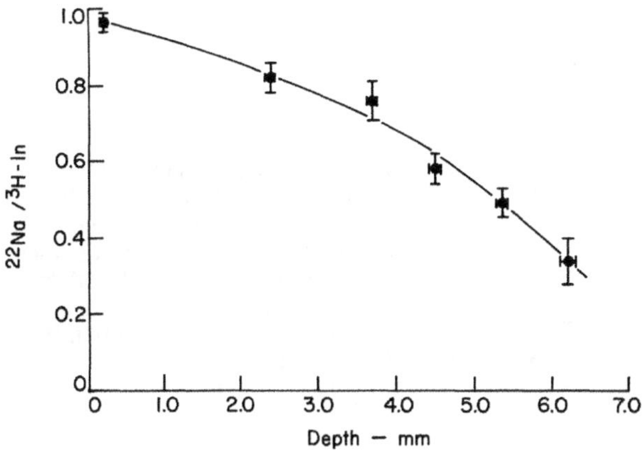

Fig. 2. Change in ^{22}Na to ^{3}H-inulin ratio in perfused fluid at different depths of insertion into the medullary collecting duct of control rats. The border between inner and outer medulla lies at approximately 4.9 mm

Table 1. ^{22}Na efflux from the lumen of the medullary collecting duct

	Control (n = 12)	Amiloride (n = 9)	ANF (n = 8)	Amil + ANF (n = 10)
Na/In ratio	0.49 ± .04	0.72 ± .05	0.72 ± .06	0.79 ± .04
MCD depth (mm)	5.36 ± .06	5.44 ± .06	5.41 ± .04	5.39 ± .04

inner medullary duct may be studied. In control animals, generally 2–3 different duct systems were perfused, and results expressed as the average change in Na/Inulin ratio with duct length in each animal. Fig. 2 shows the results of 17 such experiments. As expected, sodium efflux increased with increasing depth of insertion, about 1/2 of the labelled ion being lost in perfusion at 5–6 mm.

To determine the effect of luminal amiloride on sodium efflux in this system, ratios at a depth between 5 and 6 mm were compared for control and amiloride-containing perfusate 2×10^{-4}M) (Table 1). A significant increase ($p < 0.01$) was observed, demonstrating the expected blockade of amiloride-sensitive luminal sodium channels. Identical inhibition of sodium efflux was found when ANF (10^{-8} M) was added to perfusate (Table 1). Combination of both inhibitors had no further effect on efflux, indicating that luminal ANF indeed was capable of blocking an amiloride-sensitive sodium channel in the apical cell membrane of duct epithelium.

However, as shown in Table 2, the magnitude of the induced natriuresis was far less than that due to ANF, and amiloride did not eliminate an additional natriuretic effect of the hormone [14, 18]. Furthermore, in amiloride-treated rats ANF had an added inhibitory effect on duct transport (Fig. 3). Blockade of amiloride-sensitive sodium channels in medullary collecting duct cells, therefore, does not appear to be the sole mechanism of action of ANF in this nephron segment in vivo.

Table 2. Effect of ANF infusion on sodium excretion in normal and amiloride-treated rats[a]

	$U_{Na}V$ (nmol/min/g kidney weight) control	ANF infusion
Normal rats (n = 10)	690 ± 180	3490 ± 460
Amiloride treatment (n = 8)	2000 ± 270	3680 ± 510

[a] Data from ref's [14, 18]

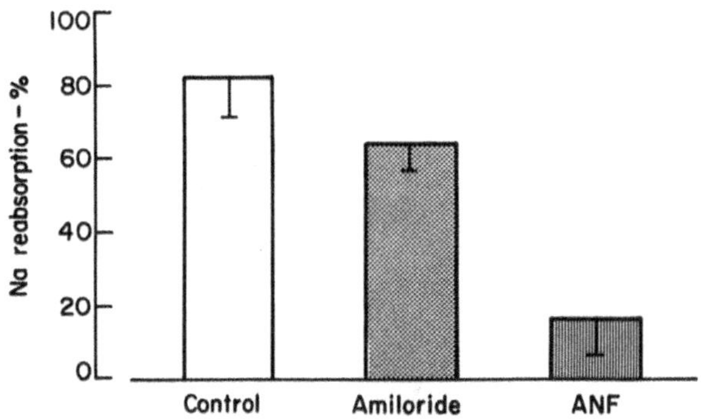

Fig. 3. Fraction of delivered sodium reabsorbed in the medullary collecting duct of control, amiloride-, and ANF-treated rats. The control value is significantly different from the other two, as is the difference between amiloride and ANF ($p < 0.05$). (Data from ref's [14, 18])

Indeed, it may be argued that ANF-induced inhibition of collecting duct transport in vivo does not involve an amiloride-like action at all. Berg et al. [1] have shown recently that luminal membranes of proximal and distal tubular epithelium are capable of degrading ANF, with no evidence of saturation even at pharmacological concentrations of the hormone. It is highly unlikely, therefore, that any filtered ANF would reach the luminal surface of the medullary collecting duct. Although this consideration does not exclude interaction of the hormone with basal receptors, producing c̄GMP which could block the sodium channel from the inside of the cell [3], again in vivo data are not in agreement with such a mechanism. A consequence of blocking amiloride-sensitive sodium entry is marked potassium reabsorption in the medullary collecting duct [15]. However, as seen in Fig. 4, intravenous ANF administration had no effect on potassium transport in this nephron segment. Thus, interaction of the hormone with a luminal amiloride-sensitive sodium channel, while demonstrable both in vitro and in vivo, may well be irrelevant to ANF natriuresis.

If this is the case, what then is the mechanism of ANF-induced inhibition of collecting duct transport? Although, as discussed above, the hemodynamic effects of the hormone as related to the traditional medullary washout hypothesis do not explain the natriuresis, it is conceivable that peritubular physical factors might act directly at the level of the medullary duct. We have speculated that an observed addition of salt and water to duct fluid during massive extracellular volume expansion could be due to a local increase in hydrostatic and/or decrease in oncotic pressure causing backflux into the lumen [9]. Indeed, attempts to raise medullary interstitial pressure by restricting renal venous outflow were associated with reduction of fractional sodium reabsorption in the duct [10]. Furthermore, Mendez et al. [7] recently documented ANF-induced rises in peritubular capillary pressures in the renal medulla, and suggested that these pressures could promote backflux of sodium-rich interstitial fluid

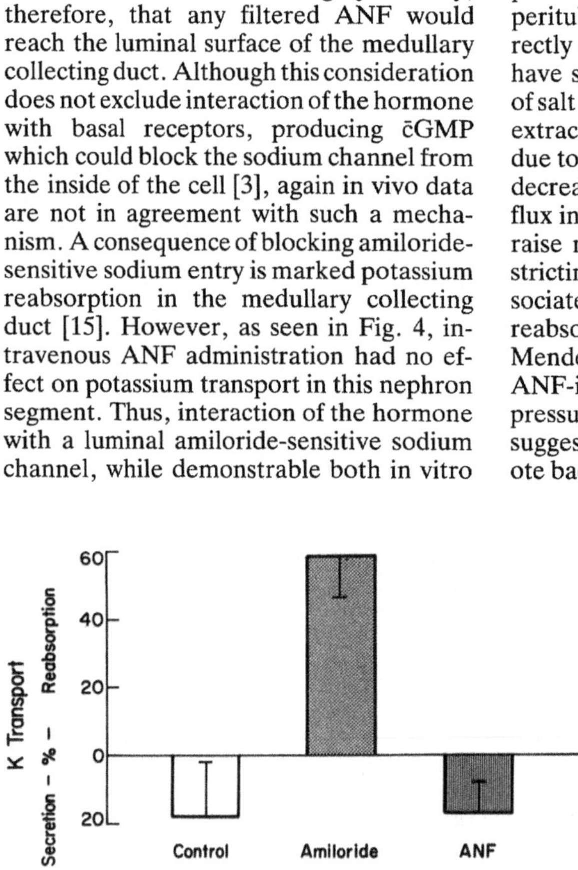

Fig. 4. Fraction of delivered potassium secreted or reabsorbed in the medullary collecting duct. The value for amiloride-treated rats is significantly different from the other two ($p < 0.01$). (Data from ref's [14, 15])

into the collecting duct lumen, thereby inhibiting net reabsorption. Such a mechanism has the appeal of simplicity, explaining ANF natriuresis on the basis of renal hemodynamic actions only. However, the existence of backflux in this part of the nephron still remains to be demonstrated. In addition, the quantitative contribution of such putative backflux to the ANF response is unknown, as is the significance of other mechanisms, such as the decrease in chloride (but not sodium!) permeability recently reported for the in vitro perfused duct [8].

Acknowledgment: Studies from our laboratory were supported, in part, by grants from the Medical Research Council of Canada and the Heart and Stroke Foundation of Ontario.

References

1. Berg JA, Hayashi M, Fujii Y, Katz AI (1988) Renal metabolism of atrial natriuretic peptide. Am J Physiol 255:F466–F473
2. Briggs JP, Steipe B, Schubert G, Schnermann J (1982) Micropuncture studies of the renal effects of atrial natriuretic substance. Pflugers Arch 395:271–276
3. Cantiello HF, Ausiello DA (1986) Atrial natriuretic factor and cGMP inhibit amiloride-sensitive Na^+ transport in the cultured renal epithelial cell line, LLC-PK_1. Biochem Biophys Res Commun 134:852–860
4. Cogan MG (1986) Atrial natriuretic factor can increase renal solute excretion primarily by raising glomerular filtration. Am J Physiol 250:F710–F714
5. Cupples WA, Sonnenberg H (1988) Load dependency of sodium chloride reabsorption by medullary collecting duct in rat. Am J Physiol 253:F642–F648
6. Goligorsky MS, Duncan RL, Westbrook S, Reinach P, Hruska KA (1987) Demonstration of a direct effect of atrial natriuretic factor on epithelium: study in cultured pig kidney cells. Min Electrol Metab 13:51–56
7. Mendez RE, Dunn BR, Troy JL, Brenner BM (1988) Atrial natriuretic peptide and furosemide effects on hydraulic pressure in the renal papilla. Kidney Internat 34:36–42
8. Sands JM, Nonoguchi H, Knepper MA (1988) Hormone effects on NaCl permeability of rat inner medullary collecting duct. Am J Physiol 255:F421–F428
9. Sonnenberg H (1975) Secretion of salt and water into the medullary collecting duct of Ringer-infused rats. Am J Physiol 228: 565–568
10. Sonnenberg H (1978) Microcatheterization studies of medullary collecting duct function in the rat kidney. In: Vogel HG, Ullrich KJ (eds) New Aspects of Renal Function. Excerpta Medica, Amsterdam Oxford, pp 175–180
11. Sonnenberg H (1988) Renal effects of atrial natriuretic factor. ISI Atlas of Science. Pharmacol 2:171–174
12. Sonnenberg H, Cupples WA, deBold AJ, Veress AT (1982) Intrarenal localization of the natriuretic effect of cardiac atrial extract. Can J Physiol Pharmacol 60:1149–1152
13. Sonnenberg H, Deetjen P (1964) Methode zur Durchströmung einzelner Nephronabschnitte. Pflugers Arch 278:669–674
14. Sonnenberg H, Honrath U, Chong CK, Wilson DR (1986) Atrial natriuretic factor inhibits sodium transport in medullary collecting duct. Am J Physiol 250:F963–F966
15. Sonnenberg H, Honrath U, Wilson DR (1987) Effects of amiloride in the medullary collecting duct of rat kidney. Kidney Internat 31:1121–1125
16. Sosa RE, Volpe M, Marion DN, Atlas SA, Laragh JH, Vaughan ED Jr, Maack T (1986) Relationship between renal hemodynamic and natriuretic effect of atrial natriuretic factor. Am J Physiol 250:F520–524
17. Wilson DR, Honrath U, Sonnenberg H (1982) Prostaglandin synthesis inhibition during volume expansion: Collecting duct function. Kidney Internat 22:1–7
18. Wilson DR, Honrath U, Sonnenberg H (1988) Interaction of amiloride and hydrochlorothiazide with atrial natriuretic factor in the medullary collecting duct. Can J Physiol Pharmacol 66:648–654
19. Zeidel ML, Seifter JL, Lear S, Brenner BM, Silva P (1986) Atrial peptides inhibit oxygen consumption in kidney medullary collecting duct cells. Am J Physiol 251:F379–F383
20. Zeidel ML, Silva P, Brenner BM, Seifter JL (1987) cGMP mediates effects of atrial peptides on medullary collecting duct cells. Am J Physiol 252:F551–F559

Mechanism of Action of Atrial Natriuretic Factor in the Adrenal Gland

T. Inagami, R. Takayanagi, K. N. Pandey, R. M. Snajdar, J. D. Corbin, and S. H. Francis

Departments of Biochemistry, Molecular Physiology and Biophysics, and Howard Hughes Medical Institute, Vanderbilt University School of Medicine Nashville, Tennessee, USA

Summary. Atrial natriuretic factor (ANF) inhibits aldosterone release from adrenal zona glomerulosa cells. The inhibition is not elicited by sodium nitroprusside which increases cGMP (cyclic 3′, 5′-guanine-monophosphate) in these cells. Permeable cGMP analogs increased aldosterone release rather than inhibiting it. These results suggested that cGMP may not mediate the action of atrial natriuretic factor. Indeed a dephosphorylation of a 240 kDa protein in plasma membrane mediated by the atrial peptide is not dependent on cGMP. In order to clarify cGMP-dependent and -independent mechanisms, two different types of receptors were separated and purified by a series of affinity chromatography. The guanylate cyclase-containing receptor was shown to have a single polypeptide chain structure of 135 kDa and highly specific for full length (greater than 24 amino acid residue) atrial peptides whereas the guanylate cyclase-free receptor was shown to be a disulfide-linked dimer of 65 kDa subunit with a lesser specificity for the structure of the effector protein.

Key words: Atrial natriuretic factor (ANF) – Adrenal zona glomerulosa inhibition of aldosterone secretion – ANF receptor – Purificaton of ANF receptor – cGMP – Sodium nitroprusside.

In 1984 ANF was found to suppress the stimulated and basal rate of aldosterone release from the adrenal gland. Teleologically, this action of ANF is in line with the general function of ANF directed to the reduction of extracellular fluid volume [1, 2, 3]. However, the action of ANF on the adrenal gland eluded numerous attempts to clarify its mechanism.

ANF exerts its effects through its interaction with ANF-specific plasma membrane receptors and its action is mediated by the production of cGMP [4, 17]. Such receptors have been found in numerous organs and tissues including vascular smooth muscle cells, vascular endothelial cells, renal glomeruli, corticomedullary regions and papilla, adrenal outer cortical layers, various regions of the brain, pituitary gland, lung, liver, intestine.

Very interesting features of ANF action is its antagonistic actions to generally hypertensinogenic actions of angiotensin II as shown in Table 1. For example, ANF dilates blood vessels, inhibits the release of vasopressin and aldosterone, directly inhibits the renal reabsorption of Na^+, the dipsogenic action, vasopressin release and hypertension elicited by centrally administered angiotensin II, and inhibits the neurotransmitter release from peripheral nerve end-

Table 1. Mutually antagonistic effects of angiotensin II and atrial natriuretic factor (ANF)

Angiotensin II	ANF
Contracts blood vessels	Inhibits the contraction
Stimulates renal Na^+ reuptake	Inhibits renal Na^+ reuptake
Stimulates aldosterone release	Inhibits aldosterone release
Stimulates vasopressin release	Inhibits vasopressin release
Stimulates water drinking	Inhibits water drinking
Inhibits renin release	Inhibits renin release
Facilitates peripheral neuro-transmission	Mildly inhibits peripheral neuro-transmission
Causes centrally mediated hypertension	No effect on central hypertension by angiotensin II

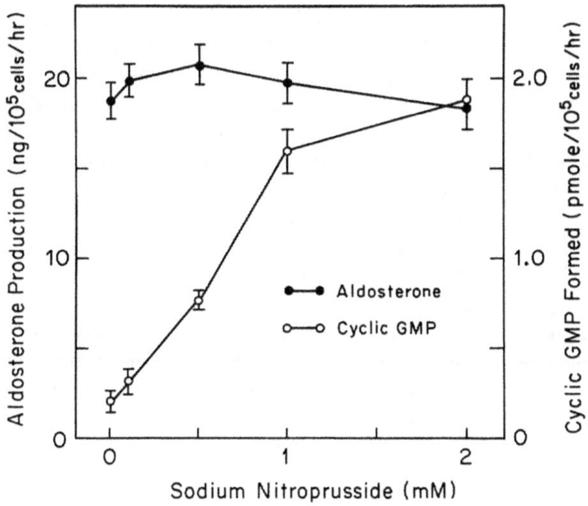

Fig. 1. Effects of sodium nitroprusside on angiotensin II-stimulated aldosterone production by adrenal glomerulosa cells of rats

ings and ganglia. The only exception to the general antagonism between angiotensin II and ANF is the inhibition of renin release by both of them although controversy still exists on the *in vivo* effect of ANF on the renin release.

In many tissue the action of ANF (atrial natriuretic factor) has been explained by the reduction of free intracellular calcium concentration, presumably mediated by cyclic GMP. However, this mechanism does not seem to apply to the inhibition of aldosterone release. Rat and bovine zona glomerulosa cells in primary culture did not show change or reduction in free Ca^{2+} concentration upon treatment with $10^{-10}-10^{7}$ M ANF which markedly reduced aldosterone production and release. On the other hand similar ANF treatment of vascular smooth muscle cells markedly reduced basal intracellular free Ca^{2+} or transient increase of Ca^{2+} concentration stimulated by angiotensin II.

We have obtained data which appears to suggest that even cGMP may not have a direct effect on the inhibition of aldosterone release. As shown in Fig. 1, cGMP (cyclic 3′, 5′-guanine-monophosphate) generated by sodium nitroprusside does not inhibit the angiotensin II induced secretion of aldosterone. Moreover, addition of permeable cGMP analogs such as 8-bromo cyclic GMP or 8-p-chlorophenylthio-cyclic GMP did not inhibit, but rather stimulated aldosterone release at a higher concentration (Table 2).

These observations suggested that cGMP may not be involved in the inhibition of aldosterone release from the adrenal cortex. We looked for an adrenal signal transduc-

Table 2. Effects of cGMP analogs on K^{+}-stimulated aldosterone release in rat glomerulosa cells

	Aldosterone release (% of control)				
Concentration (M)	cGMP	8-BR-cGMP[a]	BT_2-cGMP[b]	8-pCPT-cGMP[c]	PET-cGMP[d]
10^{-6}	106	98 102	114 107		
10^{-5}	100	101	101	122*	103
10^{-4}	97	108	97	165*	111
10^{-3}	85	131*	92	– –	
3×10^{-3}	85	161*	96	–	–

[a] 8-bromo-cyclic GMP, [b] 2′,6-dibutyryl-cGMP, [c] 8-p-chlorophenylthio-cGMP, [d] β-phenyl-1-N^2etheno-cGMP. Synthesis and characterization of these compounds will be published in Molecular Pharmacology (in press) by Francis FS, Noblett BD, Todd BW, Wells JN, Corbin JD

tion mechanism in which cGMP may not be involved in the adrenal zona glomerulosa cells.

Several proteins in plasma membranes of bovine adrenal outer cortical cells are phosphorylated upon incubation with [γ-^{32}P]-ATP. Of these phosphoproteins, ANF ($1 \times 10^{-8} \sim 10^{-7}$M) inhibited the phosphorylation of 78 kDa and 240 kDa proteins as shown in lanes 3 and 4 in panel a of Fig. 2. The 78 kDa protein was identified as protein kinase C. Similar inhibition of phosphorylation of the 78 kDa protein was also reproduced by cGMP. However, the inhibition of phoshorylation of 240 kDa protein was not effected by cGMP (Fig. 2 panel b) indicating that ANF may have cGMP independent signal transduction mechanism mediated by the 240 kDa protein associated with plasma membrane. These results indicated further detailed studies on the ANF receptors and signal transduction mechanism in the zona glomerulosa cells are essential for our understanding of the inhibition of aldosterone.

ANF binding proteins with high affinity have been demonstrated in numerous tissues. Cross-linking or photo-affinity labeling of receptors in various tissues revealed the presence of ANF receptor with apparent molecular weights of 65 000 to 70 000 and 125 000 to 140 000 [11–17]. Recent findings that purified guanylate cyclase from rat lung [6], bovine adrenal [14, 15]

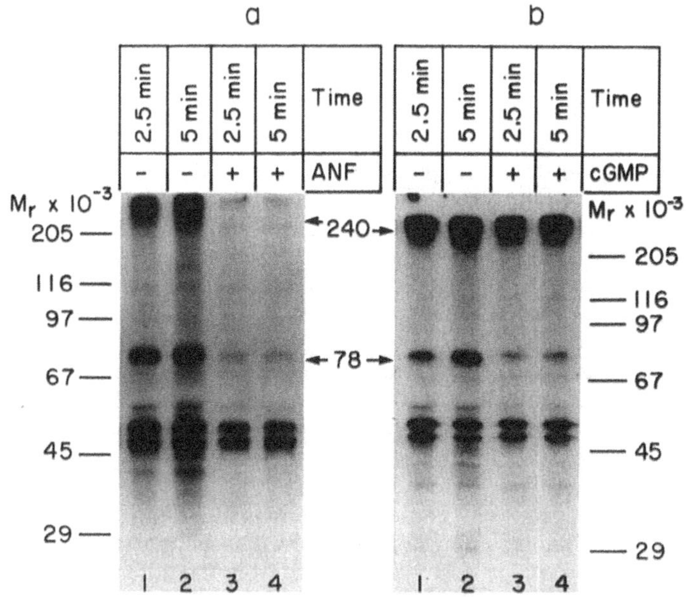

Fig. 2. a Sodium dodecylsulfate polyacrylamide gel electrophoresis (SDS-PAGE) and autoradiography of the bovine adrenal cortex membrane phosphoproteins in the absence or presence of atrial natriuretic factor (ANF). The reaction mixture was pre-incubated for 10 min in the absence (lanes 1 and 2) or the presence (lanes 3 and 4) of ANF at 4°C. In each lane 40 µg of proteins were electrophoresed in 7.5% polyacrylamide gel. The phosphorylation reaction with [γ ^{32}P] adenosine triphosphate (ATP) was allowed for indicated periods. Marker proteins are myosin, β-galactosidase, phosporylase b, bovine serum albumin, ovalbumin, and carbonic anhydrase, and their molecular weights (M_r) are shown on the left. On the right, the M_r of phosphoproteins affected by ANF are indicated with arrows. The data are representative of four experiments. **b** SDS-PAGE and autoradiography of bovine adrenal cortex plasma membrane phosphoproteins in the presence or absence of cyclic guanosine monophosphate (cGMP). The membrane preparations were pre-incubated for 10 min at 4°C in the absence or presence of cGMP. The phosphorylation reaction was allowed for indicated time periods. Samples containing 40 µg of proteins were electrophoresed in each lane in 7.5% polyacrylamide gel. The M_r of the marker proteins are shown on the right. M_r of phosphoproteins whose phosphorylation is affected by cGMP are indicated with arrows on the left. The data are representative of four experiments. Taken from Ref. [9] with permission of Biochem Biophys Res Commun

and adrenal tumor [12] plasma membranes exhibits ANF binding activity seems to support the role of cGMP as a second messenger of ANF action. As stated above, although cGMP has been known to cause vasorelaxation, it has been well documented that cGMP and its membrane-permeable analogs slightly stimulate release of aldosterone in the adrenal gland. Thus, the inhibitory role of ANF on aldosterone release cannot be explained by the ANF-dependent cGMP production. On the other hand, the stimulation of testosterone production in Leydig cells parallels with intracellular cGMP concentration [11].

These results raised the question about the relationship of the roles of the two types of receptors in mediating a variety of actions by ANF and about the possible existence of two different pathways of intracellular signal transduction mechanism of AFN action, one mediated by cGMP and the other without the intermediacy of cGMP.

To clarify the multiple pathways of ANF action, we have devised methods to purify the ANF receptors and to characterize these receptors.

Although ANF-receptor activity was relatively stable, cGMP activity was rapidly destroyed upon exposure to slightly acidic pH. In order to circumvent the lability of the cyclase activity, various media for the solubilization and chromatography of the receptor were examined.

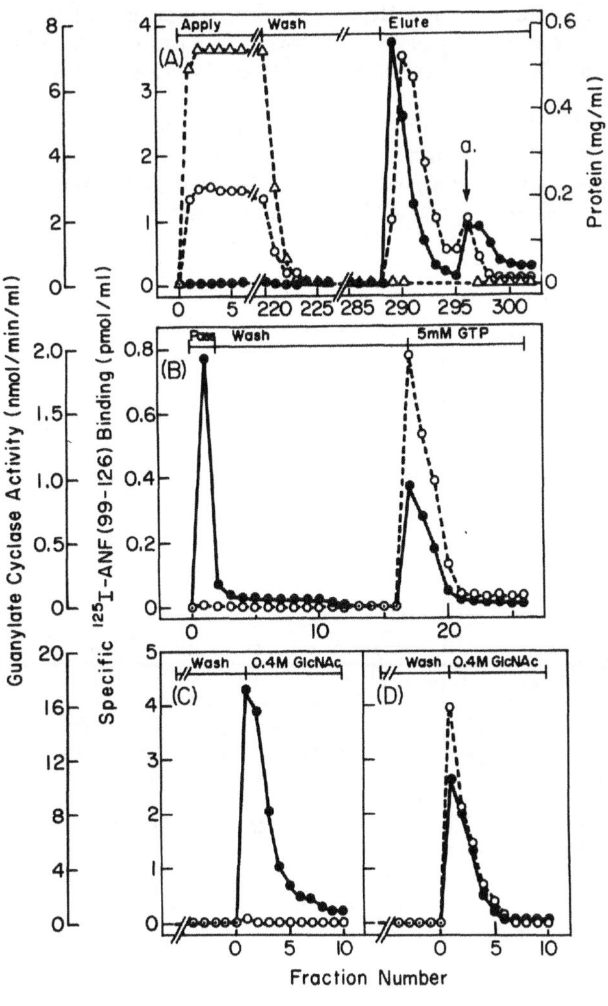

Fig. 3 A–D. Affinity chromatographic purification of atrial natriuretic factor (ANF) receptors. **A** Affinity chromatography on ANF-agarose. Open triangles indicate protein concentration; open circles indicate guanylate cyclase activity; and closed circles indicate ANF binding activity. **B** Affinity chromatography on (GTP)-agarose. Open circles and closed circles represent guanylate cyclase activity and ANF-binding activity. **C** Affinity chromatography of guanylate cyclase-free ANF receptor on wheat germ agglutinin (WGA) column. **D** Affinity chromatography of guanylate cyclase-coupled ANF receptor. Taken from Ref. [15] with permission of the Journal of Biological Chemistry

Bovine adrenal cortical outer layer cells were homogenized in a buffer containing various protease inhibitors, and plasma membrane fractions were isolated and stored frozen. The membranes were solubilized in 1% Triton X-100 in the presence of various protease inhibitors.

Receptors were purified by successive affinity chromatographic steps which included ANF-agarose, GTP-agarose (5′-guanine-triphosphate), and wheat germ agglutinin (WGA) agarose. The chromatography on ANF-agarose required special care in the elution of receptors because the receptors were very tightly bound to ANF. The application of the receptor solution was done in 10% glycerol, 0.0125% phosphatidylcholine, and 0.1% Triton X-100 at pH 7.5, whereas the elution of the receptor required 20% glycerol and 1 M NaCl combined with 0.025% phosphatidylcholine and acidification of pH to 5.5 in an acetate buffer (Fig. 3A).

The eluate was further fractionated by the GTP agarose column again in 20% glycerol, 0.025% phosphatidylcholine, and 0.1% Trition X-100. Of the two types of receptors, the one without the guanylate cyclase activity passed through the column whereas the receptor containing guanylate cyclase was retained by the column and was eluted by the buffer containing 5 mmol GTP (Fig. 3B). Both were purified further by the WGA column to homogeneity as examined by polyacrylamide gel electrophoresis (Fig. 3C and D).

Although both guanylate cyclase-containing and the cyclase-free receptors showed similar molecular weights of 135 000 by SDS-PAGE run under non-reducing conditions, the cyclase-free receptor migrated to 65 000 daltons under the reducing condition, indicating this receptor was composed of subunits.

Thus, we were able to purify two types of receptors simultaneously. The most important difference in the properties of the two types of receptors is the presence and absence of guanylate cyclase and the difference in the size.

Functional difference is also clearly recognizable as shown in Fig. 4; the guanylate cyclase-containing 135 000-dalton receptor binds ANF molecules containing more than

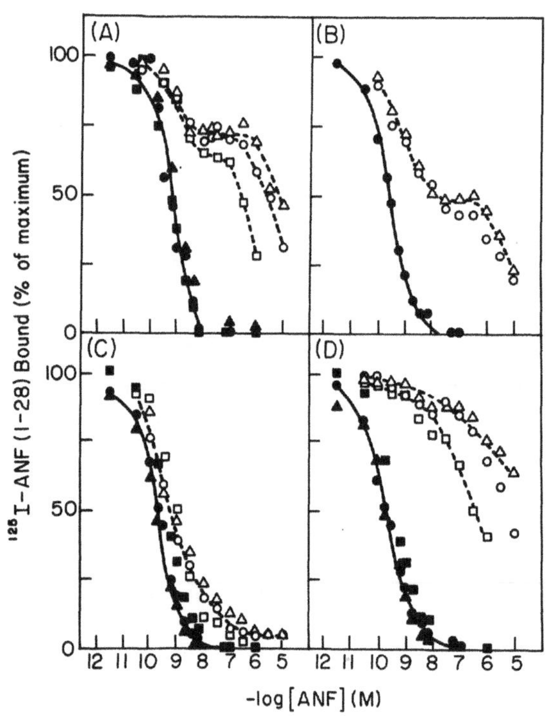

Fig. 4 A–D. Competition between ^{125}I-atrial natriuretic factor (ANF)$_{(99-126)}$ and increasing concentrations of various ANF analogs for binding to the receptor preparation from each chromatographic step. **A** The crude extract; **B** After ANF-agarose; **C** Purified guanylate cyclase-free receptor; and **D** Purified guanylate cyclase-containing receptor.
(▲):ANF$_{(96-126)}$; (●)ANF$_{(99-126)}$; (■K) ANF$_{(102-126)}$; (□K)ANF$_{99-121)}$; (○K)ANF$_{(103-123)}$; or (△K)ANF$_{(105-121)}$. Taken from Ref. [15] with permission of the Journal of Biological Chemistry

24 amino acid residues. On the other hand, guanylate cyclase-free receptors with 63 000-dalton subunits are capable of binding truncated ANF with 21 (atriopeptin I) or 17 (ring) amino acid residues. Certain tissue were responsive to the truncated ANF and may contain the cyclase-free receptors.

Vascular tissues have been shown to contain 60 000- to 70 000-dalton receptors. These findings indicate that the conversion of the large receptor to the small receptor can occur by the reduction of disulfide linkages. Whether the reversal of this process to convert 60 000-dalton cyclase-free receptor to 135 000-dalton cyclase-free receptor occurs is yet unclear. Thus, three types of receptors seem to exist in nature.

Because many types of responses induced by ANF are interpreted by cGMP, the guanylate cyclase-containing receptor may mediate the action of ANF by generating cGMP. On the other hand, the mechanism of the action of the cyclase-free receptor is not clear. Our preliminary results indicate that ANF receptors of cloned aortic smooth muscle cells are almost completely the low molecular weight cyclase-free receptor. The relaxation of aorta or artery may be mediated by cGMP. Three possible roles of the cyclase-free receptor can be envisaged: (a) It may produce cGMP through interaction with a different type of guanylate cyclase; (b) It may function without generating cGMP; and (c) It may not induce any cellular response even if ANF may be bound, and may serve as ANF-reservoir of ANF-scavenger. Clarification of precise mechanisms of the action of the two receptors will reguire further studies.

Acknowledgement: This work was supported by Research Grants HL 14192 and HL 35323 from National Institutes of Health and 84–1291 from the American Heart Association.

References

1. Atarashi K, Mulrow PJ, Franco-Saenz R, Snajdar R, Rapp J (1984) Inhibition of aldosterone production by atrial extract. Science 224:992–994
2. Chartier L, Schiffrin E, Thibault G, Garcia R (1984) Atrial natriuretic factor inhibits the stimulation of aldosterone secretion by angiotensin II, ACTH or potassium *in vitro* and angiotensin induced steroidogenesis *in vivo*. Endocrinology 115:2026–2028
3. Goodfriend TL, Elliot ME, Atlas SA (1984) Action of Synthetic atrial natriuretic factor on bovine adrenal glomerulosa. Life Sci 35: 992-994
4. Hammet P, Trembly J, Pang SC, Garcia R, Thibault G, Gutkowsk J, Cantin M, Genest J (1984) Effect of native and synthetic atrial natriuretic factor or cyclic cGMP. Biochem Biophys Res Commun 123:515–527
5. Hirose S, Akiyama F, Shinjo M, Ohno H, Murakami K (1985) Solubilization ad molecular weight estimation of atrial natriuretic factor receptor from bovine adrenal cortex. Biochem Biophys Res Commun 130: 574–579
6. Kuno T, Anderson JW, Kamisaki Y, Chang LY, Saheki DC, Leitman DC, Nakane M, Murad F (1986) Co-purification of an atrial natriuretic factor receptor and particulate guanylate cyclase from rat lung. J Biol Chem 261:5817–5823
7. Meloche S, Ong H, Cantin M, DeLean A (1986) Affinity cross-linking of atrial natriuretic factor to its receptor in bovine adrenal zona glomerulosa. J Biol Chem 261: 1525–1528
8. Misono KS, Grammer RT, Rigby JW, Inagami T (1985) Photoaffinity labeling of atrial natriuretic receptor in bovine and rat adrenal cortical membrane. Biochem Biophys Res Commun 130:994–1001
9. Pandey KN, Inagami T, Girard PR, Kuo JF, Misono KS (1987) New signal transduction mechanisms of atrial natriuretic factor: inhibition of phosphorylation of protein kinase C as a 240 kDa protein in adrenal cortical plasma membranes by cGMP dependent and independent mechanism. Biochem Biophys Res Commun 148:589–595
10. Pandey KN, Inagami T, Misono KS (1986) Atrial natriuretic factor receptor on cultured murine Leydig tumor cells: Ligand binding and photoaffinity labeling. Biochemistry 25:8467–8472
11. Pandey KN, Pavlou SN, Kovacs WJ, Inagami T (1986) Atrial natriuretic factor regulates steroidogenic responsiveness and cyclic nucleotide levels in mouse Leydig cells *in vitro*. Biochem Biophys Res Commun 138:399–404
12. Paul AK, Marala RB, Jaiswal RK, Sharma RK (1987) Co-existence of guanylate cyclase and atrial natriuretic receptor in a 180-KD protein. Science 235:1224–1226
13. Schenk DB, Phelps MN, Porter JG, Scarborough RM, McKenroe GA, Lewicki JA (1985) Identification of the receptor for atrial

natriuretic factor on cultured vascular cells. J Biol Chem 260:14887–14890

14. Takayanagi R, Inagami T, Snajdar R, Imada T, Tamura M, Misono KS (1987) Two distinct forms of receptors for atrial natriuretic factor in bovine adrenocortical cells. Purification, ligand binding and peptide mapping. J Biol Chem 262:12104–12113
15. Takayanagi R, Snajdar RM, Imada T, Tamura M, Pandey KN, Misono KS, Inagami T (1987) Purification and characterization of two types of atrial natriuretic factor receptors from bovine cortex: guanylate cyclase-linked and cyclase-free receptors. Biochem Biophys Res Commun 144:244–250
16. Vandlen RB, Arcuri KE, Napier MA (1985) Identification of a receptor for atrial natriuretic factor in rabbit aorta membranes by affinity cross-linking. J Biol Chem 260:10889–10892
17. Waldman SA, Rapoport RM, Murad F (1984) Atrial natriuretic factor selectively activates particulate guanylate cyclase and elevates cGMP in rat tissue. J Biol Chem 259:14332–14334
18. Yip CC, Laing LP, Flynn TG (1985) Photoaffinity labeling of atrial natriuretic factor receptors of rat kidney cortex plasma membranes. J Biol Chem 160:8229–9232

Atrial Natriuretic Peptide and the Renin-Angiotensin-Aldosterone-System

G. Wambach

Department of Medicine II, University of Cologne, FRG

Summary: The atrial natriuretic peptide acutely lowers arterial blood pressure and induces a natriuresis and diuresis when administered to experimental animal and man. However, the contribution of this new hormonal system in the control of sodium and water balance is unclear. Particularly, the interaction between ANP and the reninangiotensin-system is not yet defined. The present pages summarize recent data on the effect of ANP on the renin secretion both in vitro and in vivo. We then describe the impact of acute and chronic sodium loading on the plasma levels of ANP and renin in normal subjects. Finally, we discuss the modification of ANP renal action by converting enzyme inhibition. The data suggest that both systems are involved in the acute and chronic control of sodium and fluid balance.

Key words: Atrial natriuretic peptide – Renin-angiotensin-aldosterone-system

---

Introduction

Until recently, the renin-angiotensin-aldosterone system was considered to be the major hormonal regulator of sodium balance. Stimulated by a fall in blood pressure or a loss in sodium and water, this system increases arterial blood pressure and leads to a reabsorption of sodium and water by the kidney (Freeman and Davis 1983). In 1981, a natriuretic and hypotensive hormone was discovered in the atrial muscle: the atrial natriuretic peptide (ANP) (DeBold 1981). This hormone system seems to counteract the physiologic action of the renin-aldosterone system like a physiologic antagonist: at the kidney, ANP promotes natriuresis and diuresis, A II, the active component of the RAAS induces sodium retention (Seymour 1985). Angiotensin II is an important stimulator of aldosterone secretion in contrast to the inhibitory action of ANP (Campbell et al. 1985). A II has potent vasoconstrictor properties whereas ANP induces vasodilation (Winquist et al. 1984) (Fig. 1).

At the level of central nervous systems, ANP has been shown to interfere with all the central action of A II. Stimulation of water intake, salt appetite and vasopressin release induced by intraventricular administration of A II were blunted by simultaneous injection of ANP (Nakamaru et al.

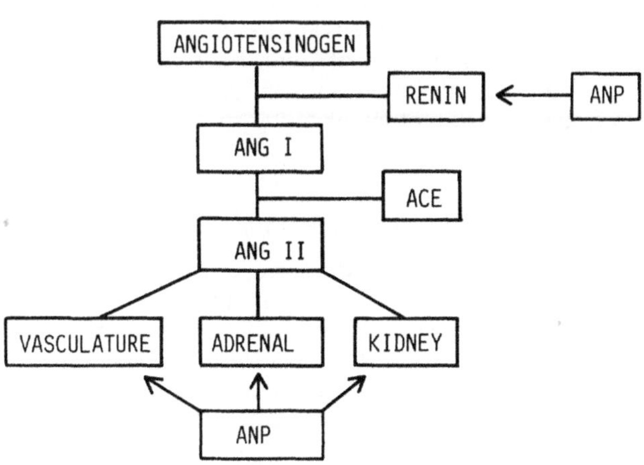

Fig. 1. Schematic drawing of the interaction between ANP and the renin-angiotensin-system

1986, Yamada et al. 1986). The interaction of both systems in the regulation of blood pressure and sodium-water homoeostasis is only partially understood (Laragh 1985).

Elevation of plasma ANP levels by acute intravenous saline infusion is demonstrated by several investigators (Sagnella 1986, Tunny et al. 1986). Controversy exists however about the effect of chronic dietary sodium loading on ANP secretion. In the rat, no difference in plasma ANP was observed during low and high salt diet (Luft et al. 1986). In normal subject, both similar and elevated plasma concentrations of ANP were measured during high salt intake compared to normal or low sodium diet (Weidmann et al. 1986, Sagnella et al. 1985). It was speculated that the ANP system reacts to acute alteration in circulating fluid volume whereas the renin-angiotensin system controls chronic adjustments of sodium homoeostasis. We therefore investigated both systems more in detail in normal subjects during acute and chronic sodium loading.

By reviewing the relationship between the atrial natriuretic peptide and the renin-aldosterone-system, we like to concentrate on three main topics:

1. Modification of renin secretion by ANP.
2. Impact of acute and chronic sodium loading on atrial natriuretic peptide and renin.
3. Effect of blockade of the renin system by ACE inhibition on the renal and adrenal action of ANP.

This review is based on our own studies and on data published by various other groups.

Modification of Renin Secretion by ANP

The secretion of renin by the juxtaglomerula cells is by itself a complex issue. At least four different mechanism are involved (Freeman and Davis 1983):

1. The baroreceptor mechanism sensing the arterial wall tension of the afferent arteriolar vessels.
2. The macula densa mechanism sensing the tubular sodium concentration.
3. The sympathetic activity.
4. Circulating endogenous angiotensin II inhibits the secretion of renin, the so called "short loop inhibition".

At least theoretically, ANP might interfere with several of this control mechanisms: ANP might induce a relaxation of the arterial wall thereby changing the baroreceptor. ANP induces an acute natriuresis and diuresis which could lead to a rise in sodium concentration at the macula densa. Finally by reducing the systemic arterial blood pressure, the renin secretion might be stimulated.

The action of ANP on renin release has been studied in in vitro experiments, in whole animals preparations and in man. Unfortunately, the results are conflicting and no final conclusions are possible at the present time.

In Vitro Effect of ANP on Renin

When incubated with kidney cortex slices, ANP inhibited basal renin release in a dose dependent manner (Obana et al. 1985). Renin secretion stimulated by isoproterenol was also reduced by ANP with an ID_{50} of 5×10^{-8} M. The renin inhibition was not Ca-dependent, however, was correlated with a stimulation of cGMP production. A similar effect of ANP on renin release was described by Kurtz using an IG-cell preparation (Kurtz et al. 1986). In this model, the action of ANP was paralleled by a rise in cGMP production and a reduction in cAMP.

In isolated afferent arterioles, no change in renin release was seen after exposure with ANP suggesting an involvement of the macula densa. More important, in an isolated perfused kidney model, Hackenthal et al. observed a constant stimulation of renin by ANP (Hackenthal et al. 1987). The stimulation of renin by ANP under these conditions was not modified by hydralazine, indomethazine and furosemide.

Studies in Whole Animal

In the anaesthetized dog, first studies reported a suppression of renin after infusion of ANP in doses of 0.1–0.3 μg/kg/min (Burnett et al. 1984, Maack et al. 1984). Similar results were obtained in conscious animals using lower ANP concentrations (Scheuer 1987).

Since this effect was not observed in the nonfiltering kidney modell, it was concluded that the modulation of renin release by ANP is mediated by a change in intratubular sodium concentration (Opgenorth et al. 1986). The effect of ANP might be different under conditions of low renal perfusion pressure (Kirchheim 1987).

Studies in Man

Similarly, several renal and vascular effects of ANP might interact in the release of renin. Weidmann described a rise in renin following administration of h-ANP in normal subjects on low sodium intake (Weidmann et al. 1986).

Cuneo and ourselves observed a significant reduction in plasma renin levels after acute administration to normal man (Cuneo et al. 1986). The inhibition of renin seems to be more constant when renin levels are high. Taken together, ANP seems to inhibit renin release by a direct mechanism and/or by changes in intratubular sodium concentration. However, the stimulation of renin under experimental conditions is of particular importance. In the whole body situation, the inhibitory effect of ANP can be modified by the action of ANP on the systemic circulation.

However, the basal secretion of renin under experimental conditions had to be taken into account. A suppresion of renin is observed primarily when renin levels are high. In addition, the hypotensive action of h-ANP may lead to a stimulation of renin.

Impact of Acute and Chronic Sodium Loading on the Atrial Natriuretic Peptide and Renin

The maintenance of sodium and fluid balance is an important physiological goal. A variety of hormonal mechanisms are involved in the sodium and volume homoeostasis. Among them, the renin-angiotensin-aldosterone-system is one of the most important regulators. The role of the atrial natriuretic peptide is a matter of great debate. Principally, the contribution of a hormone system to the sodium output is quite difficult to assess. The first step should be the measurement of blood levels of the hormone in question during variation in sodium intake. We therefore analyzed changes in plasma levels of both, ANP and renin, in normal subjects following acute saline infusion as well as during chronic dietary sodium loading.

Acute Saline Infusion

Plasma levels of ANP, renin, aldosterone and protein were measured in 7 normal subjects during a placebo experiment and following i.v. infusion of 2000 ml of normal saline administered over a period of 30 minutes.

The impact of intravenous saline infusion on plasma levels of ANP and renin in normal control subjects is outlined in Figure 2. During the control period, plasma ANP levels were constant over a period of four hours. After the infusion of 2000 ml of saline, pronounced alterations in renin and ANP levels were observed. Plasma protein concentration dropped by 0.7 g/100 ml indicating a constant expansion of intravascular volume for a period of 240 minutes. Immediately after the infusion, mean ANP plasma levels rose four-fold compared to the control period and compared to pretreatment values being significant at 60, 120 and 180 minutes. However, plasma ANP levels returned to control levels at the end of the period despite a persistent volume expansion.

In contrast, the drop in plasma renin concentration was less pronounced with a mean reduction of 50%. However, the fall in renin concentration remained constant for the period of observation. Urinary output of sodium, potassium and water remained unchanged during the control experiment. After the infusion of 2000 ml of saline, urinary sodium output rose significantly from 1.9 ± 0.5 to 11.8 ± 2.6 mmol/30 min ($p < 0.05$) and urine volume increased from 20 ± 4.7 to 104 ± 26 ml/30 min ($p < 0.01$) during the infusion period. Urinary volume and plasma ANP levels were significantly correlated ($r = 0.539$, $p < 0.001$).

These results clearly demonstrate that both renin and ANP plasma levels are altered during acute volume expansion. Studies by Hirth et al. suggest that both the acute natriuresis and the drop in renin is

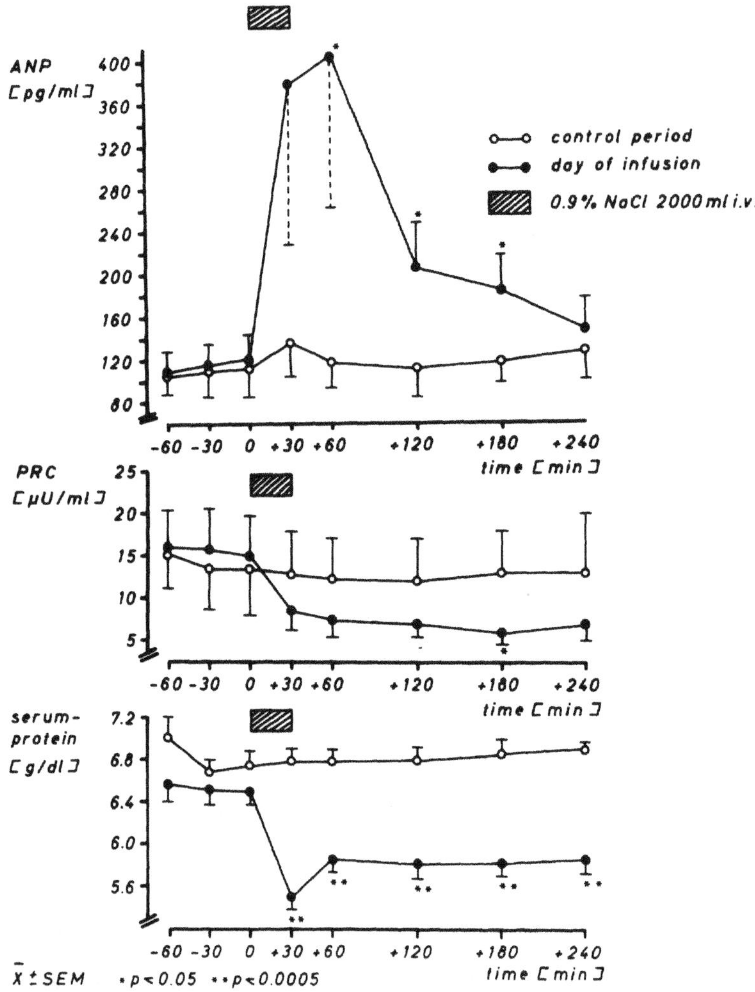

Fig. 2. Plasma levels of h-ANP and renin concentration in normal subjects following intravenous saline infusion compared to a control experiment

mediated by ANP, since pretreatment of rats with monoclonal antibodies abolished both the natriuresis and the change in renin secretion (Hirth et al. 1987).

Effect of Dietary Sodium Loading on Renin and ANP

The impact of low and high sodium intake on plasma renin concentration and plasma ANP was investigated in 11 normal subjects. At the end of a 4-day-period on low sodium (40–60 meq/day) and on the 6th day on high sodium diet (280–320 meq/day) plasma levels of renin, aldosterone and ANP were measured after an overnight rest and after 4 hours of upright posture.

A prolongued sodium loading over two weeks was conducted in 8 normal volunteers over a 15 day period. Plasma levels of renin, aldosterone and ANP as well as urinary excretion of sodium and cyclic GMP were measured on day 2, 4, 7, 10 and 15 of a high sodium intake (300–350 meq/day).

Variation in dietary sodium intake was followed by a small but significant change in ANP plasma levels. A five-fold increase in sodium intake, reflected by a rise in urinary

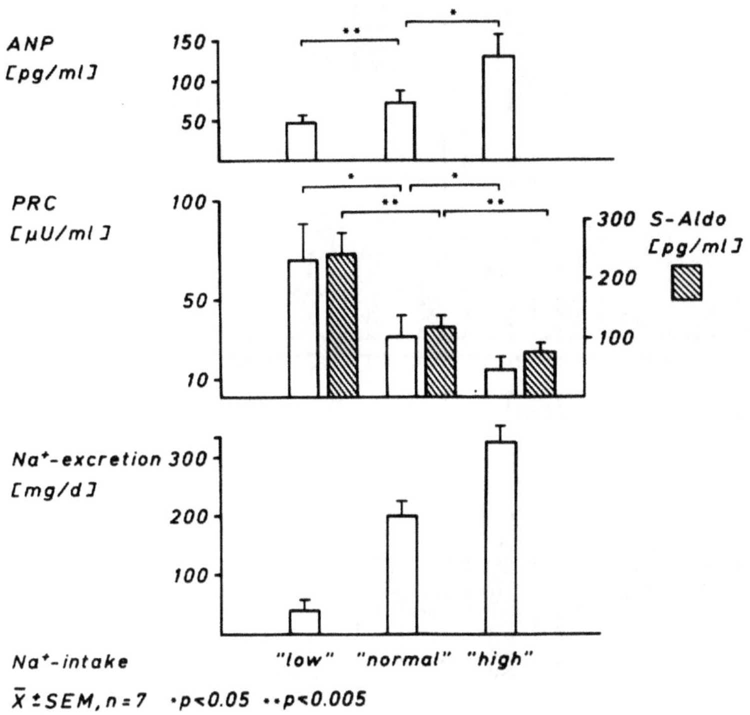

Fig. 3. Plasma levels of h-ANP and renin during chronic variations in dietary sodium intake in normal subjects

sodium from 25 ± 4 to 326 ± 32 meq/d was paralleled by a rise in ANP from 49 ± 7 to 128 ± 38 pg/ml at 8:00 and from 38 ± 4 to 72 ± 13 pg/ml at noon. PRC was lowerd by high sodium intake from 69.8 ± 19.8 to 14.4 ± 6.5 μU/ml and from 79.0 ± 13.2 to 13.4 ± 4.2 μU/ml at 8:00 and at 12:00 respectively (Fig. 3).

The effect of prolonged sodium loading on plasma levels of ANP and renin was investigated in a separate study. Sodium excretion averaged 36.4 ± 9.5 meq/day at the end of low sodium intake. Urinary sodium output rose up to 402 ± 43 meq/d with a slight decline on day 15. Plasma ANP levels almost paralleled the changes in urinary sodium excretion with significant elevated concentrations on day 4, 7, 10 and 15. Reciprocal changes were found in renin values. Plasma renin concentrations averaged 100.7 ± 26.7 μU/ml during low sodium intake. High sodium diet resulted in a substained suppresion in PRC. The minimum in renin levels was found on day 4 parallel with a maximal rise in sodium excretion and plasma ANP concentration. At day 15, ANP levels remained elevated and PRC was suppressed compared to low sodium intake. Elevation of plasma ANP during prolongued sodium loading seems to reflect a stimulated biological activity of the peptide. This is supported by the elevation of urinary cGMP excretion during this 2-week-period.

In summary, the atrial natriuretic peptide and the renin system are affected by both acute and chronic sodium loading. The stimulation of plasma ANP and the suppression of renin levels is more pronounced during acute saline loading. However, significant elevation of plasma ANP is seen up to 15 days on high sodium intake. More important, the elevation in urinary cGMP during high sodium intake in healthy subjects supports the biological action of stimulated plasma ANP levels. This must be investigated more in detail by additional approaches in the future.

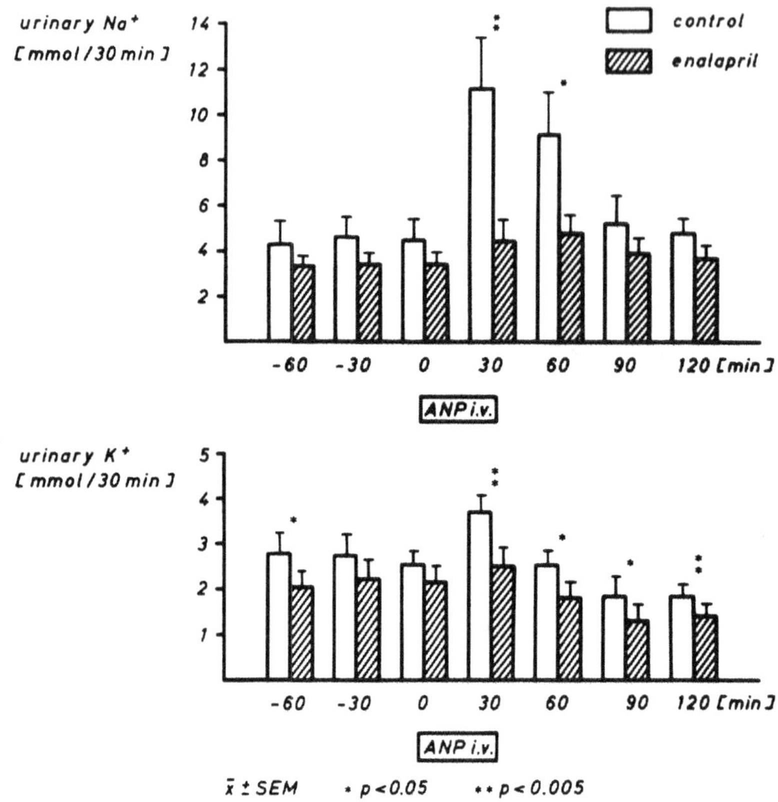

Fig. 4. Modification of renal action of exogenous h-ANP in normal subjects after blockade of the renin-angiotensin-system by enalapril treatment

Effect of Blockade of the Renin System by ACE Inhibition on the Renal and Adrenal Action of ANP

We also investigated the interaction between ANP and the renin-angiotensin-system by comparing the renal effects of exogenous ANP before and after inhibition of angiotensin I-converting-enzyme. 1–28-hANP (0.1 µg/kg/min) was infused i.v. into 10 normal subjects over 30 minutes both during a control period and following ACE inhibition with enalapril (3 × 2.5 mg p.o.). During the control infusion, urinary excretion of sodium rose from 4.5 ± 0.8 to 11.2 ± 2.2 meq/30 min and the urine volume rose from 32 ± 14 to 115 ± 34 ml/30 min. This increment in urinary volume and sodium output was almost completely abolished by ACE-inhibition (Fig. 4).

The stimulation of urinary cGMP excretion by ANP infusion was not altered by ACE-inhibition. However, the systolic and diastolic blood pressure was significantly reduced by enalapril. This acute experiment suggests that the renin-angiotensin supports the natriuretic action of ANP at the kidney. This synergistic effect might be mediated by the rise in renal perfusion pressure induced by angiotensin II. Interactions of both systems at the renal tubular levels are also possible. According to Harris et al. ANP has no direct effect on the proximal tubule, however the peptide inhibits the Na^+-uptake induced by angiotensin II (Harris et al. 1987).

References

Burnett JC, Granger JP, Opgenorth TJ (1984) Effects of synthetic atrial natriuretic factor on renal function and renin release. Am J Physiol 247:F863–F866

Campbell WB, Currie MG, Needleman P (1985) Inhibition of aldosterone biosynthesis by atriopeptins in rat adrenal cells. Circ Res 57: 113–118

Cuneo RC, Espiner EA, Nicholls MG, Yandle TG, Joyce StL, Gilchrist NL (1986) Renal, hemodynamic, and hormonal responses to atrial natriuretic peptide infusions in normal man, and effect of sodium intake. J Clin End Met 63:946–953

DeBold AJ, Borenstein HB, Verress AT, Sonnenberg H (1981) A rapid and potent natriuretic response to intravenous injection of atrial myocardial extract in rats. Life Sci 28:89–94

Freeman RH, Davis JO (1983) Factors controlling renin secretion and metabolism. In: Genest et al. (eds) Hypertension, McGraw-Hill, New York, p 225

Hackenthal E (1987) ANF und Reninsekretion. Untersuchungen an der isoliert perfundierten Rattenniere. In: Kreye/Bussmann (Hrsg) ANP – Atriales natriuretisches Peptid und das kardiovaskuläre System. Steinkopff, Darmstadt

Harris PJ, Thomas D, Morgan TO (1987) Atrial natriuretic peptide inhibits angiotensin-stimulated proximal tubular sodium and water reabsorption. Nature 326:697–698

Kirchheim HR, Ehmke H, Persson P (1987) Wirkung von ANP auf die druckabhängige Reninfreisetzung am wachen Hund. In: Kreye/Bussmann (Hrsg) ANP – Atriales natriuretisches Peptid und das kardiovaskuläre System. Steinkopff, Darmstadt

Kurtz A, Bruna RD, Pfeilschifter J, Taugner R, Bauer C (1986) Atrial natriuretic peptide inhibits renin release from juxtaglomerular cells by a cGMP-mediated process. Proc Natl Acad Sci USA 83:4769–4773

Laragh JH (1985) Atrial natriuretic hormone, the renin-aldosterone axis, and blood pressure-electrolyte homeostasis. The New Engl J Med 313:1330–1340

Luft FC, Sterzel RB, Lang RE, Trabold EM, Veelken R, Ruskoaho H, Gao Y, Ganten D, Unger T (1986) Atrial natriuretic factor determinations and chronic sodium homeostasis. Kidney Int 29:1004–1010

Maack T, Marion DN, Camargo MJE, Kleinert HD, Laragh JH, Vaughan ED Jr, Atlas SA (1984) Effects of auriculin (atrial natriuretic factor) on blood pressure, renal function and the renin-aldosterone system in dogs. Am J Med 77:1069–1075

Nakamaru M, Takayanagi R, Inagami T (1986) Effect of atrial natriuretic factor on central angiotensin II-induced responses in rats. Peptides 7:373–375

Obana K, Naruse M, Naruse K, Sakurai H, Demura H, Inagami T, Shizume K (1985) Synthetic rat atrial natriuretic factor inhibits in vitro and in vivo renin secretion in rats. Endocrinology 117:1282–1284

Opgenorth TJ, Burnett JC jr., Granger JP, Scriven TA (1986) Effects of atrial natriuretic peptide on renin secretion in non-filtering kidney. Am J Physiol 250:F798–F801

Sagnella GA, Markandu ND, Shore AC, MacGregor GA (1986) Effects of changes in dietary sodium intake and saline infusion on immunoreactive atrial natriuretic peptide in human plasma. Lancet II:1208–1211

Sagnella GA, Markandu ND, Shore AC, MacGregor GA (1986) Raised circulating levels of atrial natriuretic peptides in essential hypertension. Lancet I:179

Scheuer DA, Thrasher TN, Quillen EW Jr, Metzler CH, Ramsay DJ (1987) Atrial natriurretic peptide blocks renin response to renal hypotension. Am J Physiol 251:R423–R427

Seymour AA (1985) Renal and systemic effects of atrial natriuretic factor. Clin Exper Theory Practice A 7:887–904

Tunny TJ, Gordon RD, Klemm SA, Hamlet StM (1986) Effects of acute volume expansion on atrial natriuretic peptide levels in normal subjects, primary aldosteronism and low renin essential hypertension. J Hypertension [Suppl 6] 4:S509–S511

Weidmann P, Hellmueller B, Uehlinger DE, Lang RE, Gnaedinger MP, Hasler L, Shaw S, Bachmann C (1986) Plasma levels and cardiovascular, endocrine, and excretory effects of atrial natriuretic peptide during different sodium intakes in man. J Clin Endocrin Metab 62:1027–1036

Winquist RJ, Faison EP, Nutt RF (1984) Vasodilator profile of synthetic atrial natriuretic factor. Eur J Pharmacol 102:169–173

Yamada T, Nakan K, Morii N, Itoh H, Shiono S, Sakamoto M, Sugawara A, Saito Y, Ohno H, Kanai A, Katsura G, Eigyo M, Matsushita A, Imura H (1986) Central effect of atrial natriuretic polypeptide on angiotensin II-stimulated vasopressin secretion in conscious rats. Eur J Pharmacol 125:453–456

Interaction between ANP and the Sympathetic Activity

J. Holtz

Institut für Angewandte Physiologie und Balneologie, University of Freiburg, FRG

Summary: Three types of mutual interactions between ANP and the sympathetic activity have been identified: 1) Adrenergic atrial stimulation enhances regulated atrial ANP release; 2) the hemodynamic effects of exogenous ANP are blunted by reflex activation of sympathetic activity; 3) ANP has inhibitory actions on sympathoadrenal activity in vivo.

The direct adrenergic stimulation of regulated atrial ANP release is mediated via activation of β- and α_1-adrenoceptors; it interfers with indirect effects of sympathetic activity affecting mechanical stimuli of atrial ANP release (i.e.: diastolic atrial distension and frequency of atrial contraction).

The reflex modulation of sympathetic activity during ANP-induced hypotension and the direct ANP-induced sympathoinhibition counteract each other during exogenous ANP application, but they act in concert during elevations of atrial filling, which releases ANP and concomitantly activates sympathoinhibitory reflexes. ANP can inhibit the sympathoadrenal system by several mechanisms: by activation of mechanosensitive vagal type C afferents eliciting sympathoinhibitory reflexes, by activating ANP binding sites on sympathetic ganglia and on CNS areas outside the bloodbrain barrier, and by inhibiting norepinephrine release from postganglionic nerve terminals and epinephrine release from the adrenal medulla.

The sympathoinhibition by ANP is not attenuated by prolonged elevations of circulating ANP during development of congestive heart failure, when other ANP effects are reduced due to target organ desensitation. Thus, the relative importance of the sympathoinhibition within the broad spectrum of ANP effects is augmented during prolonged ANP exposure.

Key words: ANP – Sympathetic activity

The cardiac hormone ANP (atrial natriuretic peptide) is regarded very often as an endogenous antagonist to the renin-angiotensin system. This antagonism does not occur at the level of cell membrane receptors and it does not apply strictly to all effects of these two hormonal systems (e.g.: not for the effects of the two systems on glomerular filtration pressure in the kidney). However, it offers a useful guideline to bring the multiple actions of the atrial hormone into a functional perspective.

Three types of interactions between the renin-angiotensin system and the sympathetic activity are known: 1) the renal sympathetic nerve activity is an important stimulator of renal renin release; 2) the acute hemodynamic actions of pharmacological doses of angiotensin injections into the intact organism are blunted by blood pressure buffering reflexes, including withdrawal of sympathetic activity; 3) circulating angiotensin as well as angiotensin produced locally in organs of the circulation augments sympathetic activity by various mechanisms.

These three types of mutual interactions will be considered here in the context with the functional angiotensin-antagonist ANP and the sympathetic activity.

Stimulation of ANP-Release by Sympathetic Activity?

The circulating hormone α-ANP (or ANP_{99-126}) consists of 28 aminoacids and is formed from a larger storage form, the Pro-ANP (or ANF_{1-126}). This originates from the translation product PrePro-ANP (or Pre-ANF_{1-126}) after cleavage of an N-terminal signal peptide. The message for this PreProANP occurs in various extracardiac organs such as brain, vessels, kidneys, testes and adrenals, but the heart is the sole identified source releasing the hormon α-ANP in measurable amounts into the circulation (for reviews see De Bold 1985; Genest et al. 1988; Holtz et al. 1987a). Within the heart, the prohormone is formed in the myocytes, but the secretory pathway of the hormone appears differently regulated in atrial and ventricular myocytes.

In ventricular myocytes, the peptide is probably secreted by a pathway referred to as "constitutive", which means that products are relased once they are built up, without substantial accumulation in storage organelles and withouth modulation of the release from such storage sites by secretagogues (Kelly 1985). Estimated from the tissue levels of ANP-mRNA, the rate of prohormone synthesis is very low in adult ventricular myocardium (roughly 1/100 of atrial myocardium), but can undergo substantial augmentation during chronic cardiac overload and development of ventricular hypertrophy (Genest et al. 1988; Holtz et al. 1987a). In such states, the bulk of ventricular tissue represents a large ANP-forming capacity, but its contribution to the circulating ANP plasma levels has not yet been assessed quantitatively. Presently it is unknown, whether the sympathetic innervation can directly modify the synthesis and constitutive release of the hormone in ventricular myocardium.

In atrial myocytes, the formed prohormone is stored in abundant amounts (De Bold 1985; Forssmann et al. 1983) in the atrial secretory granules. This is the hallmark for a "regulated pathway", in which the granular content is available for rapid release, triggered by specific signals (Kelly 1985). The first mechanism to be identified, stimulating "regulated release" of ANP from the atrial granules, was stretch of the cardiac atria (Dietz 1984; Lang et al. 1985). This identification substantially contributed to our understanding of ANP as a "cardiac unloading" hormone (Holtz et al. 1987a). Preliminary experimental evidence indicated that this "regulated" atrial ANP-release could be mediated or modified by augmentations of the intracellular Ca^{2+} concentration (Ruskoaho et al. 1985; Saito et al. 1986) and therefore should be subject to direct modulation by the autonomic innervation of atrial myocytes.

Using isolated, superfused rat atria under mechanically controlled conditions with monitoring of ANP-immunoreactivity in the effluent, Schiebinger and associates (Schiebinger and Linden 1986a; Schiebinger and Linden 1986b; Schiebinger et al. 1987) were able to elegantly demonstrate mechanic and direct autonomic influences on regulated atrial ANP release as outlined in Figure 1. Their experiments (and those of others, Sonnenberg and Veress 1984) showed that the sympathetic transmitter norepinephrine augments ANP release by activation of β- and α_1-adrenoceptors, and

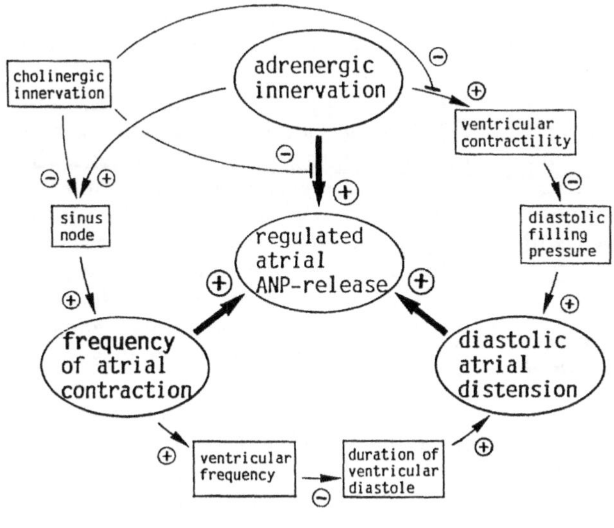

Fig. 1: Direct and indirect effects of adrenergic innervation on regulated ANP release from cardiac atria. Three direct stimuli of regulated ANP release have been identified in vitro. In situ, however, direct sympathetic stimulation must interfere with indirect effects resulting from changes in atrial mechanics.

that this adrenergically augmented release can be attenuated by muscarinic receptor stimulation (Schiebinger et al. 1987).

The cellular mechanisms, by which enhanced distension of atrial cells on the one hand and inotropic stimulation on the other hand result in regulated atrial ANP release, is under intensive study presently. Probably, an augmented intracellular availability of Ca^{2+} is the common intracellular signal in both cases. Cellular distension could activate mechanosensitive ion channels (as have been identified in endothelial cells, Lansman et al. 1987; Olesen et al. 1988), atrial stretch stimulates the phosphatidyl-inositol turnover (von Harsdorf et al. 1988), and finally, a stretch-induced activation of cardiac membrane adenylate cyclase is under study presently. Thus, the available information indicates that atrial cellular distension and positive inotropic stimulation by adrenoceptor activation cause a rise in regulated ANP release by sharing parts of the cellular pathway for signal transduction. However, the regulation of ANP synthesis in the atria and in the ventricles is less understood, effects of sympathetic activity on the rate of synthesis are unknown.

The parallel direct effect of distension and of adrenergic stimulation on ANP release in vitro does not mean that an enhanced sympathetic activity is a stimulator of ANP release in vivo. Due to the positiv inotropic adrenergic effects on the ventricles, the diastolic atrial distension can be diminished with enhanced sympathetic activity in the intact circulation. Thus, direct stimulatory effects and indirect inhibition due to changes in atrial geometry must interfere in a not yet predictable manner (Fig. 1), the net result may vary with changing hemodynamic conditions. This is probably the reason why conclusions on the role of autonomic innervation for ANP release, which were derived from studies in vivo, differed substantially.

Attenuation of Responses to Exogenous ANP by Reflex-modulation of Sympathetic Activity

In studies with ANP infusions in healthy humans without any pretreatment, infusion rates of at least 0.02 μg/kg/min ANP are necessary to obtain any significant acute hemodynamic or endocrine effects (Holtz et al. 1987a). These infusion rates result in approximately 10-fold elevations in plasma ANP levels, which is higher than any physiologic change in endogenous ANP levels. This dose-response relationship might be misunderstood as an argument against a physiological role of endogenous ANP release. However, in animal experiments it was shown that significant hemodynamic effects of atrial peptides can be unmasked, if buffering reflexes are suppressed by pretreatment with ganglionic blockade (Holtz et al. 1986).

A similar unmasking of the vasodilator potency of physiological plasma levels of atrial peptides can be achieved in humans by localized application of small dosages of ANP, which are small enough not to induce systemic effects or reflex responses. During infusion of α-ANP into the brachial artery of healthy probands, forearm blood flow and forearm venous plasma ANP concentration were measured (Bolli et al. 1987), but no systemic hemodynamic effects and no reflex responses were induced (this was controlled by analyzing vascular resistance in the contralateral forearm and by monitoring heart rate, blood pressure, plasma catecholamines and plasma renin activity during the protocol). With this approach, a dose-dependent forearm vasodilation by ANP was obtained (Bolli et al. 1987). The local ANP infusion rate causing halfmaximal dilation resulted in a forearm venous ANP concentration, which was 3.6-fold the basal level, and a 10% increase in forearm blood flow was related to a 50% increase in forearm venous ANP. These local venous ANP changes are well within the variations of endogenous plasma ANP levels, which occur physiologically in healthy humans.

These studies illustrate that the effects of exogenous ANP application, given systemically into the intact organism, must be blunted by blood pressure buffering reflexes and by autonomic counterregulation. Experiments designed to quantify directly this counterregulatory activation of sympathetic activity during exogenous ANP application identified a further action of the cardiac hormone: the inhibitory influence on the sympathetic nervous system.

Inhibition of Sympathoadrenal Activity by ANP

Initially, such an inhibition could be tentatively derived from experiments in intact animals, which typically demonstrated no or only minimal tachycardia during arterial hypotension induced by infusions of high ANP dosages. Further hints for such an inhibition were obtained later from analyses of urinary catecholamine excretion under the influence of ANP in rats (Debinski et al. 1986a; Debinski et al. 1986b). Finally, direct evidence was obtained by monitoring catecholamine plasma kinetics during ANP infusions in dogs (Holtz et al. 1987b), by electrical recordings of postganglionic sympathetic activity in rats and dogs (Imaizumi et al. 1987; Koyama et al. 1986; Schultz et al. 1988; Thorén et al. 1986), and by analyzing reflexes in healthy humans (Ebert and Cowley Jr 1988; Takeshita et al. 1987).

Figure 2 shows the effects of ANP-infusion on the release rate of norepinephrine and epinephrine into the plasma. These release rates are calculated from measurements of plasma concentrations of labelled and unlabelled catecholamines during infu-

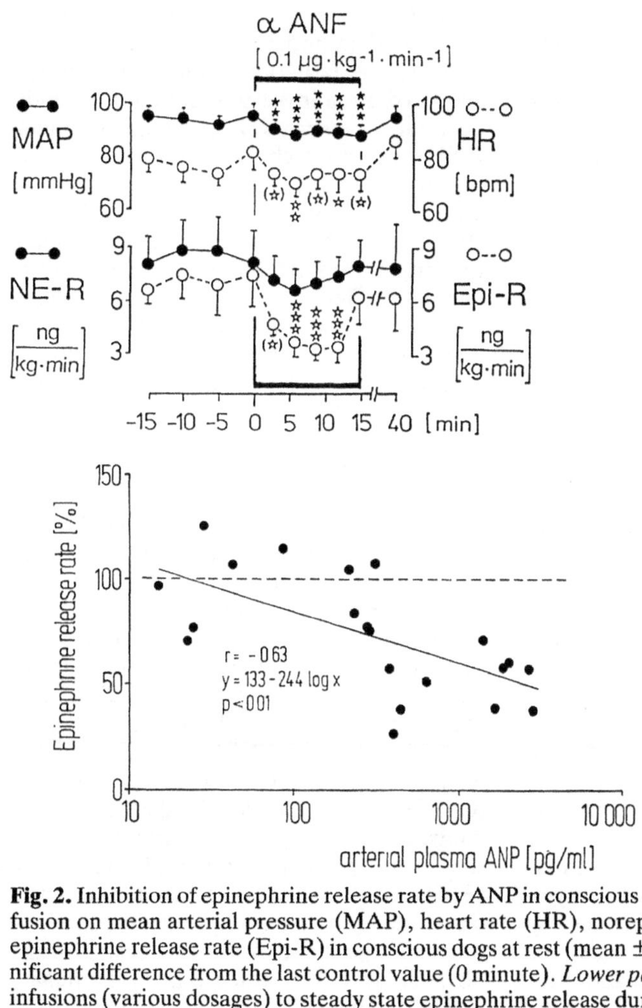

Fig. 2. Inhibition of epinephrine release rate by ANP in conscious dogs. *Upper panel:* Effect of ANP infusion on mean arterial pressure (MAP), heart rate (HR), norepinephrine release rate (NE-R), and epinephrine release rate (Epi-R) in conscious dogs at rest (mean ± SEM; n = 9). Asterisks indicate significant difference from the last control value (0 minute). *Lower panel:* Relation of plasma ANP during infusions (various dosages) to steady state epinephrine release during these infusions (as percentage of control release). The arterial plasma ANP concentration at the 100% intercept (i.e.: no change in epinephrine release) is 23 pg/ml, which is within the range of basal AP levels in these dogs (40 ± 6 pg/ml). Data from Holtz et al. 1987b.

sions of labelled catechols in tracer amounts, as described earlier (Esler et al. 1979). These assessments of catechol kinetics indicate, whether a change in plasma catecholamines results from changes in the catecholamine clearance from the plasma or from a change of catecholamine release into the plasma. Thus, these release rates, sometimes also referred to as "spillover rates" into the plasma, are better indicators of overall sympathoadrenal activity than the mere plasma concentrations of catechols. During infusions of a high ANP dosage in dogs, the epinephrine release rate declines significantly (Fig. 2a), and the threshold for this ANP-induced inhibition of epinephrine release is probably close to physiological ANP plasma levels in dogs (Fig. 2b). The heart rate and the norepinephrine release rate do not increase during the ANP-induced hypotension in the conscious dogs at rest (Fig. 2a), while similar hypotensions induced by the venodilator nitroglycerin or by the arteriolar dilator hydralazin result in significant elevations of release rate and heart rate in the same dogs (Holtz et al. 1987b).

These demonstrations of ANP-induced absolute inhibition of epinephrine release and relative inhibition of norepinephrine release indicated a global sympathoadrenal inhibition by ANP in the intact organism. Later, they were confirmed and extended by electrical recordings of postganglionic sympathetic nerve activity in lumbar, splanchnic and renal nerves (Imaizumi et al. 1987; Koyama et al. 1986; Schultz et al. 1988; Thorén et al. 1986). These studies demonstrated substantial reductions of postganglionic spike activity during ANP application, when the baroreceptor afferents were interrupted. This means that the direct sympatho-inhibitory action of ANP must interfere with sympatho-stimulation due to baroreceptor unloading during the hypotension resulting from the vascular and renal ANP actions.

This sympatho-inhibition by ANP and its interference with reflex-mediated sympatho-stimulation is demonstrable also in humans, although an ANP-induced decline in plasma epinephrine levels was seldom observed. Only two placebo-controlled small studies are available, demonstrating transient epinephrine declines, one with normotensives (Richards et al. 1985a) and one with hypertensives (Richards et al. 1985b). It is very difficult to document consistent intervention-induced declines of basal epinephrine levels in humans: the basal levels are low and the scatter is huge relative to these basal levels, and large spontaneous fluctuations occur during longer placebo-protocols (Richards et al. 1988). Inhibitory effects of ANP on sympathetic reflexes are more clearly demonstrable (Ebert and Cowley Jr, 1988; Takeshita et al. 1987). Under ANP-infusions, heart rate or plethysmographically measured forearm vasoconstriction increased less in response to baroreceptor unloading (Ebert and Cowley Jr 1988) or to lower body negative pressure (Takeshita et al. 1987) than under control conditions.

However, in another study, forearm vasoconstriciton in response to lower body negative pressure was potentiated under ANP and the tachycardia in response to baroreceptor unloading was not attenuated under ANP (Volpe et al. 1988). In this study, the ANP infusion rate was higher than in the studies demonstrating an inhibitory ANP effect on sympathetic activation, and an high priming dose of ANP was given before the start of ANP-infusions (Volpe et al. 1988). Thus it is possible that the inhibitory effect of ANP is demonstrable only in a certain dose range, and that other changes induced by higher ANP dosages result in enhanced reflex responses.

This typical interference between ANP-induced sympathoadrenal inhibition and reflex sympathetic activation (triggered by the other ANP-effects) renders comparisons of studies with varying protocols and dosages often very difficult. However, this interference is also demonstrable in studies from the same laboratory and with identical dosage: 25 ng/kg/min ANP i.v. in healthy subjects inhibited baroreceptor reflex tachycardia (Ebert and Cowley Jr 1988), but enhanced basal sympathetic activity as assessed from plasma norepinephrine levels (Ebert et al. 1988). This interference is a consequence of the unphysiological application of high exogenous dosages. During physiological ANP release from the heart, stimulated by an increase of atrial pressure, this same stimulus concomitantly triggers reflex attenuations of sympathetic activity.

Thus, neural cardiopulmonary afferents and the cardiac hormone can act in concert, complementing each other, in order to reduce sympathetic activity and to normalize elevated cardiac filling.

Mechanisms of ANP-Induced Sympathoadrenal Inhibition

Several sites for a putative inhibitory influence of ANP on sympathetic activity have been identified experimentally. In the chromaffine cells of the adrenal medulla, membrane binding sites for ANP and the synthesis of the prohormone have been demonstrated (Morel et al. 1988; Mukoyama et al. 1988; Pruss and Zamir 1987), indicating not only endocrine, but also paracrine or autocrine actions of ANP in this organ. Endocrine or autocrine actions of ANP, resulting in inhibited catecholamine synthesis and in reduced neuronal excitability, can also occur in peripheral sympathetic ganglia (Cheung 1988; Debinski et al. 1987a; Debinski et al. 1987b; Gutkind et al. 1987). Further potential targets for circulating ANP, possibly involved in its sympatho-inhibitory action, are neuronal binding sites in areas of the central nervous system outside of the blood-brain barrier, which are involved in fluid and electrolyte balance (Mantyh et al. 1987). Furthermore, ANP has been shown to inhibit stimulus-induced norepipherine release from sympathetic nerve endings in vitro (MacKay and Cheung 1987; Nakamaru and Inagami 1986) and in vivo (Zukowska-Grojec et al., 1986), although this inhibition was not observed in all studies on peripheral sympathetic neurotransmission. Studies from several laboratories are available on the activation of depressor reflexes by ANP (Imaizumi et al. 1987; Schultz et al. 1988; Thorén et al. 1986). This activation is thought to result from an ANP-induced increase in the activity of mechanosensitive atrial vagal C-fibres.

Relevance of Sympathoadrenal Inhibition?

Up to now, only tentative speculations are possible in answer to this question. However, two aspects should be considered here briefly: the potential role of reduced epinephrine release into the plasma for subsequent sympathetic neurotransmission, and the persistence of ANP-induced sympathoadrenal inhibition during development of congestive heart failure with chronically elevated ANP plasma levels.

In humans, there is good evidence that circulating epinephrine is taken up into postganglionic sympathetic nerve endings, that it is released subsequently during sympathetic activation as cotransmitter from these terminals, and that the co-released epinephrine enhances norepinephrine release by activating prejunctional β-adrenoceptors (Floras et al. 1988; Nezu et al. 1985). Such a longacting augmentation of sympathetic neurotransmission is demonstrable with plasma epinephrine levels occuring during sympathoadrenal activation (Floras et al. 1988). Therefore, small attenuations of medullary epinephrine release by ANP, as documented in dogs (Fig. 2) and occasionally in humans (Richards et al. 1985a; 1985b) do have the potential of attenuating sympathetic neurotransmission subsequently.

In congestive heart failure, the reflex control of sympathetic activity by cardiopulmonary blood volume is severely disturbed. Therefore, we studied whether the hormonal control of sympathetic activity via ANP is disturbed also (Holtz et al. unpublished). This was done in a canine model of low output failure, induced by chronic ventricular tachycardia, as described previously (Riegger et al. 1988). After two weeks of ventricular pacing at a rate of 265 min^{-1}, aortic flow in the conscious dogs at rest had declined by 37%, while plasma ANP was elevated 13-fold, plasma renin activity 9-fold, and norepinephrine release rate 2.3-fold, respectively. In this state of low output failure with enhanced neuroendocrine activity, ANP-infusions no longer lowered plasma renin activity (as was the case under control conditions) and a true vascular nonresponsiveness to ANP (up to 0.3 μg/kg/min) was demonstrable, but the sympathoadrenal inhibition by ANP was not at all affected. After two weeks of pacing, the ANP-induced inhibition of epinephrine release was not attenuated compared to control conditions, and a significant inhibition of norepinephrine release was observed

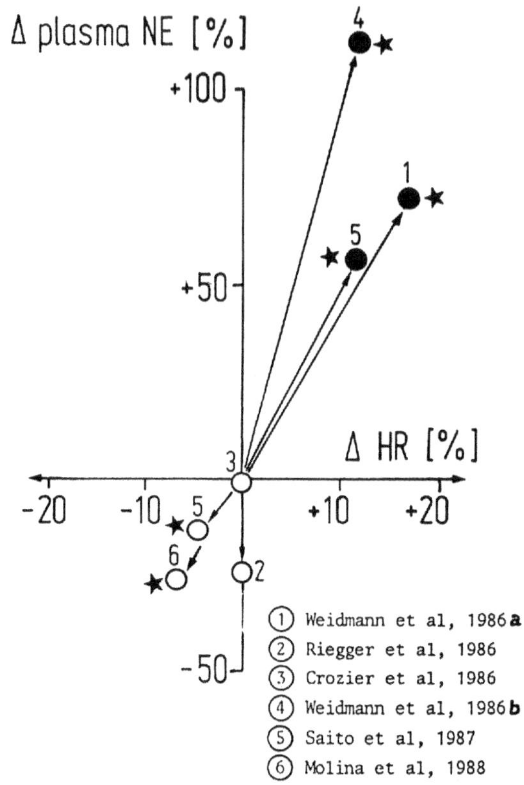

Fig. 3: Acute effects of ANP-infusions (≈ 0.1 μg/kg/min or more) on indices of sympathetic activity in healthy humans (closed circles) and in patients with congestive heart failure (open circles).

Abbreviations: Δ HR: change in heart rate; Δ plasma NE: change in plasma norepinephrine. Asterisks indicate significant changes of plasma norepinephrine. In healthy humans, sympathoexcitation is triggered during hypotension resulting from the ANP-induced vasodilation and volume contraction. In congestive heart failure, indices of sympathetic activity tend to change in the opposite direction with ANP infusions (while systemic ANP effects are attenuated). Mimicking the systemic ANP effects by infusions of sodium nitroprusside in patients with heart failure does not lower plasma norepinephrine levels, indicating a direct inhibition of sympathetic activity by the infused ANP. However, conclusive evidence for this interpretation is not yet available.

under ANP infusion (while the same ANP-dosage lowered blood pressure without changing norepinephrine release rate under control conditions, as shown in Figure 2a).

This preserved inhibition of sympathoadrenal activity by ANP during prolonged augmentation of endogenous ANP release contrasts with the disappearance of ANP actions on plasma renin and on the vascular system. This contrast demonstrates that the reduction in target organ responsiveness is not uniform during prolonged exposure to high ANP plasma levels in dogs. A shift within the spectrum of different ANP actions occurs, enhancing the relative importance of the sympathoinhibition. And the available data indicate that a similar shift might occur also during prolonged ANP exposure in humans during the development of congestive heart failure (Fig. 3).

Such a shift within the spectrum of ANP actions during prolonged exposure to high ANP plasma levels could be relevant for the chronic effects of drugs, which enhance the halflife of endogenous ANP by inhibiting ANP degradating enzymes, for the effects of sustained therpeutic ANP infusions (e.g.: for hemodynamic unloading of the failing heart in the intensive care unit), and, finally, for the regulation of sympathoadrenal activity during progression of heart failure. The threshold plasma concentration of ANP, inducing sympathoadrenal inhibition, is probably close to physiological plasma levels in dogs (Fig. 2b), but this threshold is not yet known in humans. Therefore, no definitive conclusions on the physiological, pathophysiological and therapeutic relevance of the sympathoinhibition by ANP in humans are possible at present. The sympathoinhibition is probably the least analyzed among the different actions of the new cardiac hormone. This must not necessarily reflect its biological importance.

References

Bolli P, Müller FB, Linder L, Raine AEG, Resink TJ, Erje P, Kiowski W, Ritz R, Bühler FR (1987) The vasodilator potency of atrial natriuretic peptide in man. Circulation 75:221–228

Cheung DW (1988) Atriopeptin III depresses the excitability of sympathetic neurones. Biochem Biophys Res Commun 154:411–416

Crozier IG, Ikram H, Gomez HJ, Nicholls MG, Espiner EA, Warner NJ (1986) Haemodynamic effects of atrial peptide infusion in heart failure. Lancet II:1242–1245

DeBold AJ (1985) Atrial natriuretic factor: a hormone produced by the heart. Science 230: 767–770

Debinski W, Kuchel O, Buu NT, Garcia R, Cantin M, Genest J (1986a) Involvement of the adrenal glands in the action of the atrial natriuretic factor. Proc Soc Biol Med 181:318–324

Debinski W, Kuchel O, Garcia R, Buu NT, Racz K, Cantin M, Genest J (1986b) Atrial natriuretic factor inhibits the sympathetic nervous activity in one-kidney, one-clip hypertension in the rat. Proc Soc Biol Med 181:173–177

Debinski W, Gutkowska J, Kuchel O, Racz K, Buu NT, Cantin M, Genest J (1987a) Presence of an atrial natriuretic factorlike peptide in the rat superior cervical ganglia. Neuroendocrinology 46:236–240

Debinski W, Kuchel O, Buu NT, Cantin M, Genest J (1987b) Atrial natriuretic factor partially inhibits the stimulated catecholamine synthesis in superior cervical ganglia of the rat. Neurosci Lett 77:92–96

Dietz JR (1984) Release of natriuretic factor from rat heart-lung preparation by atrial distension. Am J Physiol 247:R1093–R1096

Ebert TJ, Cowley Jr AW (1988) Atrial natriuretic factor attenuates carotid baroreflex-mediated cardioacceleration in humans. Am J Physiol 254:R590–R594

Ebert TJ, Skelton MM, Cowley Jr AW (1988) Dynamic cardiovascular responses to infusions of atrial natriuretic factor in humans. Hypertension 11:537–544

Esler M, Jackman G, Bobik A, Kelleher D, Jennings, G, Leonard P, Skews H, Korner P (1979) Determination of norepinephrine apparent release rate and clearance in humans. Life Sci 25:1461–1470

Floras JS, Aylward PE, Victor RG, Mark AL, Abboud FM (1988) Epinephrine facilitates neurogenic vasoconstriction in humans. J Clin Invest 81:1265–1274

Forssmann WG, Hock D, Lottspeich F, Henschen A, Kreye VAW, Christmann M, Reinecke M, Metz J, Carlquist M, Mutt V (1983) The right auricle of the heart is an endocrine organ: cardiodilatin as a peptide hormone candidate. Anat Embryol 168:307–313

Genest J, Cantin M, Anand-Srivastava MB, Cusson JR, De Lean A, Garcia R, Gutkowska J, Hamlet P, Kuchel O, Larochelle P, Nemer M, Schiffrin EL, Schiller PW, Thibault G, Tremblay J (1988) The atrial natriuretic factor: its physiology and biochemistry. Rev Physiol Biochem Pharmacol 110:1–145

Gutkind JS, Kurihara M, Castrén E, Saavedra JM (1987) Atrial natriuretic peptide receptors in sympathetic ganglia: biochemical response and alterations in genetically hypertensive rats. Biochem Biophys Res Commun 149:65–72

von Harsdorf R, Lang R, Fullerton M, Smith AI, Woodcock EA (1988) Right heart dilatation increases inositol-(1, 4, 5)trisphosphate accumulation. Implications for the control of atrial natriuretic peptide release. FEBS Letters 233: 201–205

Holtz J, Stewart DJ, Elsner D, Bassenge E (1986) In vivo atrial peptide-venodilation: minimal potency relative to nitroglycerin in dogs. Life Sci 39:2177–2184

Holtz J, Münzel T, Bassenge E (1987a) Das natriuretische Vorhofhormon im Menschen. Z Kardiol 76:655–670

Holtz J, Sommer O, Bassenge E (1987b) Inhibition of sympatho-adrenal activity by atrial natriuretic factor in dogs. Hypertension 9:350–354

Imaizumi T, Takeshita A, Higashi H, Nakamura M (1987) α-ANP alters reflex control of lumbar and renal sympathetic nerve activity and heart rate. Am J Physiol 253:H1136–H1140

Kelly RB (1985) Pathways of protein secretion in eukaryotes. Science 230:25–32

Koyama S, Nishida Y, Hosomi H, Abe Y (1986) Participation of baroreceptor reflexes in blood pressure and sympathetic nerve responses to a synthetic human atrial natriuretic peptide in anesthetized dogs. Eur J Pharmacol 127:43–48

Lang RE, Thölken H, Ganten D, Luft FC, Ruskoaho H, Unger T (1985) Atrial natriuretic factor – a circulating hormone stimulated by volume loading. Nature 314:264–266

Lansman JB, Hallam TJ, Rink TJ (1987) Single stretch-activated ion channels in vascular endothelial cells as mechanotransducers? Nature 325:811–813

MacKay MJ, Cheung DW (1987) Inhibition of neuromuscular transmission in the guinea-pig saphenous artery by atriopeptin II. Can J Physiol Pharmacol 65:1988–1990

Mantyh CR, Kruger L, Brecha NC, Mantyh PW (1987) Localization of specific binding sites for atrial natriuretic factor in the central nervous system of rat, guinea pig, cat and human. Brain Res 412:329–342

Molina CR, Fowler MB, McCrory S, Peterson C, Myers BD, Schroeder JS, Murad F (1988) Hemodynamic, renal and endocrine effects of atrial natriuretic peptide infusion in severe heart failure. J Am Coll Cardiol 12:175–186

Morel G, Chabot JG, Garcia-Caballero T, Gossard F, Dihl F, Belles-Isles M, Heisler S (1988) Synthesis, internalization, and localization of atrial natriuretic peptide in rat adrenal medulla. Endocrinology 123:149–158

Mukoyama M, Nakao K, Morii N, Shiono S, Itoh H, Sugawara A, Yamada T, Saito Y, Arai H, Imura H (1988) Atrial natriuretic polypeptide in bovine adrenal medulla. Hypertension 11:692–696

Nakamaru M, Inagami T (1986) Atrial natriuretic factor inhibits norepinephrine release evoked by sympathetic nerve stimulation in isolated perfused rat mesenteric arteries. Eur J Pharmacol 123:459–461

Nezu M, Miura Y, Adachi M, Adachi M, Kimura S, Toriyabe S, Ishizuka Y, Ohashi J, Sugawara T, Takahashi M, Noshiro T, Yoshinaga K (1985) The effects of epinephrine on norepinephrine release in essential hypertension. Hypertension 7:187–195

Olesen SP, Clapham DE, Davies PF (1988) Haemodynamic shear stress activates a K+ current in vascular endothelial cells. Nature 331:168–170

Pruss RM, Zamir N (1987) Regulated expression of atrial natriuretic peptide-like immunoreactivity in cultured bovine adrenomedullary chromaffin cells. Neurochem Int 11:299–304

Richards AM, Ikram H, Yandle TG, Nicholls MG, Webster MWI, Espiner EA (1985a) Renal, haemodynamic, and hormonal effects of human alpha atrial natriuretic peptide in healthy volunteers. Lancet I:545–549

Richards AM, Nicholls MG, Espiner EA, Ikram H, Yandle TG, Joyce SL, Cullens MM (1985b) Effects of alpha-human atrial natriuretic peptide in essential hypertension. Hypertension 7:812–817

Richards AM, Tonolo G, Montorsi P, Finlayson J, Fraser R, Inglis G, Towrie A, Morton JJ (1988) Low dose infusions of 26- and 28-amino acid human atrial natriuretic peptides in normal man. J Clin Endocrinol Metab 66:465–472

Riegger GAJ, Kromer EP, Kochsiek K (1986) Human atrial natriuretic peptide: Plasma levels, hemodynamic, hormonal, and renal effects in patients with severe congestive heart failure. J Cardiovasc Pharmacol 8:1107–1112

Riegger GAJ, Elsner D, Kromer EP, Daffner C, Forssmann WG, Muders F, Pascher EW, Kochsiek K (1988) Atrial natriuretic peptide in congestive heart failure in the dog: plasma levels, cyclic guanosine monophosphate, ultrastrucutre of atrial myoendocrine cells, and hemodynamic, hormonal, and renal effects. Circulation 77:398–406

Ruskoaho H, Toth M, Lang RE (1985) Atrial natriuretic peptide secretion: synergistic effect of phorbol ester and A23187. Biochem Biophys Res Commun 133:581–588

Saito Y, Nakao K, Morii N, Sugawara A, Shiono S, Yamada T, Itoh H, Sakamoto M, Kurahashi K, Fujiwara M, Imura H (1986) Bay K 8644, a voltage-sensitive calcium channel agonist, facilitates secretion of atrial natriuretic polypeptide from isolated perfused rat hearts. Biochem Biophys Res Commun 138: 1170–1176

Saito Y, Nakao K, Nishimura K, Sugawara A, Okumura K, Obata K, Sonoda R, Ban T, Yasue H, Imura H (1987) Clinical application of atrial natriuretic polypeptide in patients with congestive heart failure: beneficial effects on left ventricular function. Circulation 76: 115–124

Schiebinger RJ, Linden J (1986a) Effect of atrial contraction frequency on atrial natriuretic peptide secretion. Am J Physiol 251: H1095–H1099

Schiebinger RJ, Linden J (1986b) The influence of resting tension of immunoreactive atrial natriuretic peptide secretion by rat atria superfused in vitro. Circ Res 59:105–109

Schiebinger RJ, Baker MZ, Linden J (1987) Effect of adrenergic and muscarinic cholinergic agonists on atrial natriuretic peptide secretion by isolated rat atria. Potential role of the autonomic nervous system in modulating atrial natriuretic peptide secretion. J Clin Invest 80:1687–1691

Schultz HD, Gardner DG, Deschepper DF, Coleridge HM, Coleridge JCG (1988) Vagal C-fiber blockade abolishes sympathetic inhibition by atrial natriuretic factor. Am J Pyhsiol 255:R6–R13

Sonnenberg H, Veress AT (1984) Cellular mechanism of release of atrial natriuretic factor. Biochem Biophys Res Commun 124: 443–449

Takeshita A, Imaizumi T, Nakamura N, Higashi H, Sasaki T, Nakamura M, Kangawa K, Matsuo H (1987) Attenuation of reflex forearm vasoconstriction by α-human atrial natriuretic peptide in men. Circ Res 61:555–559

Thorén P, Mark AL, Morgan DA, O;Neill TP, Needleman AP, Brody MJ (1986) Activation of vagal depressor reflexes by atriopeptins inhibits renal sympathetic nerve activity. Am J Physiol 251:H1252–H1259

Volpe M, De Luca N, Bigazzi MC, Vecchione F, Lembo G, Condorelli M, Trimarco B (1988) Atrial natriuretic factor potentiates forearm reflex vasoconstriction induced by cardiopulmonary receptor deactivation in man. Circulation 77:849–855

Weidmann P, Hasler L, Gnädinger MP, Lang RE, Uehlinger DE, Shaw S, Rascher W, Reubi FC (1986a) Blood levels and renal effects of atrial natriuretic peptide in normal man. J Clin Invest 77:734–742

Weidmann P, Hellmueller B, Uehlinger DE, Lang RE, Gnaedinger MP, Hasler L, Shaw S, Bachmann C (1986b) Plasma levels and cardiovascular, endocrine, and excretory effects of atrial natriuretic peptide during different sodium intakes in man. J Clin Endocrinol Metab 62:1027–1036

Zukowska-Grojec Z, Haass M, Kopin IJ, Zamir N (1986) Interactions of atrial natriuretic peptide with the sympathetic and endocrine systems in the pithed rat. J Pharm Exp Ther 239:480–487

Atrial Peptides in the Endocrine Control of Fluid and Cardiovascular Homeostasis

D. J. Ramsay, C. H. Metzler, D. A. Scheuer, T. N. Thrasher

University of California, San Francisco, California, USA

Summary.

1. The effects of ANP on the baroreflex control of hormonal systems which control fluid and cardiovascular homeostasis were studied in conscious dogs.
2. Infusion of ANP, in contrast to other hypotensive maneuvers, did not result in tachycardia or increases in plasma renin activity, ACTH or vasopressin secretion.
3. The renin response to local decreases in renal perfusion pressure obtained by abdominal aortic constriction was prevented by infusion of ANP at low rates.
4. ANP does not completely block renin secretion in situations where there is increased renal sympathetic nerve activity, e.g. thoracic caval constriction. Infusion of ANP and propanolol together, however, does completely block rening secretion under these circumstances.
5. The most sensitive effect of ANP is to block angiotensin II stimulation of aldosterone secretin.
6. As ANP is released in response to small increases in atrial pressure and acts to reduce blood pressure and salt and water retention, it may have a physiological role to prevent over-expansion of blood volume.

Key words: Atrial natriuretic peptide – Vasopressin – Renin – ACTH – Aldosterone – Blood pressure

For many years it has been known that increases in left and right atrial pressures initiate vagal afferent activity which inhibits vasopressin, ACTH and renin secretion. Thus loading low pressure cardiopulmonary baroreceptors activates mechanisms which limit the ability of the renin/angiotensin/aldosterone system and vasopressin to expand volume and to increase arterial blood pressure. The discovery of a hormone secreted by the heart, atrial natriuretic peptide (ANP), which causes natriuresis, diuresis and arterial hypotension raises exciting possibilities that there may be a complementary endocrine system which also prevents overexpansion of body fluids, circulatory, congestion and hypertension (Laragh 1985). As ANP is secreted in response to increases in atrial pressure (Ledsome et al. 1985; Metzler et al. 1986), and as its ability to inhibit renin, aldosterone and vasopressin secretion has been reported by a number of laboratories it would seem to be a natural candidate for this hypovolemic, hypotensive function.

It is of interest that raised plasma ANP levels have been described in a number of animal models of congestive cardiac failure (Freeman et al. 1985; Winaver et al. 1986). Also, patients with heart failure show elevated plasma levels, and the increase in these levels is correlated with the severity of failure (Raine et al. 1986). As venous congestion and increased atrial volumes are the hallmark of congestive heart failure, it is not surprising that plasma ANP levels are elevated if the normal relationship between atrial stretch and ANP release is preserved. The possible utility of plasma ANP measurement as an index of the severity of congestive cardiac failure is a subject of current interest.

Baroreflex Function

Our own interest in ANP has centered on its possible role in the physiological regulation of fluid and electrolyte balance, particularly renin, aldosterone, ACTH and vasopressin. Additionally, vasopressin and angiotensin have been implicated more directly in cardiovascular control. We therefore set out to determine the effects of lowering arterial blood pressure with ANP on plasma

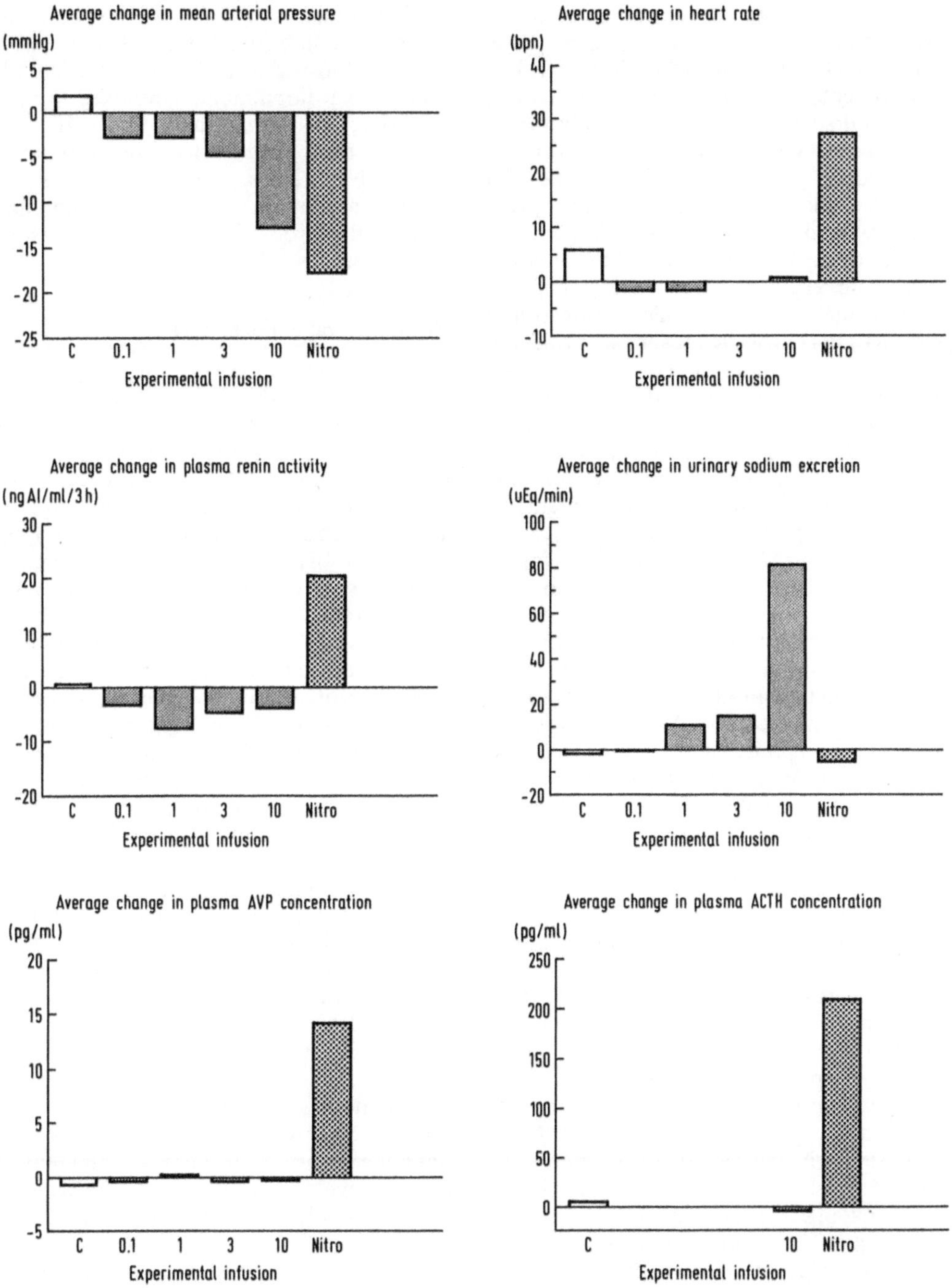

Fig. 1. The effects of infusions of ANP (1–23) at various doses in microg/min (solid) and sodium nitroprusside (hatched) on various cardiovascular and hormonal variables

vasopressin, renin and ACTH, compared with sodium nitroprusside, an agent often employed to assess baroreflex function. The experiments were carried out in conscious, trained dogs well acclimated to laboratory procedures. Various doses of ANP titrated to produce graded reductions in arterial pressure, and infusions of sodium nitroprusside adjusted to match the largest reduction in blood pressure, were tested on separate days. The results are shown in Fig. 1.

Infusions of nitroprusside demonstrated the vigorous baroreflex responses typical of arterial hypotension. There was brisk reflex tachycardia, and marked increases in plasma concentrations of vasopressin, renin and ACTH. These compensations are physiologically appropriate, and would normally result in homeostatic adjustments to return blood pressure to normal.

The effects of ANP infusion are obviously different. There are no increases in hormone levels – indeed there is a trend for plasma renin activity to be reduced. The reflex tachycardia is muted. In some way, when reduction in arterial blood pressure occur in the presence of ANP, the expected baroreflex responses to that fall in pressure do not occur or are significantly blunted.

One possibility might be that ANP interfers with secretion of the various hormones at the organ level. We have determined the effects of systemic administration of ANP on the vasopressin response to raising plasma osmolality with hypertonic NaCl in dogs (Metzler et al. 1987). In these experiments, plasma vasopressin levels were identical when ANP 1–28 at 20 ng/Kg/min was infused compared with controls. In another series of experiments, 10 times the dose of ANP was infused, again with no effect. Drinking responses to intravenous NaCl were similarly unaffected by systemic ANP. This contrasts with work showing that intracerebroventricular ANP injections do block drinking and vasopressin responses to a number of stimuli (Samson 1987). As ANP – and now brain natriuretic peptide (BNP) – has been identified in many regions of the brain, presumably there are central receptors to the peptide which are inaccessible to blood-borne peptide (Itoh et al. 1988).

In general, therefore, the results in fig. 1 seem to indicate a role for ANP in blunting cardiovascular and hormonal responses to arterial hypotension. This is in keeping with the hypothesis that ANP can act as an adjunct to cardiopulmonary reflexes to prevent overexpansion of body fluids. If atrial pressure rises, both vagal afferent discharge and ANP release inhibit vasopressin, ACTH and renin secretion to minimize further fluid retention and atrial pressure increases.

Physiological Role of ANP

Many laboratories have studied the effects of infusions of ANP into whole animals to investigate its natriuretic and hypotensive effects (Bie et al. 1988; Burnett et al. 1984; Metzler et al. 1987). In many of these studies, infusion rates have been high and anesthetized acutely prepared animals have been used. In an attempt to determine infusion rates necessary to produce acute natriuretic and cardiovascular effects, we have infused ANP (1–28) into conscious trained dogs. In our laboratory, natriuresis during one hour of infusion reaches significance between 10 and 25 ng/Kg/min. Bie et al. 1988, report a threshold for natriuresis at an infusion rate of 12.5 ng/Kg/min. These infusions raise plasma levels of ANP 3–8 fold. It is therefore important to assess if such levels can be achieved by endogenous secretion under physiological conditions.

We have reported that increases in right or left atrial pressure increase plasma ANP levels in conscious dogs (Metzler et al. 1986). In these experiments, plasma ANP increased to levels in excess of 300 pg/ml with changes in atrial pressures ranging from 1 to 14 mmHg. The relationship between increased right atrial pressure and plasma ANP was particularly sensitive, as has been reported by others. Thus increased plasma levels of ANP can be triggered by small, physiological elevations in right atrial pressure.

Mild volume expansion also results in elevated plasma ANP in conscious dogs. We have shown that by the 5th day of treatment with DOCA (15 mg/day, s.c.), plasma ANP increased to 91 $\pm$ 14 pg/ml from control levels of 42 $\pm$ 8 pg/ml in a population of dogs (Metzler et al. 1987). This correlated with approximately a 10% increase in extracellular fluid volume. It was of great interest in these experiments to find that the day of sodium 'escape' from the DOCA treatment correlated with the increased plasma ANP and occured before blood pressure was significantly increased (day 8). Furthermore, there was a 3.9 fold increase in ANPmRNA in the left atrium and 6.7 fold increase in the right atrium as shown by blot-hybridization analysis. Although this is still controversial, it is tempting to argue that raised ANP is involved in the DOCA escape phenomenon (Greenwald et al. 1988).

Results of giving ANP together with other natriuretic agents are even more striking. For example, infusion of ANP at 5 ng/Kg/min has little effect on sodium excretion. However, if this dose of ANP is infused together with hypertonic NaCl in conscious dogs, the natriuretic effect of the hypertonic NaCl is greatly enhanced. The potentiation of the hypertonic NaCl induced natriuresis was 70%. Although the mechanisms of the potentiation has not been elucidated, it draws attention to the importance of studying interactions of ANP with other systems during natriuresis.

Plasma Renin Activity

There have been a number of observations which have shown that ANP lowers plasma renin activity (Burnett et al. 1984, Freeman et al. 1985). However, the mechanism of the inhibition and its physiological significance are not clear. We therefore decided to study the effects of a low dose of ANP (5 ng/Kg/min) on the plasma renin response to graded

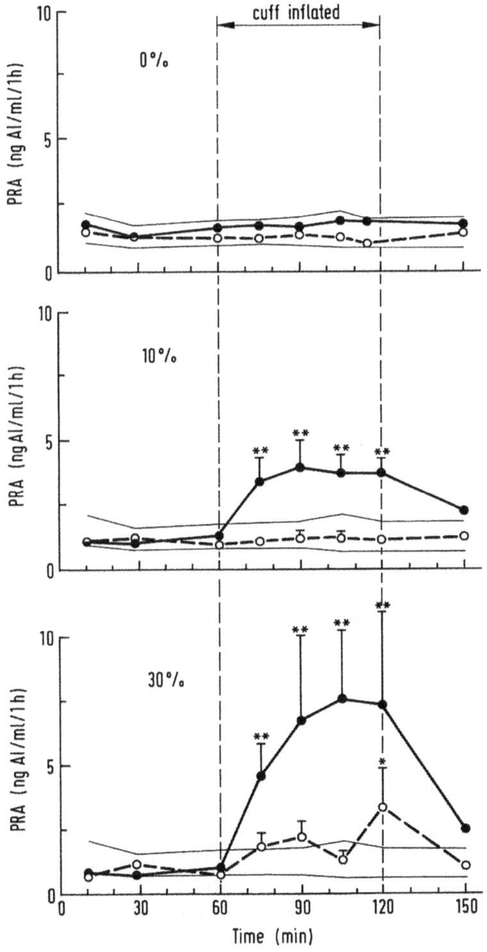

Fig. 2. Plasma renin activity in response to 0, 10 and 30% reductions in renal perfusion pressure, during infusion of ANP (1–28) at 5 ng/Kg/min (broken line) or vehicle (solid line). Dotted lines show 95% confidence limit of PRA during time control. * $P < 0.05$, ** $P < 0.01$

reductions in renal perfusion pressure. Dogs were prepared with inflatable cuffs around the abdominal aorta just above the origin of the renal arteries (Scheuer et al. 1987). The cuff was then inflated to reduce renal perfusion pressure by 0, 10 or 30% in the pressure or absence of ANP (1–28) infusions.

The results are shown in Fig. 2. The effects of the ANP infusion are dramatic. Even though renal perfusion pressure is reduced by 30%, the normal plasma renin response is almost entirely eliminated. This low rate of infusion of ANP elevated plasma levels by only 35 pg/ml, well within the range which can be achieved physiologically.

The mechanism of the inhibition of the normal renin response to reduced renal perfusion is likely to be direct on the kidney. This low dose of ANP has no effect on measured cardiovascular variables. The influ-

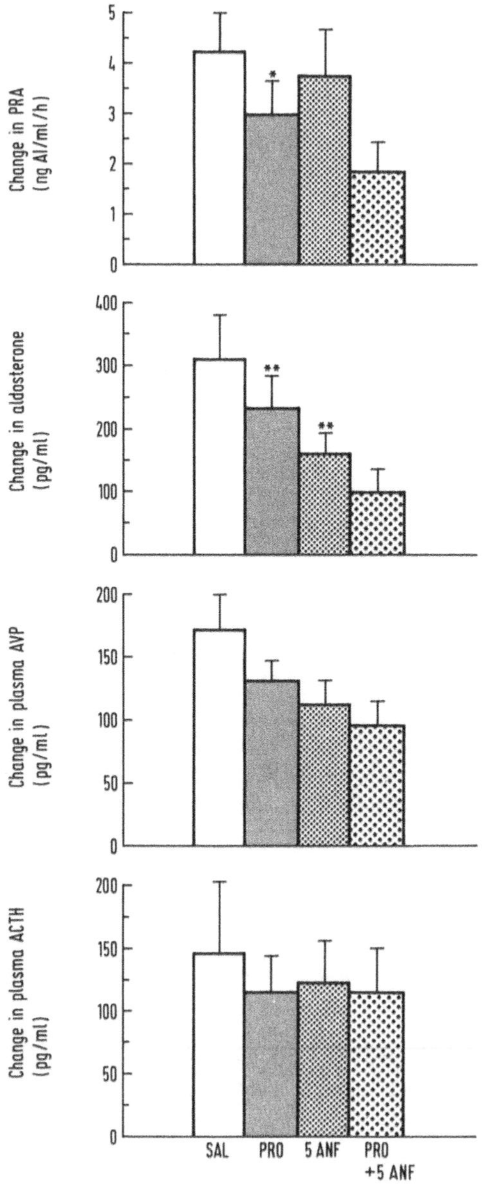

Fig. 3. Integrated change in plasma renin activity, plasma aldosterone, plasma AVP and plasma ACTH during caval constriction. Open: saline vehicle control, solid: propranolol infusion, slashed: ANF infusion at 5 ng/Kg/min. croshatched: propranolol and ANF combined. * $P < 0.05$, ** $P < 0.01$

ence of renal sympathetic nerves is unlikely to be significant, as resting renal sympathetic tone in conscious dogs is low, and the raised systemic pressure which accompanies suprarenal cuff inflation will decrease sympathetic activity further. It is of interest to note that increases in left atrial pressure, which result in ANP release, block the renin secretion response to arterial hypotension, even when the kidneys are denervated (Lee et al. 1984, 1985). Thus the inhibition of the increase in PRA which normally accompanies a fall in renal perfusion is caused by a small elevation in plasma ANP and may have important physiological consequences.

Thoracic Caval Constriction Experiments

The underlying hypothesis stated at the beginning of this paper was that ANP can act to prevent over expansion of volume by in-

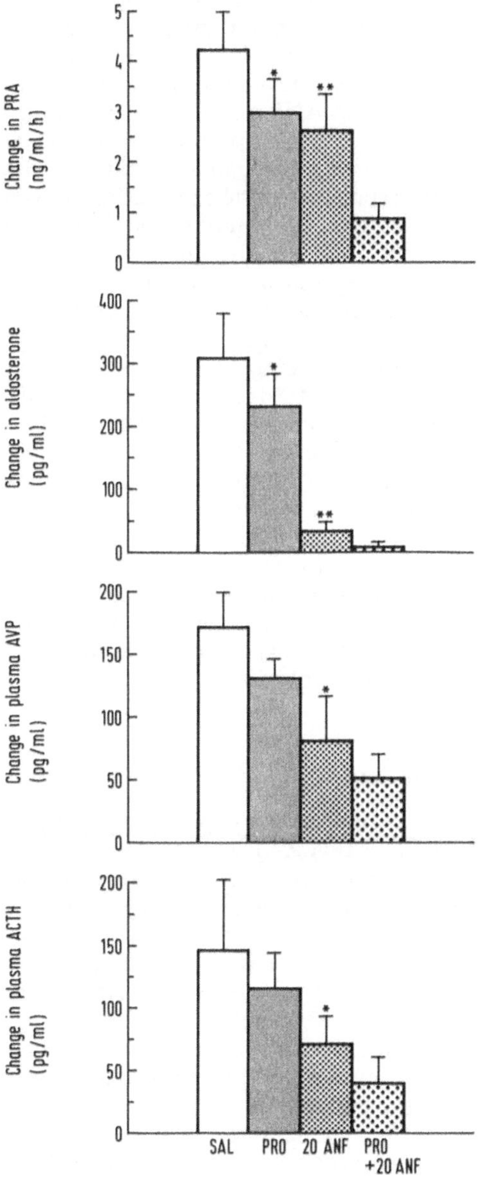

Fig. 4. Integrated change in plasma renin activity, plasma aldosterone, plasma AVP and plasma ACTH during caval constriction. Open: saline vehicle control, solid: propranolol infusion, slashed: ANF infusion at 20 ng/Kg/min. croshatched: propranolol and ANF combined. * $P < 0.05$, ** $P < 0.01$

hibiting baroreflex stimulated vasopressin, renin and ACTH secretion. The present series of experiments was designed to test the proposition directly by examining the effects of ANP infusions on secretion of these hormones (Scheuer et al., in press). Dogs were prepared with inflatable cuffs around the thoracic part of the inferior vena cava, and studied while conscious on subsequent occasions following recovery from surgery (Thrasher et al. 1982). The effects of sufficient caval cuff inflation to reduce mean arterial blood pressure by 25% was tested. The results in Fig. 3 show the marked stimulation of renin, aldosterone, vasopressin and ACTH during the 30 min of cuff inflation. The unloading of cardiopulmonary and arterial baroreceptors have been shown to contribute to the hormone secretion (Kozlowski et a. 1975; Thames et al. 1981; Morita et al. 1986; Lee et al. 1986).

In order to test the effects of reflex induced sympathetic stimulation of renin secretion, the cuff inflation treatment was repeated in the presence of a maximally effective dose of propranolol (500 micro g/Kg d, 1-propranolol i.v. followed by 7.0 micro g/Kg/min). Using a 2×2 multifactorial design, the results in Fig. 3 show a main effect of propranolol to reduce plasma renin – and thus aldosterone – levels in response to cuff inflation, whereas it was without effect on vasopressin and ACTH. Infusion of ANP alone at 5 ng/Kg/min had no significant effects on renin, vasopressin ACTH levels. The effect of combining propranolol and ANP infusion were no greater than the effect of propranolol alone, and thus, there was no interaction between the two factors.

However, of particular interest in these experiments was the ability of the ANF treatment to reduce plasma aldosterone independent of any reduction in PRA. A number of laboratories have reported that ANF inhibits angiotensin II stimulated aldosterone secretion from the adrenal cortex (Aguilera, 1987). The present demonstration that an elevation of plasma ANP of only 36 pg/ml can have this effect on aldosterone in conscious dogs shows the potential physiological significance of the effect. A reduction in plasma aldosterone should lead to increased sodium excretion. As many laboratories, including our own, have measured sodium excretion during ANP administration for only comparatively short periods (up to 60 min), and as renal responses to reductions in plasma aldosterone may take 1–2 hours to become apparent, natriuretic potency of ANP in whole animal studies may have been underestimated.

The results of experiments with infusion of 20 ng ANP/Kg/min are shown in Fig. 4. This infusion rate produces plasma concentrations of 190 pg/ml, at the high end of the physiological range in conscious dogs. At this dose of ANP, there was a significant inhibition of the renin response to caval constriction. However, it is important to note that there were no interactive effects of propranolol and ANP on PRA. Furthermore, the combination of propranolol blockade and ANF infusion completely blocked the renin response to caval constriction. Given the fact that both reflex and intrarenal mechanisms are involved in renin secretion in response to caval constriction, these results indicate that ANP must act on intrarenal mechanisms to inhibit renin secretion.

The other striking effect of the results of ANP infusion at 20 ng/Kg/min is the significant blunting of vasopressin and ACTH responses to caval constriction. Thus at these higher rates of ANP infusion, the baroreflex responses of these hormones to caval constriction are inhibited. Thus, taking the results shown in Fig. 1 and those with caval constriction, in conscious dogs there is good evidence that ANP attenuates baroreflex mediated hormonal responses to hypotension and hypovolemia.

Conclusions

These results are in support of the general hypothesis that ANP acts to inhibit the recognized baroreflex mediated hormonal responses to hypovolemia and hypotension. From our results, the most sensitive mechanism to ANP is angiotensin II stimulated aldosterone secretion. At higher plasma levels of the peptide, effects of direct ANP inhibition of renin secretion become evident, even in the presence of increased renal sympathetic nerve activity. Blunting of baroreflex initiated vasopressin and ACTH secretion is also significant.

In intact animals, the plasma levels of ANP simulated by infusion, which show inhibition of baroreflex-stimulated hormone secretion, can be achieved with small increases in atrial pressures and thus atrial stretch. Thus in situations where where there are excessive hormonal and cardiovascular responses to hypovolemia, ANP can be viewed as a physiological control, or 'off-signal' to prevent overexpansion of body fluids. The importance of this 'protective' function of ANP in such conditions as congestive cardiac failure needs assessment.

References

Aguilera G (1987) Differential effects of atrial natriuretic factor on angiotensin II and ACTH-stimulated aldosterone secretion. Endocrinol 120:229–304

Bie P, Wang BC, Leadley RJ, Goetz KL (1988) Hemodynamic and renal effects of low-dose infusion of atrial peptide in awake dogs. Am J Physiol 254:R161–R169

Burnett JC Jr, Granger JP, Opgenorth TJ (1984) Effects of synthetic atrial natriuretic factor on renal function and renin release. Am J Physiol 247:F863–F866

Freeman RH, Davis JO, Vari RC (1985) Renal response to atrial natriuretic factor in conscious dogs with caval constriction. Am J Physiol 248:R495–R500

Greenwald JE, Sakata M, Michener ML, Sides SD, Needleman P (1988) Is atriopeptin a physiological or pathophysiological substance. J Clin Invest 81:1036–1041

Itoh H, Nakao K, Yamada I, Shirakami G, Kangawa K, Minamino N, Matsuo H, Imura H (1988) Andipsogenic action of a navel peptide, brain natriuretic peptide, in rats. Eur J Pharmacol 150:193–196

Kozlowski S, Szczepanska-Sadowska E (1975) Mechanisms o hypovolemic thirst and interaction between hypovolemia, hyperosmolality and the antidiuretic system. In: Peters G, Fitzsimons JT, Peters-Haefeli L (eds) Control mechanisms of drinking. Springer, New York, pp 25–35

Laragh JH (1985) Atrial natriuretic hormone, the renin-aldosterone axis and blood pressure-electrolyte homeostasis. N England J Med 313:1330–1337

Ledsome JR, Wilson N, Courneya CA, Rankin AJ (1985) Release of atrial natriuretic peptide by atrial distension. Can J Physiol Pharmacol 63:739–744

Lee ME, Thrasher TN, Ramsay DJ (1984) Elevated cardiac pressure inhibits renin release after arterial hypotension in conscious dogs. Am J Physiol 247:R953–R959

Lee ME, Thrasher TN, Ramsay DJ (1985) Mechanisms of inhibition of renin secretion by increased left atrial pressure. Am J Physiol 248:R641-R644

Lee ME, Thrasher TN, Keil LC, Ramsay DJ (1986) Cardiac receptors, vasopressin and corticosteroid release during arterial hypotension in dogs. Am J Physiol 251:R614–R620

Metzler CH, Gardner DG, Keil LC, et al. (1987) Increased synthesis and release of atrial peptide during mineralocorticoid escape in conscious dogs. Am J Physiol 252:R188–192

Metzler CH, Lee ME, Thrasher TN, Ramsay DJ (1986) Increased right or left atrial pressure stimulates release of atrial natriuretic peptide in conscious dogs. Endocrinology 119: 2396–2400

Metzler CH, Keil LC, Ramsay DJ (1987) Atrial peptide infusion does not inhibit the water intake or vasopressin responses to hypertonic saline infusion in conscious dogs. Fed Proc 46:1075

Metzler CH, Thrasher TN, Ramsay DJ (1987) Role of atrial peptides in the physiological regulation of endocrine systems in conscious dogs. In: Brenner BM, Laragh JH (eds) Biologically action peptides. Plenum Press, New York, pp 311–315

Morita H, Manders WT, Skelton MM et al. (1986) Vagal regulation of arginine vasopressin in conscious dogs. Am J Physiol 251:H19–H23

Raine AEG, Erne P, Burgisser E, Mullen FB, Bolli P, Burkart F, Buhler FR (1986) Atrial natriuretic peptide and atrial pressure in patients with congestive heart failure. N Engl J Med 315:533–537

Samson WK (1987) Atrial natriuretic factor and the central nervous system. Clin Endocrinol Metab 16:145-159

Scheuer DA, Thrasher TN, Quillen EW, Ramsay DJ (1987) Atrial peptide blocks renin release during renal hypotension in conscious dogs. Am J Physiol 252:R423–R428

Scheuer DA, Thrasher TN, Keil LC, Ramsay DJ (1989) Mechanism of inhibition of renin response to hypotension by atrial natriuretic factor. Am J Physiol 257:R194–R203

Thames MD, Schmid PG (1981) Interaction between carotid and cardiopulmonary baroreflex in the control of plasma ADH. Am J Physiol 241:H434–440

Thrasher TN, Keil LC, Ramsay DJ (1982) Hemodynamic, hormonal and drinking responses to reduced venous return in the dog. Am J Physiol 243:R354–362

Winaver J, Hoffman A, Burnett JC, Haramati A (1986) Hormonal determinants of sodium excretion in rats with experimental high output heart failure. Am J Physiol 254:R776–R784

Natriuretic Hormones: Endogenous Na-K-ATPase Inhibitor(s) and Atrial Natriuretic Peptide

H. J. Kramer, H. Meyer-Lehnert, and H.-G. Predel

Medizinische Poliklinik, University of Bonn, FRG

Summary. After the original demonstration of endogenous sodium pump inhibitor(s) in the plasma of acutely fluid volume expanded animals and man, numerous studies have confirmed the presence of ouabain-like factors (OLF) in plasma, urine, cerebrospinal fluid and various tissues. Some of these factors represent well-known endogenous compounds which in vitro reveal inhibition of Na-K-ATPase, displacement of ^{3}H-ouabain and cross-reaction with a digoxin antibody. Small M.W. sodium pump inhibitors (OLF), which may be of hypothalamic origin, were also detected in various animal models of hypertension and in hypertensive patients and may play a role especially in the pathophysiology of volume-dependent hypertension. Our results show that OLF increases basal and vaso-pressin-stimulated intracellular Ca^{++} release in rat vascular smooth muscle cells in culture and in human platelets similar to the newly discovered endothelin. In plasma and urine natriuretic activities were demonstrated by bioassay whose activity may vary with changes in body sodium balance. We found that they are associated with small peptide(s) with a M.W. of approximately 680 Da. It is, however, not yet clear whether the two biological properties, namely sodium transport inhibition and natriuretic activity, reside in one single compound. A number of circulating Na-K-ATPase inhibitors is certainly not identical with a humoral natriuretic factor. Nevertheless, there is increasing evidence for multiple interactions between OLF and the atrial natriuretic peptide (ANP). Interestingly, recent observations in conscious animals point to a crucial role of a natriuretic factor of non-cardiac origin in the natriuresis of ECFV expansion whose release is also dependent on atrial stretch. These findings represent a new challenge to identify the putative endogenous natriuretic hormone and OLF, respectively, which may act in concert with ANP as regulators of body fluid volume and arterial pressure.

Key-words: Natriuretic Hormone – Endogenous Na-K-ATPase Inhibitor – Atrial Natriuretic Peptide

Introduction

The idea of a Natriuretic Hormone dates back indirectly to Homer Smith in 1956 [36] and first experimental evidence for a blood-borne natriuretic factor was provided by the classical cross-circulation experiment by de Wardener et al. [44]. Since then a number of investigators including ourselves continued to characterize, to isolate and to identify such a natriuretic factor. In 1969, we first characterized the natriuretic factor as an endogenous inhibitor of the Na-K-ATPase enzyme present in a small molecular weight plasma fraction which was also natriuretic when tested in a bioassay [25]. Ten years later this observation was confirmed and extended by Gruber et al. [13] when they found that this factor which emerged during acute extracellular fluid volume (ECFV) expansion cross-reacted with a digoxin antibody. Within this same time period Haddy et al. [14] presented evidence that volume-dependent hypertension is associated with an inhibition of active vascular smooth muscle cell sodium transport and that the plasma of volume-dependent hypertensive animals contains an inhibitor of active cellular sodium transport. Based on these observations de Wardener and MacGregor [43] have put forward the hypothesis that an endogenous Na-K-ATPase inhibitor participates in the pathogenesis of arterial hypertension. However, during the subsequent search by many investigators for a potential role of an endogenous digitalis-like substance (DLS) in body fluid volume regulation and in hypertensive as well as in other states of disturbed sodium balance, the use of such different terms as digitalis (DLS)- or ouabain-like substance (OLS), sodium transport inhibitor (STI) and Natriuretic Hormone as synonyma as well as the use of assay methods such as the digoxin radioimmunoassay to measure digoxin-like immunoreacting activity (DLIA) have rather contributed to more confusion than to result in a final chemical identification of this substance(s). Although many authors assume that the endogenous Na-K-ATPase inhibitor is also natriuretic, there is no definite answer yet whether these two biological properties, namely inhibition of active sodium transport and natriuretic activity, are shared by one single compound. It rater appears that there is a number of different endogenous Na-K-ATPase inhibitors present in the circulation which may not be identical with a humoral natriuretic substance.

In contrast, the discovery of Atrial Natriuretic Peptide(s) (ANP) by de Bold et al. [3] has led to the identification of a potent natriuretic and vasorelaxant system which has no effect on the Na-K-ATPase enzyme. Its physiological and pathophysiological roles, however, are still questionable. The following short review will summarize and compare the presently available information on these two endogenous natriuretic and vasoactive systems, namely their site of origin, chemical properties, biological effects, mechanisms of action, physiological and pathophysiological implications and their potential interaction with each other.

Site of Origin

With regard to their *site of origin* it is well-known that circulating ANP is released mainly from the cardiac atria (Lit. see Ref. [21]). In contrast, the Natriuretic Hormone is secreted presumably from the hypothalamic area. There are ample in vitro- and in vivo-data to support this assumption [15, 17, 31, 37]. The stimuli for the release of the Natriuretic Hormone are an increase in cerebrospinal fluid sodium concentration and/or a rise in plasma (and interstitial) fluid volume. We originally hypothesized that the Natriuretic Hormone is released from the hypothalamus via a signal from low pressure receptors located in the heart atria [24]. Later in this review we will come back to the potential interaction between these atrial receptors and the hypothalamic release of a Natriuretic Hormone.

Biological Actions

With regard to their hemodynamic and renal actions, ANP acts on the systemic vasculature as a vasorelaxant agent [21], whereas the Natriuretic Hormone has been shown to possess sodium transport inhibitory (STI) activity and will thereby indirectly result in enhanced vascular sensitivity to endogenous vasoconstrictors [20]. Its role as a contributing factor to the development of systemic arterial hypertension has been demonstrated experimentally in a number of animal models of hypertension by Haddy et al. [14]. Both hormones, ANP and the Natriuretic Hormone, however, have on property in common, namely their potent natriuretic activities [21, 27] (Fig. 1).

Physico-Chemical Properties

With respect to the *physico-chemical properties* of the Natriuretic Hormone we [20] and others [31, 42] have suggested that this hormone is a peptide with a molecular weight (M.W.) of approximately 500 Da. This was based on the passage of membrane filters with defined M.W. cut-off points and on the finding of an inactivation of its natriuretic activity by proteolytic enzymes [27]. We also found that the Na-K-ATPase inhibitor in the plasma of volume-expanded animals is inactivated by chymotrypsin suggesting that this activity also relates to a peptidic compound [19]. A series of different compounds were recently identified as endogenous sodium transport inhibitors in the plasma and urine of animals and men. Thus, Cloix et al. [5] have described a steroid with a M.W. of 432 Da as an endogenous inhibitor of Na-K-ATPase. Recently, Masugi et al. [29] have identified a very unstable peroxide-like substance which inhibits the Na-K-ATPase enzyme in vitro and has a M.W. of approximately 600 Da. Tamura et al. [38] first published the in vitro-inhibitory effects of non-esterified fatty acids on the Na-K-ATPase enzyme whose concentration rises with acute volume expansion. In uremic patients Dasgupta et al. [8] observed recently the presence of a digoxin-like immunoreacting substance with a M.W. of 532 Da, but the authors have not identified the chemical structure of this compound. Finally, Goto et al. have isolated from the urine of human subjects [12] as well as from the plasma of dogs [11] a ouabain-displacing peptide with a M.W. of 343 Da. Thus, there is a number of endogenous Na-K-ATPase inhibitors whose relation to the Natriuretic Hormone is unknown since the identification of most of these compounds is based solely on in vitro-assays demonstrating an inhibition of the Na-K-ATPase enzyme. Therefore, interpretation must carefully consider the type of assay used to demonstrate such endogenous compounds. Nevertheless, we have shown that one of the properties of the natriuretic material is that it binds to a digoxin antibody [18] and that the Na-K-ATPase inhibitor apparently also reacts with this antibody [23].

The material which we isolated from the urine of salt-loaded human subjects through gelfiltration, subsequent immunoprecipitation with the digoxin antibody and thereafter purified by repetitive reverse-phase high performance liquid chromatography (HPLC) is an at least as potent natriuretic factor as is the ANP (Fig. 1). One major difference relates to its longer duration of action which extents to about three hours [27], whereas the natriuresis after bolus injection of ANP lasts only a few minutes [21].

Our preliminary data suggest that this material which was isolated from the urine by gel filtration, immunoprecipitation and reverse-phase HPLC is a small weak acidic peptide with a M.W. of approximately 680 Da and an isoelectric point at a pH of approximately 5. Amino acid analysis of the purified fraction(s) (kindly performed by Dr. Liddiard, Darmstadt, and Prof. Dr. Fahrenholz, Frankfurt) revealed the amino acid compositions listed in Table 1 [27].

The urine fraction which is natriuretic also inhibits the Na-K-ATPase enzyme in vitro in a manner similar to ouabain with a 50% enzyme inhibition obtained with an amount equivalent to a 0.8 minute urine collection period. This same fraction also displaces ^{3}H-ouabain from its binding sites, i.e. the Na-K-ATPase enzyme, in an identical manner as ouabain [23].

Mechanisms of Action

Regarding the *mechanisms of action* there are major differences at the *renal tubular*

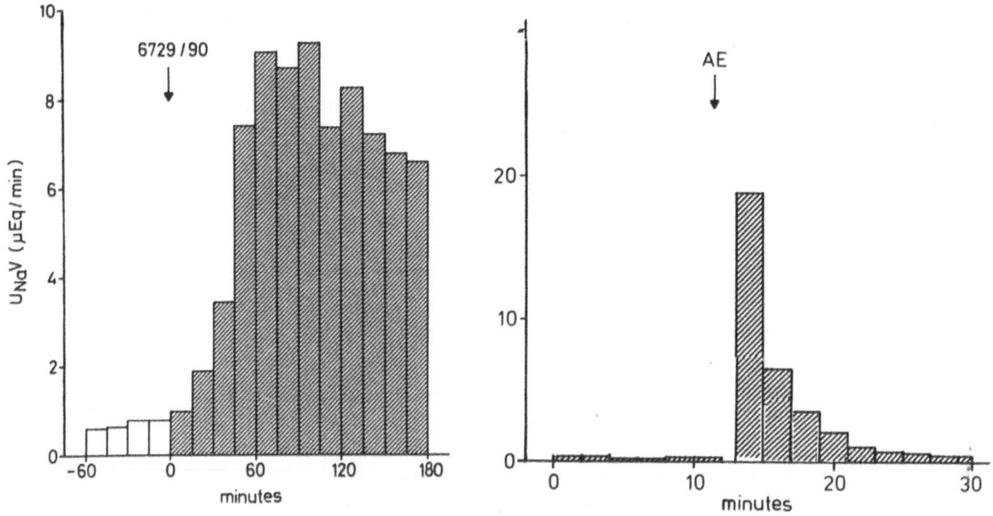

Fig. 1. Onset and time course of natriuresis after bolus i.v. injection of purified natriuretic material from the urine of salt loaded healthy subjects (6729/90) and of atrial extract (AE) from one rat heart. Bioassays were performed in conscious rats

Table 1. Natriuretic hormone. Preliminary amino acid composition of the small M.W. substance(s) associated with the natriuretic activity isolated from the urine by gel chromatography and reversed-phase HPLC (A) and including an immunoprecipitation step using a digoxin antibody (B)

	A		B	
	rel. values (nmol)	molar ratio	rel. values (nmol)	molar ratio
Asp	2.2	1	0.5	1
Glu	2.5	1	0.8	2
Gly	4.8	2	1.0	2
Ser	4.6	2	0.4	1
(Phe)	(4.8)	(2)	–	–
estimated	M.W.	~640 Da (970 Da)		~680 Da

level between ANP and the Natriuretic Hormone. Whereas the former stimulates intracellular cGMP synthesis [21] but may also act at distal tubular sites by inhibiting the amiloride-sensitive sodium channel [4], the latter presumably inhibits active distal tubular sodium reabsorption in the cortical and/or medullary collecting duct, a tubular site which is most sensitive to ouabain [9], by depressing the activity of the Na-K-ATPase enzyme through binding to its E2-P configuration [15]. At the *vascular level* the vasorelaxant effect of ANP results from suppression of intracellular Ca^{++} release by its stimulation of cGMP synthesis [30], but an activation of the Na/K/Cl-cotransport has also been demonstrated in the presence of ANP [33]. On the contrary, the Natriuretic Hormone is presumed to cause an increase in vascular sensitivity to endogenous vasoconstrictors by inhibiting active sodium transport and thereby to raise intracellular Ca^{++} [20] Inhibition of 5-hydroxytryptamine reuptake was also observed in the presence of the Na-K-ATPase inhibitor [5]. We have recently shown that the ouabain-like inhibitor which we have isolated from the urine of salt-loaded healthy subjects increases basal intracellular Ca^{++}-concentration and also potentiates vasopressin-induced intracellular Ca^{++} release in vitro in cultured vascular smooth muscle cells [41]. Thus, there are quite opposite effects of ANP and the Natriuretic Hormone on free intracellular Ca^{++} as the ultimate step for contraction-relaxation of the vascular smooth muscle cell.

Pathophysiological Roles

Altered plasma concentrations of ANP and of Natriuretic Hormone were found in a variety of pathophysiological states [20, 21]. Increased levels of Natriuretic Hormone, STI, or DLIA were observed in experimental and clinical hypertension [14, 20, 22], in pregnancy [39], in newborns [40], and in chronic renal failure [28]. We found low Natriuretic Hormone activities in patients with congestive heart failure, decompensated liver cirhosis, and in non-uremic patients with the nephrotic syndrome [20]. However, the interpretation of some of these findings must be cautious especially when these data represent DLIA measured in crude plasma extracts with a radioimmunoassay for digoxin. This appears to be an insensitive method to detect specific natriuretic factors or endogenous Na-K-ATPase inhibitors [26, 28].

Interactions of Natriuretic Hormone and ANP

Preliminary observations suggest home potential interactions between the Natriuretic Hormone and ANP. Thus, it has been shown by Crabos et al. [7] that ANP inhibits in vitro the release of the sodium transport inhibitor from cultured brain tissue. ANP was also shown to raise plasma DLIA in vivo [35]. Hue et al. [16] suggested that ouabain and a ouabainlike factor may stimulate calcium-dependent ANP release from isolated rat atria and Bloch et al. [2] demonstrated that ouabain induces the secretion of proatrial natriuretic peptide by rat atrial cardiocytes. Finally, it has been suggested that ANP release during acute ECFV expansion is related to basal activity of the sodium transport inhibitor [32].

Conclusion

To conclude with the introductory remark that, whereas there is relatively firm data for a physiological and pathophysiological role of the yet putative Natriuretic Hormone, a role for the previously identified ANP in the physiological regulation of ECFV and blood pressure is much less settled and becomes even doubtful in the presence of recent observations [1, 10]. Thus, Sakata et al. [34] have recently shown that only in the anesthetized rat saline-induced natriuresis and diuresis depend on ANP secretion whereas in the conscious rat the natriuresis and diuresis induced by acute ECFV expansion appears "to depend on an intact right atrium and might reflect a peripheral release of a putative noncardiac diuretic substance". This seems to be true also for ECFV regulation in the conscious dog. From their experimental data Cowley et al. [6] conclude "that atrial natriuretic peptide does not normally mediate the diuretic and natriuretic response to acute physiological levels of volume expansion". In conscious dogs "either another yet unidentified substance is normally released from cardiac atria or another substance is released via the central nervous system with atrial stretch". This then is compatible with our original hypothesis regarding the release of a Natriuretic Hormone, namely that acute ECFV expansion provokes a signal from the atria to the central nervous system, an area presumably located in the AV3V-region, to release the Natriuretic Hormone. These recent findings thus represent a new challenge to finally identify chemically the Natriuretic Hormone and Na-K-ATPase inhibitor which presumably play an important role in ECFV and blood pressure regulation perhaps in concert with the short-lasting natriuretic and vasorelaxant activities of ANP whose physiological significance, however, is not yet cleary defined [1].

Acknowledgments: Part of our studies cited in this review were supported by grants from the Deutsche Forschungsgemeinschaft and from the Ministerium für Wissenschaft und Forschung des Landes Nordrhein-Westfalen, FRG (FA-2914, FA-8871, IVA6-402-046-87).

References

1. Blaine EH (1988) Role of atriopeptin in blood pressure regulation. Am J Med Sci 295:293–298
2. Bloch KD, Zamir N, Lichtstein D, Seidman CE, Seidman JG (1988) Ouabain induces secretion of proatrial natriuretic factor by rat atrial cardiocytes. Am J Physiol 255: E383–E387
3. De Bold AJ, Borenstein HB, Veress AT, Sonnenberg H (1981) A rapid and potent natriuretic response to intravenous injection of atrial myocardial extract in rats. Life Sci 28:89–94
4. Cantiello HF, Ausiello DA (1986) Atrial natriuretic factor and cGMP inhibit amiloride-sensitive Na^+ transport in the cultured renal epithelial cell line, LLC-PK_1. Biochem Biophys Res Commun 134:852–860
5. Cloix JF, Crabos M, Wainer IW, Ruegg U, Seiler M, Meyer P (1985) High yield-purification of a urinary Na pump inhibitor. Biochem Biophys Res Commun 131:1234–1240
6. Cowley AW jr, Anderas PR, Skelton MM (1988) Acute saline loading in normal and bilaterally atrial-resected conscious dogs. Am J Physiol 255:H144–H152
7. Crabos M, Ausiello DA, Haupert GT jr, Cantiello HF (1988) Atrial natriuretic peptide regulates release of Na^+-K^+-ATPase inhibitor from rat brain. Am J Physiol 254: F912–F917
8. Dasgupta A, Yeo KT, Malik S, Sandu P, Ahmad S, Kenny M (1987) Two novel endogenous digoxin-like immunoreactive substances isolated from human plasma ultrafiltrate. Biochem Biophys Res Commun 148: 623–628
9. Doucet A, Barlet C (1986) Evidence for differences in the sensitivity to ouabain of NaK-ATPase along the nephrons of rabbit kidney. J Biol Chem 261:993–995
10. Goetz KL, Wang BC, Geer PG, Leadley RJ jr, Reinhardt HW (1986) Atrial stretch increases sodium excretion independently of release of atrial peptides. Am J Physiol 250:R946–R950
11. Goto A, Yamada K, Ishii M, Yoshioka M, Ishiguro T, Eguchi C, Sugimoto T (1988) Presence of digitalis-like factor in mamma-

lian plasma. Biochem Biophys Res Commun 152:322–327
12. Goto A, Yamada K, Ishii M, Yoshioka M, Ishiguro T, Sugimoto T (1988) The effects of urinary digitalislike factor on cultured vascular smooth muscle cells. Hypertension 11:645–650
13. Gruber KA, Whitaker JM, Buchalew VM jr (1980) Endogenous digitalis-like substance in plasma of volume-expanded dogs. Nature 287:743–745
14. Haddy FJ, Pamnani MB, Clough DL (1980) Volume overload hypertension: a defect in the sodium-potassium pump? Cardiovasc Rev Rep 1:376–385
15. Haupert GT jr, Sancho JM (1979) Sodium transport inhibitor from bovine hypothalamus. Proc Natl Acad Sci USA 76:4658–4660
16. Hu JO, Mondorf RW, Lang RE (1988) Inhibition of cardiac Na/K ATPase stimulates atrial natriuretic peptide (ANP) release. 12th Scient Meet Int Soc Hypertension, Abstract No 1234
17. Jandhyala BS, Lokhandwala MF, Kivlighn SD, Ansari AF, De Feo ML (1987) Intracisternal administration of pergolide, a dopamine receptor agonist, triggers the release of an inhibitor of ouabain-sensitive sodium, potassium-dependent adenosine triphosphatase and enhances vascular reactivity in anaesthetized dogs. Clin Sci 73:183–188
18. Klingmüller D, Weiler E, Kramer HJ (1982) Digoxin-like natriuretic activity in the urine of salt-loaded healthy subjects. Klin Wochenschr 60:1249–1253
19. Kramer HJ (1976) Natriuretic activity in plasma following extracellular volume expansion. In: Kaufmann W, Krause HD (eds) Central nervous system control of Na^+ balance – relations to the renin-angiotensin system. Thieme, Stuttgart, pp 126–133
20. Kramer HJ (1981) Natriuretic Hormone – a circulating inhibitor of sodium- and potassium-activated adenosine triphosphatase. Its potential role in body fluid and blood pressure regulation. Klin Wochenschr 59: 1225–1230
21. Kramer HJ (1988) Atrial natriuretic hormones. Minireview. Gen Pharmacol 19: 747–753
22. Kramer HJ, Bäcker A, Krück F (1977) Antinatriferic activity in human plasma following acute and chronic salt loading. Kidney Int 12:214–222
23. Kramer HJ, Bäcker A, Weiler E, Liddiard C (1986) Studies on ouabain-like endogenous natriuretic factors in human urine. Inhibition of Na-K-ATPase and ^{3}H-ouabain binding. Klin Wochenschr 64:760–766
24. Kramer HJ, Gonick HC, Krück F (1972) Natriuretisches Hormon. Klin Wochenschr 50:893–897
25. Kramer HJ, Gonick HC, Paul W, Lu E (1969) Third factor: inhibitor of Na-K-ATPase? 4th Int Congr Nephrology, Abstracts I (Free communications), p 373
26. Kramer HJ, Heppe M, Pennig J, Kipnowski J, Klingmüller D, Düsing R, Krück F (1985) Relation of endogenous digoxin-like immunoreacting activities to salt balance and renal function in man. Klin Wochenschr 63 [Suppl III]:107–110
27. Kramer HJ, Heppe M, Weiler E, Bäcker A, Liddiard C, Klingmüller D (1985) Further characterization of the endogenous natriuretic and digoxin-like immunoreacting activities in human urine: effects of changes in sodium intake. Renal Physiol 8:80–89
28. Kramer HJ, Pennig J, Klingmüller D, Kipnowski J, Glänzer K, Düsing R (1985) Digoxin-like immunoreacting substance(s) in the serum of patients with chronic uremia. Nephron 40:297–302
29. Masugi F, Ogihara T, Sakaguchi K, Tomii A, Hasegawa T, Chen Y, Azuma M, Kumahara Y (1988) Partial purification and property of plasma ouabain-like inhibitor of Na-K-ATPase in patients with essential hypertension. 12th Scient Meet Int Soc Hypertension. Abstract No 0457
30. Meyer-Lehnert H, Tsai P, Schrier RW (1987) Atrial natriuretic factor (ANF) inhibits arginine vasopressin-stimulated Ca^{++} fluxes and cell contraction in vascular smooth muscle cells. Klin Wochenschr 65 [suppl VIII]: 115–121
31. Mir MA, Morgan K, Chappell S, Lewis M, Spurlock G, Collins, P, Scanlon M (1988) Calcium retention and increased vascular reactivity caused by a hypothalamic sodium transport inhibitor. Clin Sci 75:197–202
32. Morris MJ, Pernollet MG, Meyer P, Devynck MA (1988) Is there a relationship between the stimulation of atrial natriuretic factor by acute volume expansion and the plasma digitalis-like activity? 12th Scient Meet Int Soc Hypertension, Abstract No 1109
33. O'Donnell ME, Bush EN, Holleman W, Owen NE (1987) Biologically active atrial natriuretic peptides selectively activate Na/K/Cl cotransport in vascular smooth muscle cells. J Pharmacol Exp Therap 243:822–828
34. Sakata M, Greenwald JE, Needleman P (1988) Paradoxical relationship between atriopeptin plasma levels and diuresis-natriuresis induced by acute volume expansion. Proc Natl Acad Sci USA 85:3155–3159
35. Shilo L, Pomeranz A, Rathaus M, Weiss W,

Bernheim J, Shenkman L (1988) Atrial natriuretic peptide administration to normal and salt depleted rats – effects on digoxin-like immunoreactive factor, aldosterone, ACTH, and renal function. Life Sci 42: 1855–1859
36. Smith HW (1957) Salt and water volume receptors: an exercise in physiologic apologetics. Am J Med 23:623–652
37. Takahashi H, Matsuzawa M, Okabayashi H, Suga K, Ikegaki I, Yoshimura M, Ijichi H (1986) Evidence for a digitalis-like substance in the hypothalamo-pituitary axis in rats. J Hypertension 4 [Suppl 6]:S317–S320
38. Tamura M, Kuwano H, Kinoshita T, Inagami T (1985) Identification of linoleic and oleic acids as endogenous NaK-ATPase inhibitors from acute volume-expanded hog plasma. J Biol Chem 260:9672–9677
39. Valdes R jr (1985) Endogenous digoxin-like immunoreactive factors: impact on digoxin measurements and potential physiological implications (Review). Clin Chem 31:1525–1532
40. Valdes R, Graves SW, Brown BA, Landt M (1983) Endogenous substance in newborn infants causing false-positive digoxin measurements. J Pediat 102:947–950
41. Wanning C, Meyer-Lehnert H, Kramer HJ (1989) Endogenous inhibitor of Na-K-ATPase increases intracellular free calcium (Ca^{2+} in human platelets and rat vascular smooth muscle cells. Kidney Int 35:337
42. De Wardener HE, Clarkson EM (1985) Concept of natriuretic hormone. Physiol Rev 65:658–759
43. De Wardener HE, MacGregor GA (1980) Dahl's hypothesis that a saluretic substance may be responsible for a sustained rise in arterial pressure: its possible role in essential hypertension. Kidney Int 18:1–9
44. De Wardener HE, Mills IH, Clapham WF, Hayter CJ (1961) Studies on the efferent mechanism of the sodium diuresis which follows the administration of intravenous saline in the dog. Clin Sci 21:249–258

Atrial Natriuretic Peptide: Pathophysiological and Clinical Relevance

Atrial Natriuretic Peptide in Heart Failure*

A. J. G. Riegger,

Medizinische Universitätsklinik Würzburg, FRG

Summary. The secretion of atrial natriuretic peptide (ANP) in heart failure is increased. Its potential beneficial effects in heart failure are due to a reduction of volume and load of the heart through its vasodilatory, diuretic and natriuretic properties. In patients with severe congestive heart failure pharmacologic doses of intravenous infusions of ANP improve ventricular function by reducing pre- and afterload. In patients with heart failure ANP suppresses the secretion of aldosterone and to a small extend of cortisol leaving plasma levels of renin, norepinephrine, prostacyclin and prostaglandin E_2 unchanged. The diuretic and natriuretic effects of ANP in heart failure are however considerably attenuated. Similar results have been obtained in animal models of heart failure studying hemodynamic, neurohumoral and renal changes over a whole dose response curve using unfusion rates which increase plasma levels of ANP within the pathophysiologic and pharmacologic range.

There is evidence from animal studies in experimental models of heart failure, that ANP may be important in the pathogenesis of cardiac failure in the early phase of the disease where ANP may suppress the activity of the renin-angiotensin-aldosterone system. In later phases of heart failure these effects of ANP are overridden most likely by more severe circulatory impairment which causes an increase of vasoconstrictory mechanisms like the renin-angiotensin-aldosterone system and vasopressin. In contrast to the early phase of heart failure where peripheral vascular resistance, renal blood flow and renal vascular resistance are not increased, the activation of vasoconstrictor mechanisms increase peripheral vascular resistance and renal vascular resistance and decreases renal blood flow. The attenuation of the renal effects of ANP in heart failure are possibly due to the different hemodynamic conditions especially within the kidneys, to a reduction of specific binding sites for ANP or possibly due to a rapid degradation of ANP within the kidneys. Counter-regulating neurohumoral systems may also be important like the renin-angiotensin-system, sympathetic nerve activity and vasopressin.

Key words: Atrial natriuretic peptide – Heart failure – Hemodynamic, hormonal and renal changes

Introduction

The importance of atrial natriuretic peptide (ANP) in heart failure is due to its potential to unload the heart by reducing plasma volume, by its vasodilatory properties to reduce afterload and preload and by its inhibitory effects on vasoconstrictor and volume retaining factors like the renin-angiotensin-aldosterone system, the sympathetic nerve activity and possibly vasopressin. These effects are summarized in Fig. 1 which shows schematically the regulation and actions of ANP.

Our group (Riegger et al. 1985) and Tikkanen et al. (1985) showed that plasma levels of ANP are increased in patients with heart failure according to the severity of the disease.

* Supported by the "Deutsche Forschungsgemeinschaft"

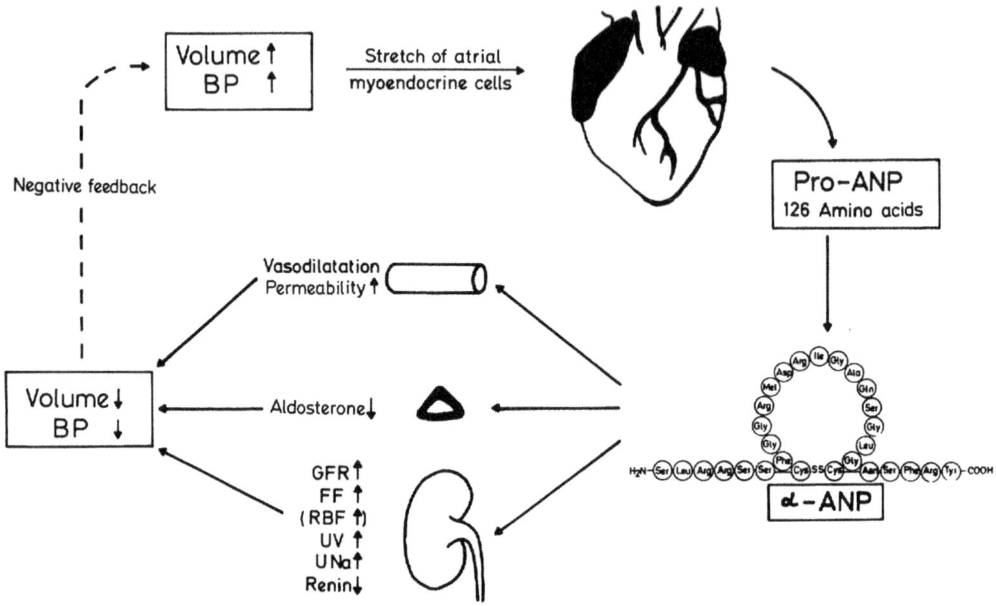

Fig. 1. ANP effects

ANP-Secretion in Heart Failure

The adequate stimulus for the secretion of ANP from the myoendocrine cells of the atria is stretch (Dietz 1984). This assumption is supported by numerous findings in patients with congestive heart failure (Dietz et al. 1986; Raine et al. 1986; Richards et al. 1986) where a linear relationship was found between right and/or left atrium pressures and plasma levels of ANP. In patients with severe heart failure however Jessup et al. (1987) were unable to demonstrate a significant correlation between right atrial pressure, pulmonary capillary pressures and the measured plasma levels of ANP.

We found in an experimental model of congestive heart failure (Riegger et al. 1987a) due to rapid right ventricular pacing, that plasma levels of ANP parallel the increase of right atrial pressure during the first week of right ventricular pacing, after 7 days however, a decrease of ANP of about 20% in plasma was observed, despite a further increase of atrial pressures. Similar results have been demonstrated in the same experimental setting by stimulating the dogs for 5 weeks in the relation of ANP plasma levels and the echocardiographically measured dimensions of the left atrium (Moe et al. 1987). These authors showed a highly significant linear correlation between the dimension of the left atrium and the secretion of ANP during the development of heart failure in the first week. This correlation however could not be demonstrated later on when even a reduction of ANP levels was found despite of a further increase of the size of the atria. The dissociation between plasma levels of ANP and atrial pressures and/or atrial dimensions may be explained by changes of the compliance of the atria, by a reduction of storage granules of the prohormone which may lead the a deficit of atrial ANP-reserve and by the fact that ANP may be also secreted by the myocardium of the ventricles in heart failure which has been demonstrated in the genetic cardiomyopathic hamster (Edwards et al. 1987) and in rats with aortocaval fistula (Lattion et al. 1986).

ANP in the Pathogenesis of Heart Failure

We studied in an animal model of congestive heart failure due to rapid right ventricular pacing (Riegger and Liebau 1982) hemodynamic, hormonal and renal changes in the early phase of heart failure. In this experiment (Holmer et al. 1987) we induced relatively mild to moderate heart failure in conscious dogs by a pacing rate of 240 beats/min. Rapid right ventricular pacing resulted in a significant decrease of cardiac output, mean arterial blood pressure and in an increase of mean pulmonary arterial pressure and mean pulmonary capillary wedge pressure. We found no changes in peripheral vascular resistance and renal plasma flow. According to the rise in right atrial pressure we found an increase of ANP and in relation to the deterioration of cardiac function an increase of sympathetic nerve activity measured by norepinephrine plasma levels. Despite a profound fall in blood pressure and in increase in sympathetic tone we found on the fourth day a significant suppression of the renin-angiotensin-aldosterone system. The most likely explanation for this and for the lack of increase of peripheral vascular resistance and decrease of renal blood flow may be the increased secretion of ANP which may have counter-balanced vasoconstrictor effects due to increased sympathetic tone and by direct action may have suppressed renin and aldosterone secretion. In an other experiment using the same experimental setting (Riegger et al. 1988) where we induced more profound circulatory impairment by increasing the heart rate to 260 beats/min and by pacing the dogs for 10 days we found despite of an increased secretion of ANP a significant increased plasma concentration of renin and a decrease of effective renal plasma flow. From these results one may conclude that ANP may be important in mild to moderate heart failure by counter-balancing vasoconstrictor mechanisms like the renin-angiotensin system, but in more severe stages of the disease with profound hemodynamic alterations these effects of ANP are no longer able to suppress vasoconstrictor, sodium and volume retaining mechanisms.

Effects of Exogenous ANP in Heart Failure

We investigated in patients with severe congestive heart failure, the effect of pharmacologic intravenous doses of ANP on hemodynamic, hormonal and renal parameters (Riegger et al. 1986). Intravenous bolus injections of alpha ANP of 50, 100 and 200 μg resulted in a dose-related reduction of systolic and diastolic blood pressure, a decrease of peripheral vascular resistance with a concomittant increase of cardiac output. High doses of ANP also reduced mean and diastolic pulmonary arterial pressure. No significant changes were observed on heart rate and right atrial pressure. Similar hemodynamic changes were found following a continuous infusion of ANP (20 μg/min). Intravenous application of ANP in patients with heart failure led to a considerable reduction of aldosterone plasma levels as well as to a small decrease of plasma cortisol. Plasma renin concentration, ACTH, norepinephrine, 6-keto-prostaglandin F_1 alpha and prostaglandin E_2 remained unchanged. The reduced diuresis, natriuresis and renal excretion of potassium in patients with heart failure were doubled by the intravenous application of ANP. Comparing these renal effects of ANP in heart failure with the efficacy of ANP using similar doses in normal volunteers or patients with essential hypertension demonstrates a considerable (about 5 to 6 times) attenuation of its diuretic and natriuretic properties. Similar hemodynamic effects after intravenous application of ANP and an attenuation of its renal effects have been demonstrated by numerous other investigators (Cody et al. 1986; Crozier et al. 1986; Saito et al. 1987).

In order to quantify the effects of ANP more precisely we performed investigations in normal dogs and in dogs with chronic congestive heart failure by infusing ANP over a whole dose-response range using infusion rates which induced plasma levels within the pathophysiological and pharmacological range (Riegger et al. 1988). Intravenous infusions of alpha-ANP (0.01, 0.03, 0.1, 0.3 and 0.6 μg/kg/min) in normal healthy dogs resulted in a significant reduction of mean arterial blood pressure, cardiac output, stroke volume and right atrial pressure. Heart rate and peripheral vascular resistance did not change. This indicates that blood pressure and cardiac output were reduced by a reduction of stroke volume due to a reduced preload. After chronic heart failure was established ANP-infusions reduced only significantly mean arterial pressure. Cardiac output, stroke volume and the elevated right atrial pressure were not changed. Similar to healthy dogs we found no changes of peripheral vascular resistance. In healthy animals we found a dose-related increase of urine flow, sodium, magnesium and calcium excretion, the renal excretion of potassium was only significantly increased at the highest infusion rate. In heart failure however, the excretory renal effects of ANP were completely abolished.

Effective renal plasma flow and glomerular filtration rate were measured at baseline and during an intravenous infusion of ANP in a concentration of 0.03 and 0.1 μg/kg/min. In healthy dogs, intravenous infusions of ANP resulted in a dose-related increase of renal plasma flow and in an increase of glomerular filtration rate which was more pronounced in relation to the augmentation of plasma flow resulting in an increased filtration fraction. In animals with heart failure, ANP showed no effects on renal plasma flow. Glomerular filtration rate and filtration fraction increased, but the increase was less than in healthy dogs.

The intravenous application of ANP was able to suppress plasma renin secretion significantly in healthy dogs; in dogs with chronic congestive heart failure, having a significantly elevated basal plasma renin secretion, ANP showed no effects on plasma levels of renin.

In conclusion, the data suggest that ANP may be important in the early phase of the pathogenesis of heart failure by counterbalancing vasoconstrictor systems like the renin-angiotensin-aldosterone system. In more severe hart failure its effects are attenuated resulting in a stimulation of the renin system. The intravenous application of ANP shows beneficial effects in patients with severe heart failure concerning hemodynamic changes, but its renal effects are considerably attenuated.

New approaches are needed for a more effective treatment of patients with heart failure by ANP which can possibly be achieved by the development of analoga of ANP or by substances which decrease the degradation of ANP, thereby increasing the endogenous production of the hormone.

References

1. Cody RJ, Atlas SA, Laragh JH, Kubo SH, Covit AB, Ryman KS, Shaknovich A, Pondolfino K, Clark M, Camargo MJF, Scarborough RM (1986) Atrial natriuretic factor in normal subjects and heart failure patients: plasma levels and renal, hormonal, and hemodynamic responses to peptide infusion. J Clin Invest 78:1362–1374
2. Crozier IG, Nicholls MG, Ikram H, Espiner EA, Gomez HJ, Warner NJ (1986) Haemodynamic effects of atrial peptide infusion in heart failure. Lancet II:1242–1245
3. Dietz JR (1984) Release of natriuretic factor from heart-lung preparation by atrial distension. Am J Physiol 247:R1093–R1096
4. Dietz R, Purgaj J, Lang RE, Schömig A (1986) Pressure dependent release of atrial natriuretic peptide (ANP) in patients with chronic cardiac disease: does it reset? Klin Wochenschr 64 (Suppl IV):42–46
5. Edwards BS, Ackermann DM, Wold LE, Burnett JC (1987) Presence of ventricular immunoreactive "atrial" natriuretic factor in heart failure. Kidney Int 31:268 (abstr.)
6. Holmer SR, Riegger AJG, Notheis WF, Kromer EP, Kochsiek K (1987) Hemodynamic changes and renal plasma in early heart failure: Implications for renin, aldosterone, norepinephrine, atrial natriuretic peptide and prostacyclin. Basic Res Cardiol 82:101–108
7. Jessup M, Scortichini D, Mintz G, Gutkowska J, Cantin M, LeJemtel T (1987) Cardiac filling pressures and atrial natriuretic factor in patients with chronic heart failure. Heart Failure 2:274–279
8. Lattion AL, Michel JB, Arnauld E, Corvol P, Soubrier F (1986) Myocardial recruitment during ANF mRNA increase with volume overload in the rat. Am J Physiol 251: H890–H896
9. Moe GW, Howard RJ, Angus C, de Bold AJ, Armstrong PW (1987) Pathophysiologic role of atrial size and pressure in the modulation of plasma natriuretic factor during evolving experimental heart failure. Circulation 76 [Suppl. IV]:IV–135 (abstr.)
10. Raine AEG, Erne P, Bürgisser E, Müller FB, Bolli P, Burkart F, Bühler FR (1986) Atrial natriuretic peptide and atrial pressure in patients with congestive heart failure. N Engl J Med 315:533–537
11. Richards AM, Cleland JGF, Tonolo G, McIntyre GD, Leckie BJ, Dargie HJ, Ball

SG, Robertson JIS (1986) Plasma alpha natriuretic peptide in cardiac impairment. Br Med J 293:409–412

12. Riegger AJG, Liebau G (1982) The renin-angiotensin-aldosterone system, antidiuretic hormone and sympathetic nerve activity in an experimental model of congestive heart failure in the dog. Clin Sci 62:465–469
13. Riegger AJG, Kromer EP, Kochsiek K (1985) Der natriuretische Vorhoffaktor bei schwerer kongestiver Herzinsuffizienz. Plasmaspiegel, hämodynamische, hormonale und renale Effekte. Dtsch Med Wochenschr 110:1607–1610
14. Riegger AJG, Kromer EP, Kochsiek K (1986) Human atrial natriuretic peptide: plasma levels, hemodynamic, hormonal, and renal effects in patients with severe congestive heart failure. J Cardiovasc Pharmacol 8:1107–1112
15. Riegger AJG, Elsner D, Kromer EP, Daffner C, Forssmann WG, Muders F, Pascher EW, Kochsiek K (1988) Atrial natriuretic peptide in congestive heart failure in the dog: plasma levels, cyclic guanosine monophosphate, ultrastructure of atrial myoendocrine cells, and hemodynamic, hormonal, and renal effects. Circulation 77:398–406
16. Saito Y, Nakao K, Nishimura K, Sugawara A, Okumura K, Obata K, Sonoda R, Ban T, Yasue H, Imura H (1987) Clinical application of atrial natriuretic polypeptide in patients with congestive heart failure: beneficial effects on left ventricular function. Circulation 76:115–124
17. Tikkanen I, Fyhrquist R, Metsärinne K, Leidenius R (1985) Plasma atrial natriuretic peptide in cardiac disease and during infusion in healthy volunteers. Lancet II:66–69

The Atrial Natriuretic Peptide in Human Hypertension

J. Genest, P. Larochelle, J. R. Cusson, and M. Cantin

Multidisciplinary Research Group on Hypertension, Clinical Research Institute of Montreal, Canada

Summary. Measurements by radioimmunoassay of the ANP C-terminal (Ser 99-Tyr 126), N-terminal (Asn 1-Arg 98), and cyclic GMP in plasma of 77 healthy subjects and 32 patients with labile hypertension but with diastolic pressures below 90 mmHg at time of blood sampling, 74 with mild hypertension and diastolic pressures between 90–104 mmHg, 16 with moderate hypertension and diastolic pressures between 105 and 114 mmHg, and 7 with severe hypertension and diastolic pressures above 115 mmHg were found to be within normal range in all groups of patients with untreated essential hypertension. In view of the reported increases in right and left atrial pressures in patients with mild and moderate hypertension, these findings suggest a hyporesponsiveness of the atria to release ANP in essential hypertension.

Key words: Atrial natriuretic peptide – Human essential hypertension – N-terminal ANP – Cyclic GMP

The atrial natriuretic peptide (ANP) is a 28 amino acid peptide released by both atria, mainly under the stimulus of increased pressure and/or stretch. There is strong evidence linking ANP to hypertension [1]. ANP abolishes and prevents the vasoconstrictor effect of the two major pressor substances, norepinephrine and angiotensin II, both on isolated strips of aorta or renal arteries as well as in vivo. It is the most powerful natriuretic and diuretic substance known, being about 500–1000 times more potent than furosemide. It inhibits aldosterone synthesis and release, both in the basal states as well as in the stimulated state. ANP decreases renin release and blocks the effects of the renin-angiotensin system. It decreases cardiac output. Its intravenous infusion for up to 12 days to 2K–1C, 1K–1C, DOCA-salt, and to Dahl's salt-sensitive hypertensive rats and to spontaneously hypertensive rats lowers blood pressure to normal levels as first demonstrated by Garcia et al. (see review in [1]).

The purpose of this work was to study the plasma levels of immunoreactive ANP measured after extraction on Sep-Pak cartridges in patients with essential hypertension of varying severity. A first study made by Larochelle, Cusson and our group in 101 untreated patients with essential hypertension showed that they had similar mean plasma IR-ANP concentrations as that of a control group and that their individual values were within the range seen in normotensive subjects [2–4]. These findings were consistent with the results of Tsuchiya et al. [5] who demonstrated normal plasma cyclic GMP levels (a marker of ANP activity) in 68 patients with essential hypertension when compared to control subjects.

Identical results of normal plasma IR-ANP levels in similar groups of patients with essential hypertension were obtained by other workers [6–15] whereas other groups reported slightly but significantly higher mean plasma IR-ANP concentration in groups of hypertensive patients undefined as to type and severity [16–23]. Even in these latter studies, plasma IR-ANP concentrations in hypertensive patients were rarely above 50 pmol/L. Since some of the latter studies included patients with severe hypertension, incipient congestive heart failure and/or receiving antihypertensive medication or since blood sampling was sometimes taken during acute hypertensive emergencies, it was felt that the occasionally high levels were the consequence of clinical complications. In view of these conflicting findings and in order to clarify the confusion, Larochelle, Cusson et al., did a second study with two large groups of patients with essential hypertension, one treated (N = 156) and the other untreated (N = 138) [24]. In this study, the C-terminal ANP (Ser 99-Tyr 126), the N-terminal ANP

(Asn 1-Arg 98) and cyclic GMP were also measured simultaneously in the same plasma samples by radioimmunoassay. Results for C-terminal ANP are expressed in pmol/L and can be converted in picogram/mL by multiplying them by 3.06.

Subjects

Seventy-seven healthy subjects served as normotensive controls, and 32 patients with labile hypertension but with distolic pressures below 90 mmHg at the time of blood sampling, 74 with mild hypertension and diastolic pressures between 90–104 mmHg, 16 with moderate hypertension and diastolic pressures between 105–114 mmHg, and 7 with severe hypertension and diastolic pressures above 115 mmHg were studied. None of these hypertensive patients received any medication or the latter had been withdrawn for at least 3 weeks prior to blood sampling. In some instances, two measurements were obtained from the same subjects and patients at different intervals and on a few occasions one of the three parameters was not measured because of technical reasons. This explains the few discrepancies in the number of results versus the number of patients. In addition, another group of 92 patients with moderate and severe essential hypertension but receiving various antihypertensive drugs was similarly studied. At the time of blood sampling, blood pressure was controlled in 16 patients (diastolic pressure below 90 mmHg) and uncontrolled in 76, 51 of whom had diastolic pressures below 105 mmHg, 15 below 115 and 10 above 115.

All control subjects and treated and untreated hypertensive patients had normal biochemical profiles and physical examination, thus eliminating significant degrees of renal or cardiac impairment. None presented signs of secondary hypertension. Forty percent of untreated hypertensive patients and 48% of treated patients had echocardiographic evidence of left ventricular hypertrophy.

Results

The overall results of these two groups of patients in comparison to the control subjects are described in Table 1 and in Fig. 1. The distribution of individual values obtained in the control subjects and the various subgroups of patients with essential hypertension divided according to their diastolic pressures at the time of blood sampling are described in Table 2 and in Fig. 2.

Plasma C-terminal ANP (Ser 99-Tyr 128), N-terminal (Asn 1-Arg 98) and cyclic GMP are within normal range in all patients with untreated essential hypertension and there is no significant difference when the mean value of each group is compared to that of control subjects with the exception

Table 1. Second Study 1988 – Plasma ANF in essential hypertension

	Normotensive subjects (N = 77)	Essential hypertension untreated (N = 97)	Essential hypertension treated (N = 76)
Age (years)	49 ± 2	46 ± 2	54 ± 1[d]
Weight (kg)	64.0 ± 1.4	75.7 ± 1.7[b]	76.2 ± 1.8[b]
SBP (mm Hg)	116 ± 2	159 ± 2[b]	170 ± 3[b,d]
DBP (mm Hg)	71 ± 1	100 ± 1[b]	102 ± 1[b]
Plasma:			
Aldosterone (pmol/L)	333 ± 19	372 ± 19	494 ± 47[a,c]
cGMP (nmol/L)	4.7 ± 0.2	5.0 ± 0.3	7.1 ± 0.5[b,e]
C-ANP (SER 99-TYR 126) (pmol/L)	11.5 ± 0.7	10.5 ± 0.6	17.9 ± 1.2[b,e]
N-ANP (ASN 1-ARG 98) (pmol/L)	580 ± 35	488 ± 20[a]	895 ± 67[b,e]

[a] "p" < 0.02; [b] "p" < 0.0001, versus normotensive subjects; [c] "p" < 0.02; [d] "p" < 0.001; [e] "p" < 0.0005, versus untreated patients (Larochelle et al. 1988)

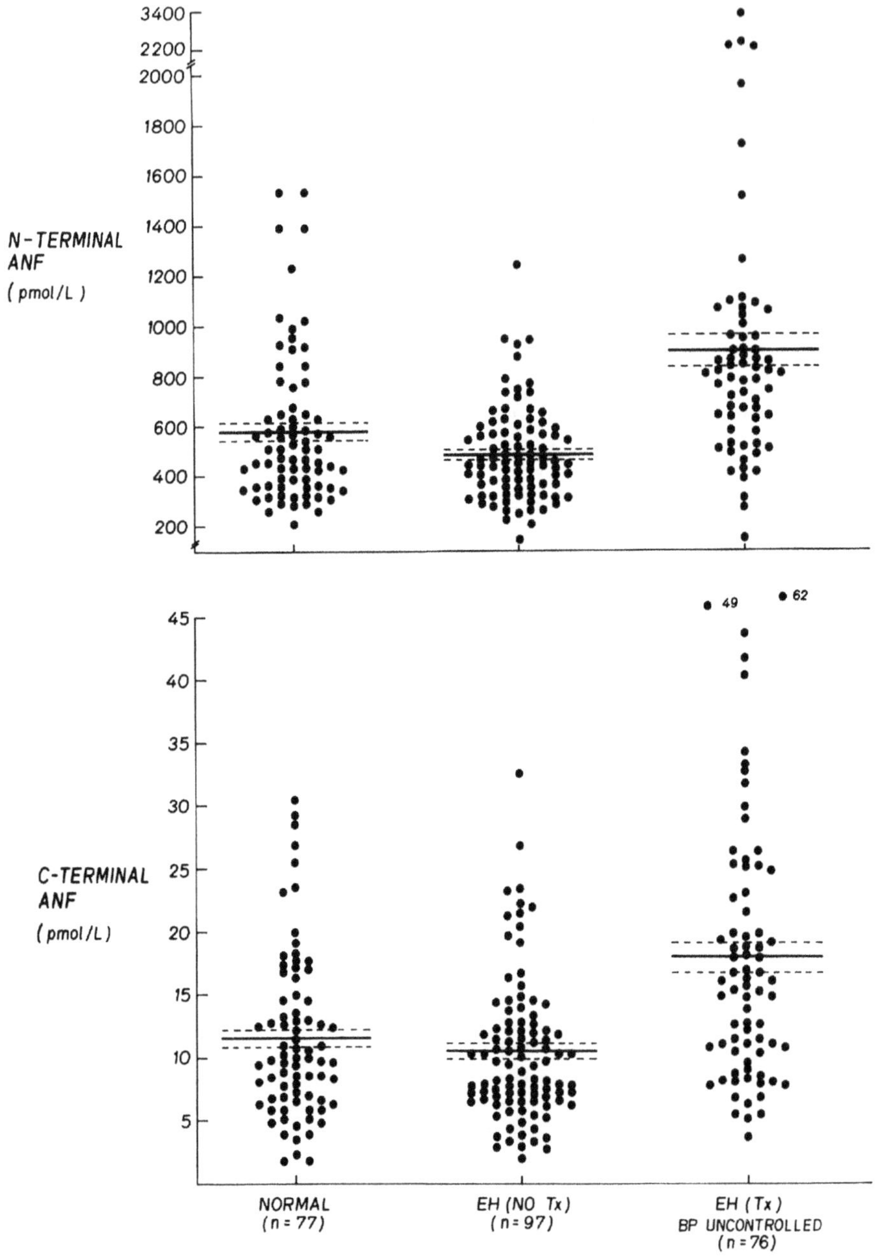

Fig. 1. Individual results of the C-terminal ANP (Ser 99-Tyr 126) and of the N-terminal ANP (Asn 1-Arg 98) in the control subjects and in the two groups of untreated and treated (Tx) patients. In the latter group, the blood pressure was not controlled to normal levels despite the medication given at the time of blood sampling. Note the absence of any significant difference between the untreated group when compared to that of the control subjects

Table 2. Plasma concentrations of GMP, C-terminal SER 99-TYR 126, N-terminal ASN 1-ARG 98 ANP in untreated and treated groups of patients with essential hypertension

	Sub-groups according to diastolic P.	N	AGE (years)	cGMP (nmol/L)	C-ANP (SER 99-TYR 126) (pmol/L)	N-ANP (ASN 1-ARG 98) (pmol/L)
Control Subj.	90 mm Hg	77	49 ± 2	4.7 ± 0.2	11.5 ± 0.7	580 ± 35
Essential ht untreated	90 mm Hg	32	47 ± 3	5.4 ± 0.6	12.4 ± 1.5	444 ± 23
	90–104	74	46 ± 1	5.4 ± 0.4	9.8 ± 0.6	443 ± 23
	105–114	16	46 ± 3	4.2 ± 0.4	12.4 ± 2.0	446 ± 52
	115	7	40 ± 3	4.1 ± 1.2	11.4 ± 1.6	481 ± 82
Treated	90	16	54 ± 3	4.7 ± 1.9	10.2 ± 1.0	684 ± 86^a
	90–104	51	53 ± 1	6.5 ± 0.5^a	15.3 ± 1.1^b	774 ± 46^b
	105–114	15	54 ± 3	6.9 ± 1.3^a	22.0 ± 3.8^b	953 ± 201^b
	115	10	59 ± 2	7.1 ± 1.1^a	25.4 ± 4.5^b	1304 ± 241^b
MEAN ± SEM; ^{a,b} "p": ANOVA between groups:				0.004	0.0001	0.0003

(Larochelle et al. 1988)

that the mean N-terminal ANP concentration is slightly but significantly ("p" < 0.02) lower in the untreated essential hypertensive group when compared to that of control subjects (Table 2). In the untreated hypertensive patients, left ventricular hypertrophy was not associated with higher plasma levels of either C-terminal ANP or of N-terminal ANP and of cyclic GMP.

On the other hand, a significant mean increase of all three parameters was found in the group of 76 hypertensive patients receiving antihypertensive drugs and with diastolic pressures still above 90 mmHg (Table 2). Even in the treated group under medication but with diastolic pressures below 90 mmHg, the mean plasma values of the N-terminal ANP (Asn 1-Arg 98) are slightly but significantly increased. As illustrated in Fig. 1, only a few patients had values of C-terminal ANP and of N-terminal ANP above the normal range.

Discussion

These findings indicate that plasma IR-ANP is within normal range in essential hypertension and that the factors which can be responsible for increased concentrations are 1) antihypertensive medication without adequate control of blood pressure, 2) significant left ventricular hypertrophy associated with severe hypertension, as pointed out by Montorsi et al. [25], 3) severe hypertension accompanied by symptoms or signs of renal or congestive heart failure.

Nevertheless, it is difficult to reconcile our results with those reported recently by Sagnella et al. [26] who have used a similar method for measurement of plasma IR-ANP in 106 patients with uncomplicated essential hypertension and without clinical and biological evidence of renal or heart failure and who found a mean plasma ANP concentration in hypertensive patients of 6 pmol/L in comparison to 3 in 47 normotensive subjects. Also Sugawara et al. [17] studied 34 patients with untreated essential hypertension, 14 of whom were in WHO stage 2, and 7 in stage 3. Mean plasma ANP levels in these patients was 30 pmol/L in comparison to age-matched normotensive controls in whom plasma ANP levels were 12 pmol/L. Similarly, Wambach et al. [23] reported mean plasma ANP levels of 48 pmol/L in 36 patients with essential hypertension in comparison to levels of 18 pmol/L in 31 normotensive controls.

It is of importance to note that in both studies done by Larochelle et al., plasma IR-ANP (Ser 99-Tyr 128) levels in essential hypertension were between 5 to 25 pmol/L. The plasma levels reported by the other groups, even when increased in patients with essential hypertension, showed that in almost all instances the plasma concentrations of IR-ANP were below 50 pmol/L. On the other hand, Cusson et al. [27] found that

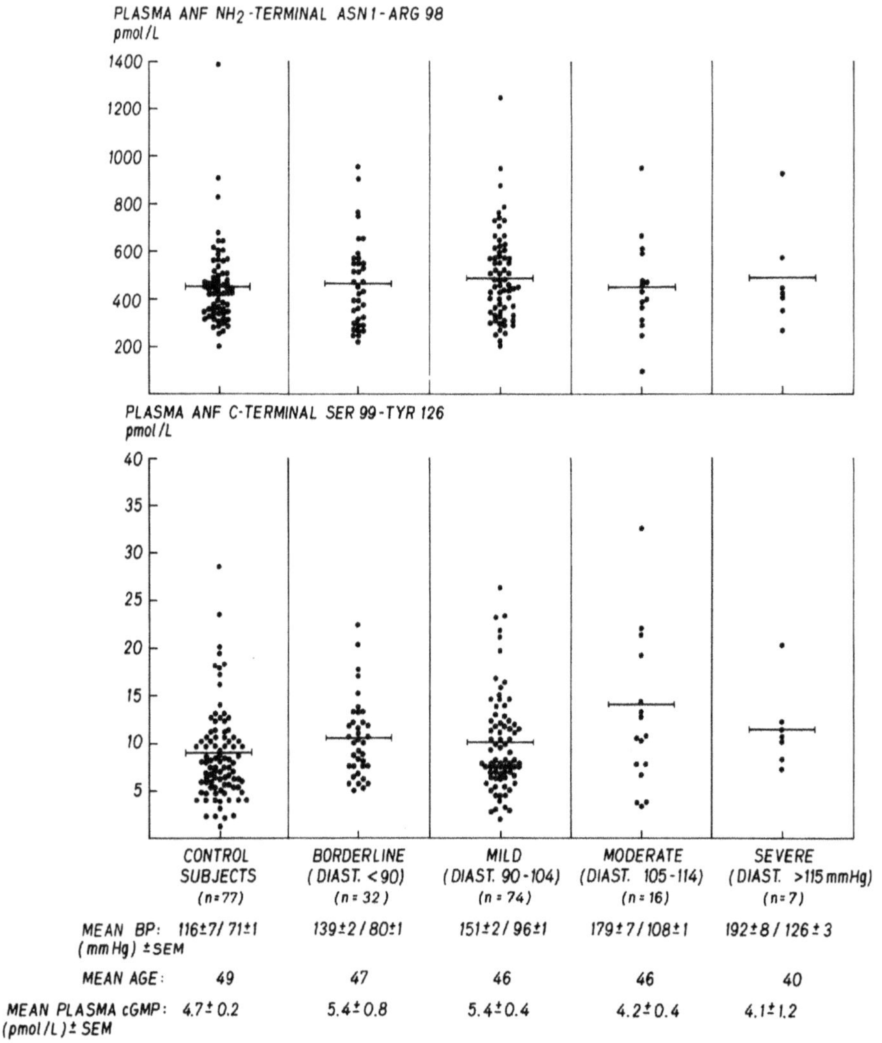

Fig. 2. Results of plasma ANP (Ser 99-Tyr 126) and of the N-terminal (Asn 1-Arg 98) in untreated patients with essential hypertension divided into groups according to their blood pressure at the time of blood sampling

infusions of plasma h-ANP 28 AA (Ser 99-Tyr 126) with plasma levels of about 80 pmol/L had no effect on blood pressure of control subjects and patients with mild essential hypertension. Hynynen et al. [28] obtained similar findings with infusions of alpha-h-ANP (50 mg/kg)/min for 30 min to 11 healthy volunteers which produced no change in mean arterial pressure despite marked natriuresis and diuresis and plasma IR-ANP levels about 100 pmol/L. Weidmann et al. [29], using higher rates of ANP infusion in 10 essential hypertensive patients with plasma levels of over 130 pmol/L, reported a significant decrease of blood pressure of 7/10 mmHg. Zimmerman et al. [30] have shown that successive increases in h-ANP infusions to conscious dogs had no effect on mean blood pressure even in the presence of significant natriuresis and plasma IR-ANP concentrations of 90 pmol/L. Only when the plasma concentration reached 170 pmol/L was there a significant decrease in systolic and diastolic blood pressures. These findings strongly suggest that the levels found or reported in patients with essential hypertension are much below those necessary to lower blood pressure when ANP is administered by intravenous infusion.

In view of the reported increases in right and left atrial pressures in patients with mild and moderate hypertension by London et al. [31] and by Ferlinz et al. [32], and of the increased pulmonary systolic and diastolic arterial pressures in patients with mild essential hypertension by Guazzi et al. [33] and by Olivari et al. [34], our findings of normal plasma IR-ANP concentration in patients with essential hypertension (concentrations which are much below those reached during the I.V. ANP infusions which produce significant lowering of blood pressure) suggest a hyporesponsiveness of the atria to release ANP in essential hypertension. Goetz [35] has calculated on the basis of his own studies in dogs and those of Raine et al. in humans [36] that there is an average increase in plasma IR-ANP concentration of 10.5 to 14 pmol/L for each 1 mm increase in left and in right atrial pressures.

In this context, it is of great interest to emphasize the recent findings reported by Jin [37] that dietary 8% NaCl loading for 12 days had no effect on the plasma IR-ANP concentration in SH-rats, whereas it induces significant ("p" < 0.01) increase in WKY rats, suggesting again a hyperresponsiveness of the atria to release ANP in SH-rats in response to salt loading.

Conclusion

The findings of normal plasma concentration of C-terminal ANP 28 AA (Ser 99-Tyr 126), N-terminal 98 AA (Asn 1-Arg 98) and of cGMP (marker of ANP activity) in patients with essential hypertension in view of the reported increased right and left atrial pressures in such patients suggest three possibilities: a) either ANP has nothing to do in the long-term control of high blood pressure in humans [38] in spite of the accumulated experimental evidence, or b) there is a hyporesponsiveness of the atria to release

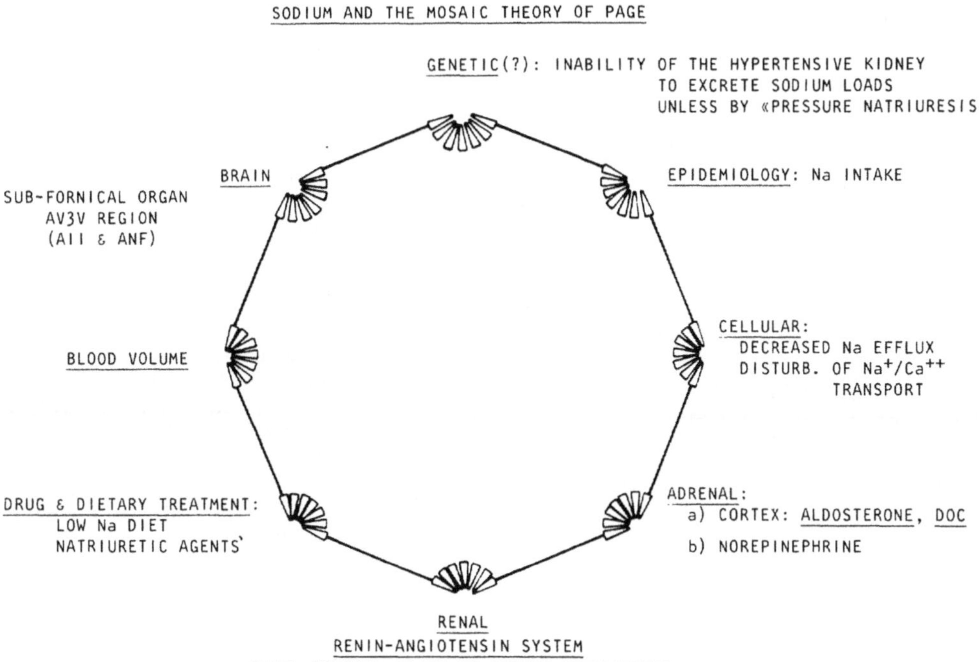

Fig. 3. Adaptation of the mosaic theory of Page to the relationship of sodium to the various aspects of hypertension

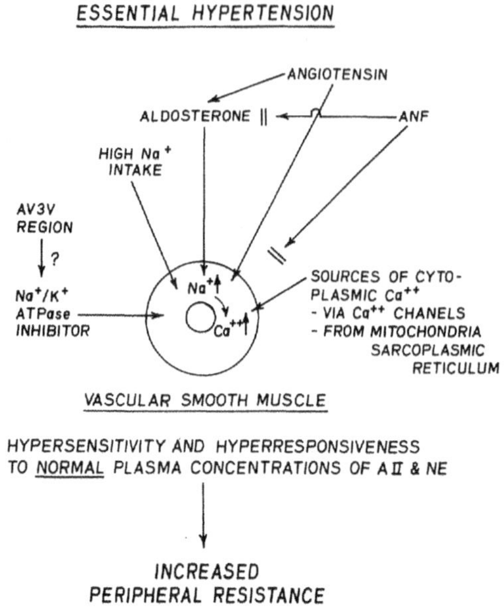

Fig. 4. Possible mechanisms leading to the hypersensivity and hyperresponsiveness of vascular smooth muscle in hypertension

ANP in essential hypertension. If this is the case, such a hyporesponsiveness is consistent with our long-held view that disturbances in sodium regulation play a central part in the mechanism of essential hypertension (Figs. 3, 4) and is compatible with: 1) a decrease in ability of the hypertensive kidney to excrete a high sodium intake or sodium load unless by increasing arterial pressure ("pressure natriuresis") [39–41], 2) a decreased inhibition of aldosterone and its inappropriately high levels of secretion and excretion and plasma concentration in patients with essential hypertension, especially during high sodium intake [42–44], 3) the increased peripheral resistance characteristic of essential hypertension due to an insufficient concentration of circulating ANP to prevent or to decrease the vasoconstrictor activity associated either with norepinephrine or with angiotensin II.

References

1. Genest J, Cantin M (eds) (1988) The atrial natriuretic factor, its physiology and biochemistry. Springer, Berlin Heidelberg New York, pp 1–145
2. Larochelle P, Cusson JR, Gutkowska J, Schiffrin EL, Hamet P, Kuchel O, Genest J, Cantin M (1987) Plasma concentration of atrial natriuretic factor in essential and renovascular hypertension. Br Med J 294: 1249–1252
3. Genest J (1986) The atrial natriuretic factor. Br Heart J 56:302–316
4. Genest J, Larochelle P, Cusson JR, Garcia R, Gutkowska J, Cantin M (1988) The atrial natriuretic factor in hypertension. Am J Med Sci 295:299–304
5. Tsuchiya S, Ogawa K, Sataka K (1980) Plasma levels of cyclic nucleotides in patients with essential hypertension. Jpn Heart J 21:803–815
6. Zachariah PK, Burnett JC, Ritter S, Strong CG (1987) Atrial natriuretic peptide in human essential hypertension. Mayo Clin Proc 62:782–786
7. Kohno M, Yasunari K, Matsuura T, Murakama K, Takeda T (1987) Circulating atrial natriuretic polypeptide in essential hypertension. Am Heart J 113:1160–1163
8. Nakaoka H, Kitahara Y, Amano M, Imataka K, Fujii J, Ishibashi M, Yamaji T (1987) Effect of β-adrenergic receptor blockade on atrial natriuretic peptide in essential hypertension. Hypertension 10:221–225
9. Naruse N, Naruse K, Obana K, Kurimoto F, Sakurai H, Honda T, Higashida T, Demura H, Inagami T, Shizume K (1986) Immunoreactive alpha-human atrial natriuretic polypeptide in human plasma. Peptides 7:141–145
10. Andersson OK, Persson B, Aurell M, Granerus G, Wysocky M, Hedner J, Hedner T (1986) Basal and stimulated levels of immunoreactive atrial natriuretic peptide (α-hANP) levels in relation to central venous pressure, renal and central hemodynamics and sodium excretion in normotensive and hypertensive man. J Cardiovasc Pharmacol 8:1300
11. Hedner T, Hedner J, Towle AC, Hartford M, Ljiungram S, Wikstrand J, Berglund G (1986) Plasma atrial natriuretic peptide (ANP) in patients with mild to moderate hypertension. J Cardiovasc Pharmacol 8:1299
12. Nishiuchi T, Saito H, Yanasaki Y, Saito S (1986) Radioimmunoassay for atrial natriuretic peptide: Method and results in normal subjects and patients with various diseases. Clin Chim Acta 159:45–47
13. Nozuki M, Mouri T, Itoi K, Takahashi K, Totsune K, Saito T, Yoshinaga K (1986) Plasma concentrations of atrial natriuretic peptide in various diseases. Tohoku J Exp Med 148:439–447

14. Yamaji T, Ishibashi M, Sekihara H, Takabu F, Nakaoka H, Fujii J (1986) Plasma levels of atrial natriuretic peptide in primary aldosteronism and essential hypertension. J Clin Endocrin Metab 63:815–818
15. Nilsson P, Lindholm L, Schersten B, Horn R, Melander A, Hesch RD (1987) Atrial natriuretic peptide and blood pressure in a geographically defined population. Lancet I:883–885
16. Sugawara A, Nakao K, Sakamoto M, Morii N, Yamada T, Itoh H, Shiono S, Imura H (1985) Plasma concentration of atrial natriuretic polypeptide in essential hypertension. Lancet II:1426–1427
17. Sugawara A, Nakao K, Kono T, Morii N, Yamada T, Itoh H, Shiono S, Saito Y, Mukoyama M, Arai H, Imura H (1988) Atrial natriuretic factor in essential hypertension and adrenal disorders. Hypertension 11 [Suppl I]:212–216
18. Sagnella GA, Markandu ND, Shore AC, MacGregor GA (1986) Raised circulating levels of atrial natriuretic peptides in essential hypertension. Lancet I:179–181
19. MacGregor GA, Sagnella GA, Markandu ND, Shore AC (1986) Raised plasma levels of atrial natriuretic peptide in untreated essential hypertension. J Cardiovasc Pharmacol 8:1301
20. Richards AM, Tonolo G, Davidson G (1986) Plasma atrial natriuretic peptide in essential hypertension. Proceedings, Council for High Blood Pressure Research, American Heart Association, Hypertension 8:826
21. Arendt RM, Stangl E, Zahringer J, Liebisch DC, Herz A (1985) Demonstration and characterization of alpha-human atrial natriuretic factor in human plasma. FEBS Lett; 189:57–61
22. Iimura O, Shimamoto K, Ando T, Ura N, Ishida H, Nakagawa M, Yokoyama T, Fukuyama S, Yamaguchi Y, Yamaji I (1987) Plasma levels of human atrial natriuretic peptide in patients with hypertensive diseases. Can J Physiol Pharmacol 65:1701–1705
23. Wambach G, Bonner S, Stimpel M, Kaufmann W (1988) Relationship between plasma atrial natriuretic peptide and left atrial and left ventricular involvement in essential hypertension. J Hypertens 6:573–577
24. Larochelle P, Cusson JR, Thibault G, Hamet P, Genest J, Cantin M (1989) C- and N-terminal fragments of atrial natriuretic factor in essential hypertension. Hypertension (submitted for publication)
25. Montorsi P, Tonolo G, Polonia J, Hepburn D, Richards AM (1987) Correlates of plasma atrial natriuretic factor in health and hypertension. Hypertension 10:570–576
26. Sagnella GA, Markandu ND, Buckley MG, Shore AC, Sugden AL, Singer DRJ, MacGregor GA (1988) Plasma atrial natriuretic peptide in essential hypertension. Am J Hypertens 1:112–118
27. Cusson JR, Hamet P, Gutkowska J, Kuchel O, Genest J, Cantin M, Larochelle P (1987) Effects of atrial natriuretic factor in natriuresis and cGMP in patients with essential hypertension. J Hypertens 5:435–443
28. Hynynen M, Kupari M, Salmenpera M, Tikkanen I, Heinonen J, Fyhrquist F, Totterman KJ (1988) Hemodynamic effects of alpha-human atrial natriuretic peptide in healthy volunteers. J Cardiovasc Pharmacol 11: 711–715
29. Weidmann P, Hasler L, Gnädinger MP, Lang RE, Uehlinger DE, Shaw S, Rascher W, Reubi FC (1986) Blood levels and renal effects of atrial natriuretic peptide in normal man. J Clin Invest 77:734–742
30. Zimmerman RS, Schirger JS, Edwards BS, Heublein DM, Schwab TR, Burnett JC (1987) Cardiovascular renal responses to physiologic concentrations of atrial natriuretic factor (ANF). J Am Coll Cardiol 9:242A
31. London GM, Safar ME, Safar AL, Surion AC (1985) Blood pressure in the "low pressure system" and cardiac performance in essential hypertension. J Hypertens 3:337–342
32. Ferlinz J (1980) Right ventricular performance in essential hypertension. Circulation 61:157–162
33. Guazzi M, Fiorentini C, Olivari MP, Polese A (1979) Cardiac load and function in hypertension. Am J Cardiol 44:1007–1012
34. Olivari MT, Fiorentini C, Polese A, Guazzi MD (1978) Pulmonary hemodynamics and right ventricle function in hypertension. Circulation 57:1185–1190
35. Goetz KL (1987) Atrial natriuretic peptide and atrial pressure. N Engl J Med 316:485
36. Raine AE, Erne P, Bürgisser E, Müller FB, Bolli P, Burkart F, Bühler FR (1986) Atrial natriuretic peptide and atrial pressure in patients with congestive heart failure. N Engl J Med 315:533–537
37. Jin H, Chen YF, Yang RH, Ming QC, Oparil S (1988) Impaired release of atrial natriuretic factor in NaCl-loaded spontaneously hypertensive rats. Hypertension 11:739–744
38. Greenwald JE, Sakata M, Michener ML, Sides SD, Needleman P (1988) Is atriopeptin a physiological or pathophysiological substance? Studies in the autoimmune rat. J Clin Invest 81:1036–1041
39. Guyton AC, Coleman TG, Young DB, Lohmeier TE, De-Clue JW (1980) Salt-balance and long-term blood pressure control. Ann Rev Med 13:15–27

40. Tobian L, Lange J, Magraw S, Coffee K (1974) Body sodium and hypertension, sodium retention by "hypertensive kidneys". Trans Assoc Am Phys 87:225–232
41. Tobian L, Johnson MA, Lange J, Magraw S (1975) Effect of varying perfusion pressures on the output of sodium and renin and the vascular resistance in kidneys of rats with "post-salt" hypertension and Kyoto spontaneous hypertension. Circ Res 36 [Suppl I]:I-162–I-170
42. Genest J, Nowaczynski W, Kuchel O, Boucher R, Rojo-Ortega JM, Constantopoulos G, Ganten D, Messerli F (1976) The adrenal cortex and essential hypertension. Recent Progr Horm Res 32:377–427
43. Collins RD, Weinberger MH, Dowdy AJ, Nokes GW, Gonzales CM, Luetscher JA (1970) Abnormally sustained aldosterone secretion during salt-loading in patients with various forms of benign hypertension: Relation to plasma renin activity. J Clin Invest 49:1415–1426
44. Luetscher J, Beckerhoff R, Dowdy AJ, Wilkinson R (1972) Incomplete suppression of aldosterone secretion and plasma concentration in hypertensive patients on high sodium intake. In: Genest J, Koiw E (eds) Hypertension '72. Springer, Berlin Heidelberg New York, pp 286–292

Atrial Natriuretic Peptide: Protective Effects in Acute Renal Failure

S. G. Shaw, and P. Weidmann

Medizinische Poliklinik, University of Berne, Switzerland

Summary. Protective effects of systemic or intrarenal administration of atrial natriuretic peptide have been demonstrated in many experimental models of acute renal failure including ureteral ligation, endotoxin and renal artery clamping.

Multiple actions of the peptide appear to contribute to these beneficial effects which involve an increase in glomerular filtration pressure, alleviation of tubular obstruction, a more rapid restoration of renal blood flow and high energy phosphate levels, antagonism of catecholamines and modulation of other intrarenal or circulating regulators of renal function. The magnitude of the renal improvement produced by ANP under different conditions however, may be modified not only by the severity of the initial insult but also by factors relating to its use including the ability to maintain mean arterial pressure and blood volume, the stage at which it is administered, the total dose and duration of treatment as well as its concentration. Careful control of these parameters is necessary in order to optimise the beneficial response. These preliminary studies may provide a basis for the future potential use of atrial natriuretic peptide in clinical situations where renal function may be temporarily compromised such as cancer chemotherapy, radiodiagnostic procedures, cardiac surgery and renal transplantation.

Key words: ANP – Renal failure – Protective effects

Introduction

Interest in the potential of Atrial Natriuretic Peptide (ANP) to protect against the development of renal failure following an acute insult to the kidney derives from studies in normal animals and man showing that under certain conditions ANP can increase renal blood flow, facilitate excretion of salt and water, relax vascular and non-vascular smooth muscle and augment glomerular filtration (Weidmann et al. 1986; Ballerman et al 1985).

Not surprisingly, awareness of this favorable pharmacological profile of action rapidly prompted a series of studies of potential therapeutic effects of acute intrarenal or systemic ANP infusion during the early or maintenance phase of several experimental models of acute renal failure (ARF), (Shaw et al. 1987; Nakamoto et al. 1987; Heidbreder et al. 1986; Schafferhans et al. 1986; Capasso et al. 1987).

Despite these encouraging beginnings, the demonstration of ANP's ability to produce sustained improvements in renal function is still lacking in many of these experimental systems and initial studies of ANP's affects in the treatment of acute renal failure in man, have been somewhat disappointing. (Bozkurt et al. 1987). In this report, effects of systemic and intra-renal administration of human (1–28) ANP are described in three models of ARF. These studies show that under appropriate conditions, treatment with ANP can produce sustained improvements in renal function in these experimental models and provide some insight into several mechanisms which may contribute to the protective effects. Furthermore the data suggest several important factors which may influence the magnitude of the renal response to ANP in different experimental and clinical situations.

The three models of ARF are those induced by endotoxin, ureteral ligation and renal artery clamping which may have their clinical counterparts in forms of ARF associated with bacteremia and hepatic disease, ureteral obstruction, and the associated complications of cardiac surgery and renal transplantation respectively.

Effects of ANP in Experimental Models of ARF Induced by Endotoxin, Ureteral Ligation and Renal Artery Clamping

Endotoxemic Renal Failure

Endotoxin, a component of the cell wall of gram-negative bacteria, has been detected in elevated concentrations in serum in various clinical forms of ARF. Injection of endotoxin results in release of catecholamines and thromboxanes which have been strongly implicated in the subsequent sequence of events leading to vasoconstriction and intravascular coagulation (Bolton et al. 1978). Since this form of renal failure has been found to be refractory to preventative measures such as volume expansion, calcium channel blockade, and mannitol, which have been found effective in other models of ARF, it provided an attractive model in which to examine the range of ANP's protective effects. (Kikeri et al. 1986).

In the rat, an acute single doese of E. Coli endotoxin, (Fig. 1), induces a reversible form of oliguric renal failure characterised by a reduction in GFR and renal blood flow and a significant increase in the fractional excretion of sodium. Immediately after intravenous injection of 20 mg/Kg endotoxin in Sprague Dawley rats under pentobarbital anaesthesia, human (1–28) ANP (8 μg/ml) in 0.9% saline/1% albumin (experimental group) or saline/albumin alone (control group) was infused for three hours into the left renal artery at a rate of 20 μl/min. Urine loss was replaced by 0.9% saline. Clearance of C14 Inulin (GFR), fractional excretion of sodium ($FENa^+$), urine flow hematocrit and mean arterial pressure were monitored. In controls, 3 h after endotoxin injection, GFR in left and right kidneys was reduced from 0.43 ± 0.03 and 0.47 ± 0.04 to 0.17 ± 0.01 and 0.2 ± 0.001 ml/min/100 g respectively; urine flow, (0.23 ± 0.02 ml/h) hematocrit (42 ± 1%) and mean arterial pressure (120 ± 3 mmHg) were unaltered at this time but $FENa^+$ increased from 0.08 ± 0.02 to 1.27 ± 0.1% in the left and from 0.05 ± 0.01 to 1.2 ± 0.1% in the right kidney ($p < 0.001$). Intrarenal ANP maintained GFR in the left kidney at 81% (0.35 ± 0.02 ml/min/100 g) of baseline during the three hour infusion, while GFR in the non-ANP-infused right kidney decreased to 44% (0.21 ± 0.02 ml/min/100 g, $p < 0.001$. vs normal), $FENa^+$ in the left and right kidneys increased to 5.7 ± 0.6 and 1.0 ± 0.03% with urine flow rates of 3.4 ± 0.35 and 0.6 ± 0.05 ml/h respectively ($p < 0.001$) reflecting the natriuretic effect of ANP.

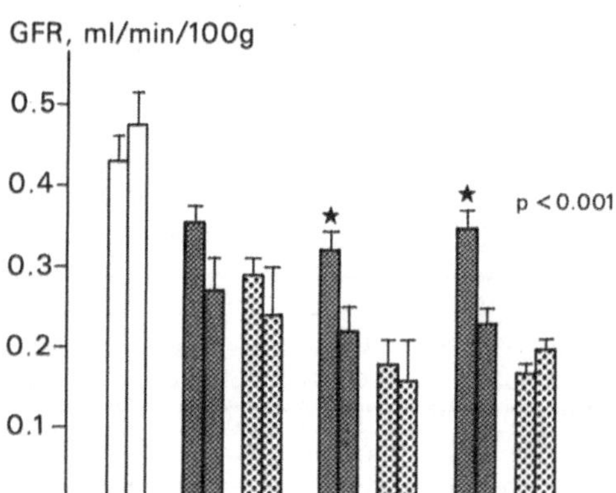

Fig. 1. Decrease in glomerular filtration rate in left and right kidneys, 1, 2 and 3 hours after bolus intravenous injection of 20 mg/Kg E. Coli Endotoxin in the rat (dotted bars) and its prevention by intra-renal infusion of human (1–28) ANP into the left renal artery (hatched bars). Normal GFR values measured in untreated left and right kidneys are shown by the open bars

Post Ureteral Obstruction

Urinary tract obstruction is a relatively common cause of acute renal failure. After unilateral obstruction a transient increase in renal blood flow occurs resulting from initial afferent arteriolar vasodilation but, as obstruction persists, blood flow decreases due to effects of the locally acting vasoconstrictor agents thromboxane A2 and angiotensin (Yarger et al. 1980). Since ANP may antagonise these compounds, its potential to improve GFR following 24 h of unilateral ureteral obstruction was assessed in the rat; a model characterised by particularly severe vasoconstriction after release of only 24 h of unilateral ureteral ligation.

Because intravenous infusion of ANP is a more convenient mode of administration than direct injection into the renal artery, the model was also used to investigate the possibility of giving ANP systemically and to evaluate ways of improving the renal response by controlling the reduction in blood volume known to be associated with systemic ANP administration. To this end, urine losses were replaced either with saline or Physiogel, a gelatine-based plasma substitute. As shown in Figure 2, GFR, urine volume and osmolar excretion in the previously obstructed control kidney measured after 3 h of systemic saline infusion was markedly depressed compared to normal. Intravenous infusion of human (1–28) ANP at 0.6 ml/h and a concentration of 12.5 μg/ml for 3 h with saline replacement of urine losses produced a small improvement in GFR but at the expense of a large fall in mean arterial pressure to a final mean value of 93 mmHg over 3 h. In contrast, ANP infusion and replacement of urine losses with Physiogel over the same length of time produced a further improvement in all three parameters and maintained mean arterial pressure at 116 mmHg.

Ischemic Renal Failure

Bilateral renal artery obstruction or obstruction of the artery of a solitary kidney leads to a severe decrease in glomerular filtration rate and often renal infarction.

In experimental models, using previously uninephrectomised or bilaterally renally intact animals, human (1–28) ANP administered systemically for 1 h, or locally as a 4 h intrarenal infusion following 45–60 min of renal ischemia, restored C14 inulin clearance rates to 50–70% of normal over the time of infusion (Shaw et al. 1987; Nakamoto et al. 1987). Histologically, kidneys treated with ANP for 4 h after ischemia displayed a markedly reduced incidence of medullary hyperremia, tubular obstruction and necrosis at 4 and 24 h compared to saline treated controls (Shaw et al. 1987).

Considered together, the data from these and previous studies suggest that ANP may be able to provide unique protection from

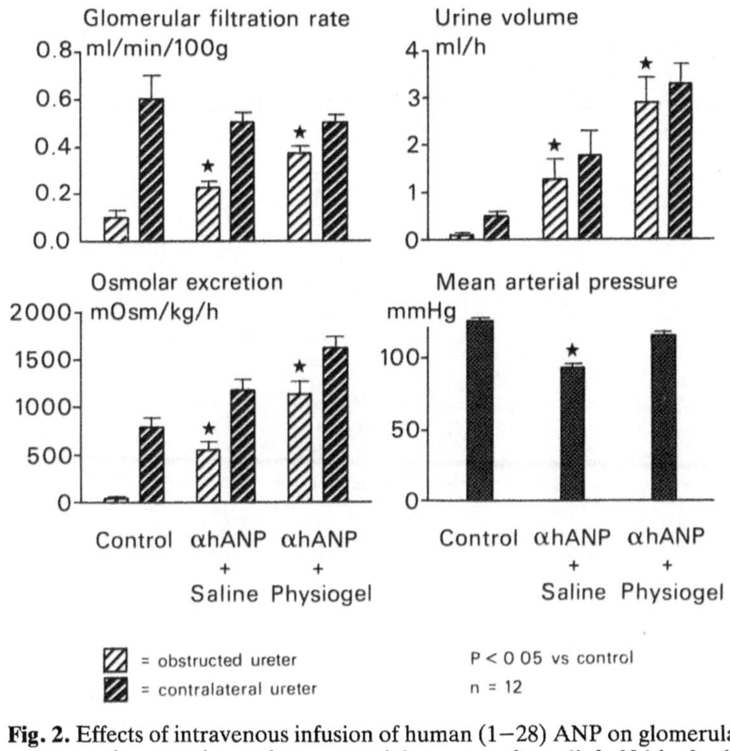

Fig. 2. Effects of intravenous infusion of human (1–28) ANP on glomerular filtration rate, urine volume, osmolar excretion and mean arterial pressure after relief of 24 h of unilateral ureteral obstruction in the rat. Urine losses were replaced either with saline or Physiogel

acute renal failure induced by a wide variety of agents and show that ANP is capable of producing sustained improvements in renal function in these models at least when given during the early stages.

Potential Mechanisms

In view of the varied pathophysiology involved in different forms of ARF and the wide range of models in which ANP has now been shown to exert a beneficial action, it is likely that multiple pharmacological actions of the peptide involving both vascular and tubular components underly its protective action. Potentially these include a more rapid restoration of renal blood flow which in the ischemic model is restored faster in ANP infused kidneys and reaches pre-ischemia levels after approximately 50 min of intrarenal perfusion (Fig. 3). High energy phosphate levels are also restored more rapidly compared to non-ANP-treated controls (Fig. 4) (Nakamoto et al. 1987). Associated accumulation of intrarenal and circulating catecholamines and activation of the renal sympathetic nerves which have been implicated in both ischemia and endotoxin mediated forms of ARF may also be prevented (Shaw et al. 1988). Potentially, catecholamines may exacerbate the severity of renal damage by causing vasoconstriction and prolonging ischemia or by contributing to the formation of oxygen free-radicals (Singal et al. 1982).

Overall, these combined actions of ANP would tend to favor a more rapid restoration of renal metabolism towards normal and limit further damage. Additional mechanisms are likely to be involved in ANP's protective effects and further investigation is needed of potential interactions with the renin/angiotensin, prostaglandin and thromboxane systems. Furthermore, a possible cyclic GMP-mediated protective effect of ANP against oxygen free-radical induced re-perfusion injury at the cellular level should also be considered (Vonruecker et al. 1988).

Factors Influencing the Response to ANP in ARF

As more information becomes available concerning effects of ANP, it is apparent that its effectiveness in ameliorating ARF in various model systems is to some extent dependent upon the severity of the initial insult and the amount of irreversible cell damage which has occurred. Consequently, ANP is not equally effective under all circumstances in restoring renal function in

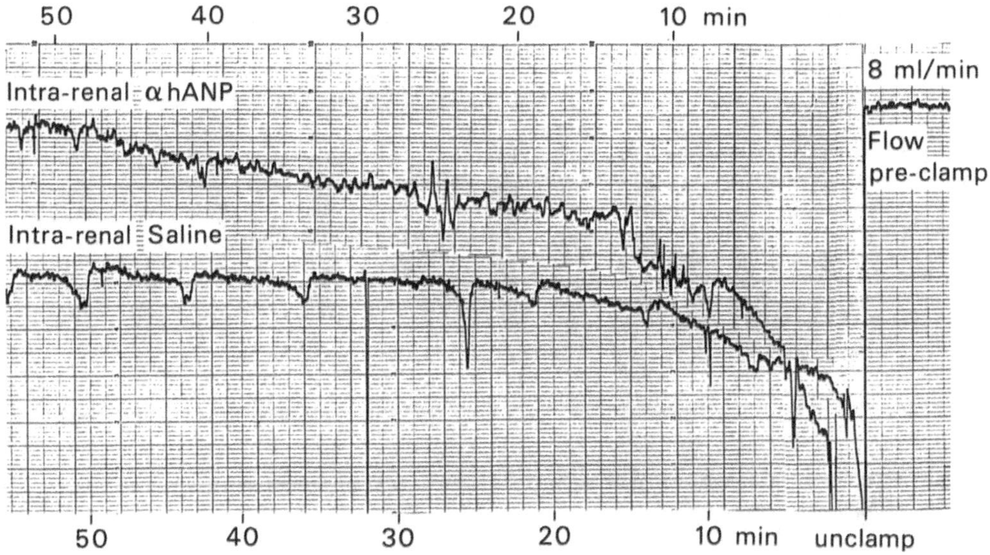

Fig. 3. Effects of intrarenal infusion of human (1–28) ANP on the recovery of renal blood flow following 45 min of renal ischemia in the rat

every form of renal failure and in some cases appears to produce little improvement (Boskurt et al.). Although in some cases part of this non-responsiveness may lie in an inability of irreversibly damaged tissue to respond to ANP, in other situations aspects of the way ANP is used may influence the renal response.

From the present data at least four important criteria can be identified which must be fulfilled if effects under experimental and clinical conditions are to be properly assessed and the beneficial response optimised.

These include the ability to maintain mean arterial pressure and blood volume, the time at which ANP is given, the dose and duration of treatment and the concentration of ANP which may be needed under different circumstances.

In the studies relating to the effects of ANP after relief of 24 h of unilateral ureteral ligation, it was apparent that the maintenance of mean arterial pressure and blood volume with Physiogel enhanced the beneficial renal response. The likely explanation for this enhanced response to systemic ANP infusion when urine is replaced by Physiogel rather than saline, is that the excretion of essentially protein-free water in response to ANP enables the oncotic pressure of the plasma to balance the usual effect of ANP which normally lowers blood volume and mean arterial pressure partly by producing a shift of water out of the vascular compartment.

In the clinical setting this factor may have several consequences in affecting the renal response to ANP. The homeostatic maintenance of peripheral resistance in the setting of volume depletion is mediated by the reflex activation of vasoconstrictor mechanisms involving the autonomic nervous system, the renin angiotensin system and possibly vasopressin. Thus, the beneficial increase in GFR in response to ANP may be counteracted by a fall in mean arterial pressure and the activation of antagonistic circulating vasoactive agents. Under these circumstances it may be inappropriate to administer ANP systemically without taking precautions against the expected decrease in MAP. If this cannot be improved by correcting volume depletion then alternative strategies should be considered. These might include the simultaneous administration of a pressor agent and renal vasodilator such as dopamine, the administration of lower doses of ANP, although this is unlikely to achieve the necessary therapeutic intra-renal concentrations, or to administer ANP directly into the renal artery as in experimental endotoxemic and ischemic renal failure.

An additional factor influencing the response to ANP may be the time at which it is administered. Figure 5, for example, shows

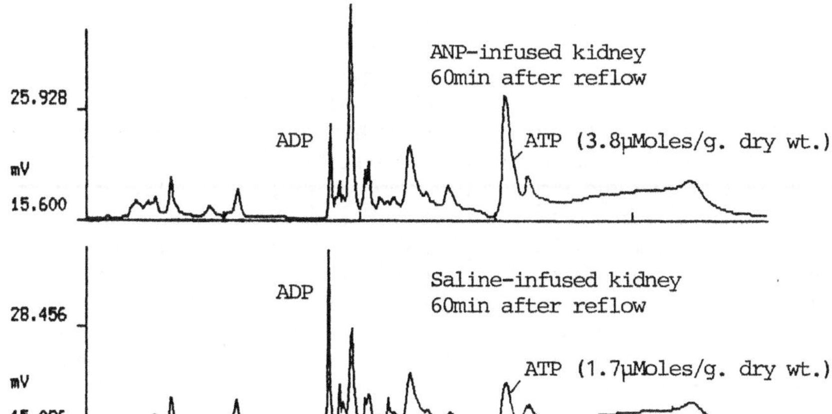

Fig. 4. HPLC profile of ATP concentrations in post ischemic rat kidneys perfused either with saline or human (1–28) ANP for 1 h following release of 45 min of renal artery occlusion

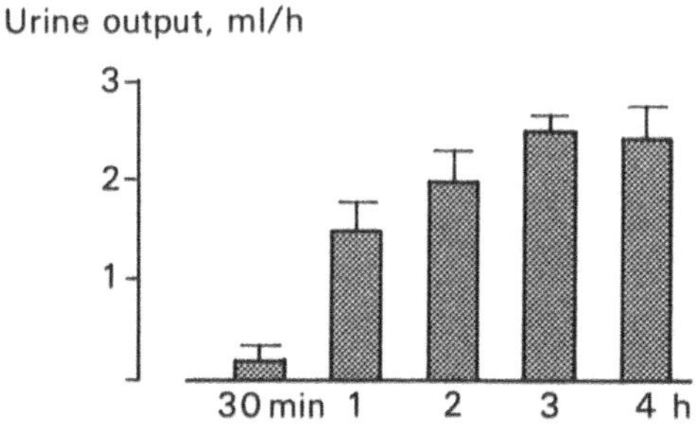

Fig. 5. The renal response to repeated intravenous bolus injection of 600 ng human (1–28) ANP in normal rats at different times following surgery for placement of ureter, carotid and jugular catheters

the response in a normal rat to the same bolus intravenous injection of 600 ng of ANP at different times after completion of surgery for placement of ureter, carotid and jugular catheters. The maximum response to the diuretic effect is markedly blunted soon after surgery and progressively improves as the equilibration time is prolonged suggesting activation of other counteractive circulating or intrarenal factors which blunt the ANP response.

Clinically this may be of considerable importance particularly if ANP is to be assessed for its beneficial effects following renal transplantation (Bozkurt et al.). Under such circumstances ANP is usually administered shortly following completion of the anastomosis and continued for a relatively short period over the time when the maximum response would be expected to be markedly blunted. In such studies it may be more beneficial to delay the time of ANP administration or at least to continue the infusion for a sufficient length of time to allow the blunting effects of surgery to subside. Considering additional therapeutic interventions, identification of the factors mediating this blunted response may offer the future possibility of combined therapy with ANP and antagonists of these systems. Alternatively, it may be that ANP needs to be given intrarenally in higher doses or continued for a period of several hours before a favorable response can be obtained.

The importance of the duration of treatment is highlighted by studies in ischemic renal failure where although systemic ANP infusion for 1 h and intrarenal infusion for 4 h improves GFR, striking differences can be seen in the histological appearance of the kidneys (Shaw et al. 1987; Nakamoto et al. 1987). It is apparent from these studies in post ischemic kidneys treated with ANP that the disappearance of medullary hyperremia and protein casts is not an instantaneous process but occurs gradually over the course of a 4 h intrarenal infusion. At the end of this period C14-inulin clearance is measured to be between 50–70% of normal. Shorter infusion times, lower doses or systemic administration of ANP results in less dramatic improvements in renal function and histology indicating that the length of time of administration, the total dose given and the severity of the insult are important factors which can influence the speed and extent of recovery.

It seems, therefore, that a critical therapeutic concentration of ANP may be needed for a critical length of time in order to prevent the development of permanent renal damage following a period of renal ischemia. Within reason, it is likely that with more severe insults it is necessary to administer ANP over longer periods of time at higher concentrations. This however, may set a limit on the use of ANP in vivo. Under some conditions the amount of ANP required for the necessary time to produce a lasting beneficial response may not be possible to achieve even with the intrarenal mode of infusion because ANP escaping into the general circulation produces uncontrolable hemodynamic effects which overide the beneficial effect. This problem may occur in the transplantation of cadaveric kidneys which have been subjected to a period of warm ischemia. One solution, however, may be to perfuse donor kidneys in vitro before transplantation with a higher concentration of ANP. A pilot study of autotransplantation in the rat suggests that such an approach may be possible (Shaw et al. 1988). Kidneys subjected to 30 min of cold ischemia then transplanted with a re-anastomosis time of 45 min of warm ischemia do not function well immediately after transplantation and are severely atrophied when assessed after three months. Perfusion in vitro with a high dose of ANP (3 μg/min for 30 min), before re-anastomosis however, appears to improve the long term survival of the graft. More extensive studies are clearly needed of this potential method of pretreatment and storage of cadaveric kidneys which may extend the usefulness of suitable organs for transplantation to those which have been subjected to a certain period of ischemia.

In summary, initial experimental studies of potential therapeutic effects of ANP in several forms of renal failure offer promising beginnings in terms of its future clinical use in intensive care units, in cancer chemotherapy and radiodiagnostic procedures and as a preventative therapy in cardiac surgery and renal transplantation. Clearly more detailed information is still needed to determine the optimum conditions for the use of ANP which, if not obtained may delay effective assessment of its clinical use in various forms of renal failure and limit the scope of this potentially important future therapeutic agent.

References

Ballermann JB, Hoover R, Karnovsky J, Brenner B (1985) Physiologic regulation of atrial natriuretic peptide receptors in rat renal glomeruli. J Clin Invest 76:2049–2056

Bolton WK, Atuk N (1978) Study of chemical sympathectomy in endotoxin-induced lethality and fibrin deposition. Kidney Int 13:263–270

Bozkurt F, Kirste G, Leipziger J, Schollmeyer P, Drexler H, Keller E (1987) Effects of human atrial natriuretic peptide on diuresis and hemodynamics in oligoanuric renal transplant recipients. Transplantation Proceedings XIX, No 5, pp 4192–4195

Capasso G, Anastasio P, Giordano D, Albaro L, Rudolfo A, Gaspare de santo N (1987) Atrial natriuretic factor increases glomerular filtration rate in the experimental acute renal failure induced by cisplatinin. In: Amerio A, Campese V, Coratelli P, Massry S (eds) Advances in experimental medicine and biology, vol 212, Acute renal failure. Plenum Press, New York, pp 285–290

Heidbreder E, Schafferhans K, Schramm G, Heidland A (1986) Toxic renal failure in the rat: beneficial effects of atrial natriuretic factor. Klin Wochenschr 64 [Suppl VI]:78–82

Kikeri D, Pennell P, Huang K, Jacob A, Richman A, Bourgoignie J (1986) Endotoxemic acute renal failure in awake rats. Am J Physiol 250:F1098–1106

Nakamoto M, Shapiro JI, Shanley PF, Chan L, Schrier R (1987) In vitro and in vivo protective effect of Antriopeptin III on ischemic acute renal failure. J Clin Invest 80:698–705

Schafferhans K, Heidbreder E, Grimm D, Heidland A (1986) Norepinephrine-induced renal failure: Beneficial effects of atrial natriuretic factor. Nephron 44:240–244

Schafferhans K, Strohmeier J, Geiger H, Bahner U, Klandwehr EP, Heidland A (1988) Contrast media induced acute renal failure protective action of atrial natriuretic peptide. Proceedings Int. Symposium "Endocrinology of the Heart" Cologne October 1988

Shaw SG, Weidmann P, Hodler J, Zimmermann A, Paternostro A (1980) Atrial natriuretic peptide protects against acute ischemic renal failure in the rat. J Clin Invest 80:1232–1237

Shaw SG, Höflin F, Peter H, Noelpp U, Studer U, Weidmann P (1988) Atrial natriuretic peptide in kidney autotransplantation: Quantitative data using radioisotope nephrography. In: Schmidt HAE, Csernay L (eds) Nuklearmedizin. Schattauer, Stuttgart, S 454–458

Shaw SG, Weidmann P, Hodler J (1988) Atrial natriuretic peptide: Effects on renal tissue catecholamines following renal ischemia. In: Brenner B, Laragh JH (eds) Amn. Soc. Hyp. Symp. Series "Advances in atrial peptide research". Raven Press, New York, pp 371–375

Singal P, Kapur N, Dhillon SK, Beamisk R, Dhalla N (1982) Role of free radicals in catecholamine-induced cardiomyopathy. Can J Physiol Pharmacol 60:1390–1397

Vonruecker A, Pella R, Bidlingmaier F (1988) Atrial natriuretic peptide protects against damage induced by hypoxia or hypochlorous acid. Proceedings Int. Symposium, Endocrinology of the heart. Cologne 1988

Weidmann P, Hasler L, Gnadinger M et al. (1986) Blood levels and renal effects of atrial natriuretic peptide in man. J Clin Invest 77:734–742

Yarger WE, Schodan DD, Harris RH (1980) Obstructive nephropathy in the rat possible roles for the renin angiotensin system, prostaglandins and thromboxanes in post-obstructive renal function. J Clin Invest 65:400–412

ANP and Volume Regulation in Liver Cirrhosis

R. Brunkhorst[1] and G. Brabant[2]

[1] Abteilung Nephrologie und [2] Abteilung Endokrinologie; Medizinische Hochschule Hannover, FRG

Summary. The possible role of atrial natriuretic peptide (ANP) in the pathogenesis of the impaired excretion of sodium and water in patients with liver cirrhosis is still controversially discussed. High concentrations of circulating ANP in most patients with cirrhosis and a normal responsiveness of ANP secretion to volume expansion support a role of the peptide as an indicator of plasma volume. The impaired diuretic and natriuretic effect of exogenous ANP suggests an impaired renal action of ANP in cirrhosis which may be a cofactor for sodium and water retention in cirrhosis.

Key words: Human atrial natriuretic peptide – Liver cirrhosis and ascites – sodium retention

The pathogenesis of ascites formation in patients with liver cirrhosis is still only incompletely understood. Two concepts are currently competing to explain the disturbed volume regulation in these patients (see Fig. 1):

The "overflow" concept of Liebermann et al. [19] proposes a sodium retention by the kidney as a primary event leading to water retention and an increase in circulating plasma volume followed by ascites formation. The mechanism eliciting renal sodium retention is unknown. A direct activation of the renal branches of the sympathetic system, of the renin-angiotensin-aldosteron-system (RAAS) and other hormonal systems has been discussed. This concept was supported experimentally by Levy et al. who could demonstrate by studies in cirrhotic dogs that sodium retention and an expansion of plasma volume precedes ascites formation [18].

In contrast, the "underfilling" theory [9, 24] proposes that primarily ascites is formed due to a decreased oncotic pressure in the plasma and an elevation of the hydrostatic portal venous pressure leading to a fluid shift into the abdominal space. The resulting decrease of the effective plasma volume secondarily activates the RAAS, the sympathetic system, prostaglandin or other vasoactive hormonal systems (Fig. 1).

Theoretical Considerations on ANP in the Volume Regulation in Liver Cirrhosis

With the characterization of atrial natriuretic peptide (ANP) as a potent diuretic and natriuretic hormone [8, 26], an important role of this peptide in the pathogenesis of ascites formation has been anticipated. According to the "overflow" concept theoretically a decrease in ANP secretion or an impairment of its effects on the kidney level should be expected if the peptide plays a role in the primary pathomechanism of ascites formation. However, if the hormone is only altered in response to the rise in plasma volume, plasma levels should be increased. Following the "underfilling" concept, due to the decreased effective plasma volume the major stimulus for ANP secretion is lacking, thus lowered circulating plasma levels could be expected. The secondary activation of other hormonal factors in the underfilling state such as catecholamines, arginine-vasopressin or the RAAS, known to directly activate ANP release, however, may obscure this pattern and lead to normal or even elevated plasma ANP levels.

ANP in Experimental Models

ANP-Plasma Levels

Several animal models have been used to investigate the role of ANP in the course of cirrhosis and of ascites formation. Lajkill et al. investigated the acute and chronic effects of bile duct ligation in rats [29]. In this model it is known, that a histologically proven cirrhosis with a significant reduction of renal sodium excretion (UNaV) occurs only in the chronic situation after six weeks. As compared to control animals investigated after six but not after two weeks of bile duct ligation a significant increase of ANP plasma levels could be observed. In another experimental model, the induction of liver cirrhosis by inhalation of tetrachlorcarbon CCl_4), histologically proven cirrhosis occurs, sodium excretion is decreased and plasma volume is increased in comparison to control rats. We could demonstrate that ANP plasma values are significantly higher in cirrhotic compared to control rats (see Fig. 2a) [5]. Similar results were obtained by studies of Olivera who investigated the ANP-response to volume expansion in cirrhotic rats [23]. Basal ANP levels were increased in cirrhotic rats but the relative stimulation to a given volume load was comparable in both groups, suggesting an intact secretory mechanism in cirrhosis.

Effect of Exogenous ANP

To test the renal responsiveness to the peptide we investigated renal blood flow (RBF), glomerular filtration rate (GFR) and UNaV in CCl_4 induced cirrhosis and in control rats basally and under intravenous application of ANP (2 μg/kg as bolus and 0.5

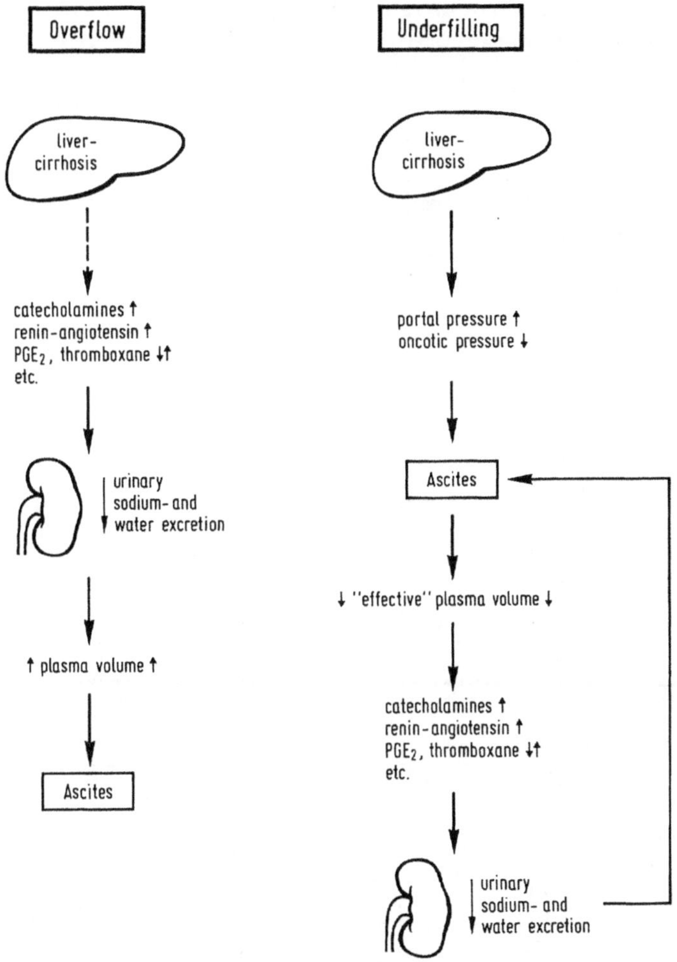

Fig. 1. Schematic drawing of the "overflow" and of the "underfilling" theory of ascites formation in liver cirrhosis

μg/kg as infusion [5]. Under basal conditions RBF, GFR, and UNaV were significantly lowered in cirrhotic rats compared to controls. Under ANP administration RBF, GFR and UNaV increased in control as in cirrhotic rats, but the effect on GFR and UNaV was significantly attenuated in cirrhotic rats (see Fig. 2b).

In summary experimental data indicate that ANP plasma levels are increased in cirrhosis, the secretory mechanism following volume stimulation is intact but the renal responsiveness to ANP seems to be impaired.

ANP in Human Cirrhosis

ANP Plasma Levels

In a great number of patients of all stages of liver cirrhosis ANP plasma levels have been investigated; however, with different techniques of measurement of ANP, different study designs (diuretic treatment, sodium restricted diet) the data obtained varied considerably [2, 6, 7, 10, 11, 13, 14, 16, 17, 20, 21, 22, 25, 27, 28]. Our results of a study in 52 patients with cirrhosis (see Fig. 3) are representative for what has been found by others, as most authors described elevated mean levels of ANP in the plasma. The wide scatter of ANP plasma concentration (see Fig. 3) demonstrates, that some of the patients have normal or even low levels of the peptide as it has been described by several other investigators [2, 6, 10, 12, 22, 28].

Elevated ANP concentrations in the plasma may be caused by increased secretion, decreased metabolism or circulation of ANP-like material, cross-reacting in some of the assay systems. Gines et al. studied in humans the secretion of ANP by measuring the ANP directly in the coronary sinus [14]. He could demonstrate a significantly elevated secretion in patients with liver cirrhosis. To further exclude the possibility of an altered peripheral extraction of the peptide Gines investigated the splachnic extraction of ANP in cirrhotic patients and in controls. No significant difference between both groups could be obeserved. The metabolism of the peptide has been further elucidated by measurement of the plasma half life of ANP. In accordance with other groups we could demonstrate a comparable plasma disappearance rate of ANP-bolus between cirrhotic patients and healthy controls. Recently Imura et al. further stressed this issue [15] by investigating the distribution of alpha and gamma ANP in these two groups. Even though ANP plasma levels were slightly but not significantly elevated in cirrhotic patients the ratio of the two peptides was identical, suggesting a normal pattern of ANP processing and secretion in cirrhosis. In contrast to congestive heart failure ANP immunoreactivity in patients with liver cirrhosis truly represents ANP as by Arendt et al. could be demonstrated using sensitive HPLC methods [1].
Summarizing these studies it seems most likely that elevated ANP plasma levels in cirrhosis are caused by an increased secretion rate of peptide.

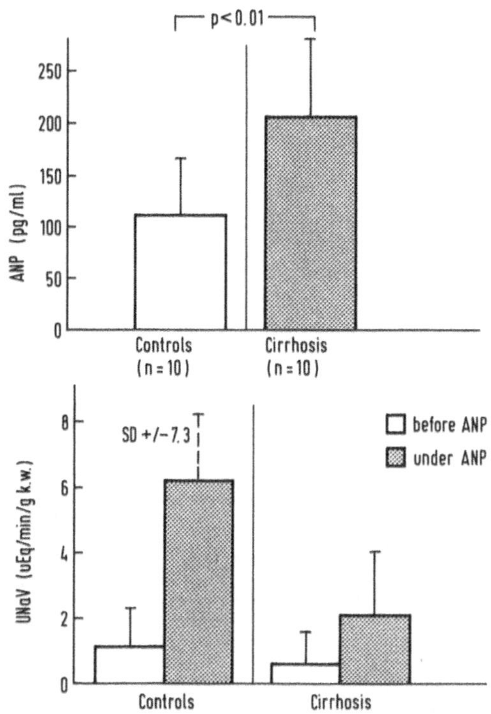

Fig. 2. a. Mean values +/− standard deviation of ANP plasma levels in control rats and in rats with CCl_4 induced liver cirrhosis. **b.** Mean values ± standard deviation of the urinary sodium excretion (UNaV) per gram kidney weight (k.w.) before and under ANP infusion in control rats (n = 9) and in rats with CCl_4 induced liver cirrhosis (n = 10)

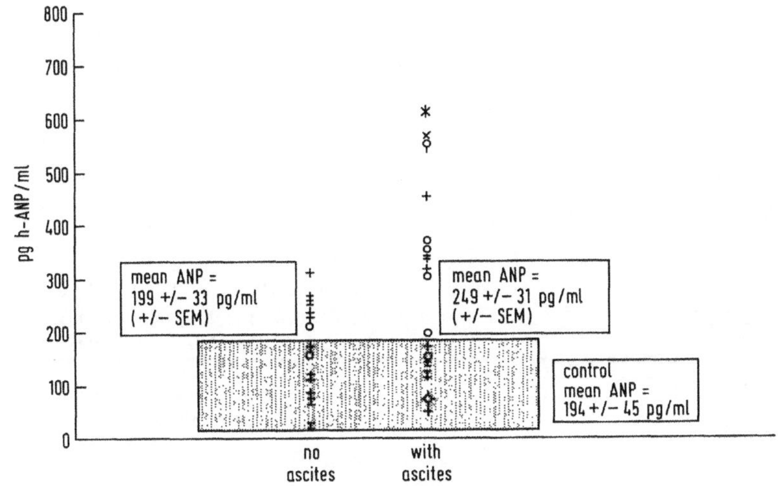

Fig. 3. Single values of ANP plasma levels in healthy volunteers (n = 32) and in patients with liver cirrhosis with (n = 28) and without ascites (n = 24)

ANP Secretion Following Volume Expansion

Several authors investigated the ANP response to acute volume expansion in patients with liver cirrhosis. Peritoneovenous shunting, a procedure known to be associated with an increase of sodium- and water excretion in patients with liver cirrhosis and ascites, acutely increases circulating plasma volume. Campbell et al. could demonstrate a severalfold, rapid increase of ANP plasma levels following this procedure in patients with cirrhosis [7].

An excellent model to compare the effect of an acute volume stimulation on ANP plasma levels between healthy and cirrhotic subjects represents the "head out water immersion" procedure [9]. In healthy persons it induces a two fold rise in plasma ANP levels. In cirrhotic patients the ANP release after one hour of water immersion was found to be impaired in patients with ascites [13]. These findings were contradicted by Epstein et al. who demonstrated an even higher ANP release in patients with ascites and edema compared to controls after head out water immersion [10]. It is important to note that Epstein reported on a good stimulation of ANP in some patients who showed an only inadaequate increase of natriuresis and diuresis after head out water immersion. Thus one might conclude that the release of ANP to a physiological volume stimulus is intact but that the renal response to ANP is impaired. The reduced increase of ANP secretion in patients with ascites as it was described by Gerbes might be explained by data of our group on the application of an ANP bolus (50 μg) prior to and after successful treatment of the ascites. As it is shown in Fig. 4 ANP plasma levels following bolus injection of the peptide are lowered compared to controls in cirrhotic patients with ascites, whereas the ANP levels were completely normalized after successful treatment of the ascites. One possible reason might be a rapid distribution of ANP into the ascites. This conclusion is supported by direct measurements of ANP-levels in the ascites [4].

Renal Effects of Exogenous ANP

In healthy subjects infusion of synthetic human ANP-28 is followed by a significant increase of natriuresis and diuresis [28, 30]. The first report on an infusion of ANP for 1 hour in a cirrhotic subject with ascites was encouraging [12] but further studies revealed a great variability in the renal response to ANP in cirrhosis. Salerno reported on a comparable increase in natriuresis and diuresis in cirrhotic patients without avid sodium retention compared to normal controls [27]. However, in cirrhotic

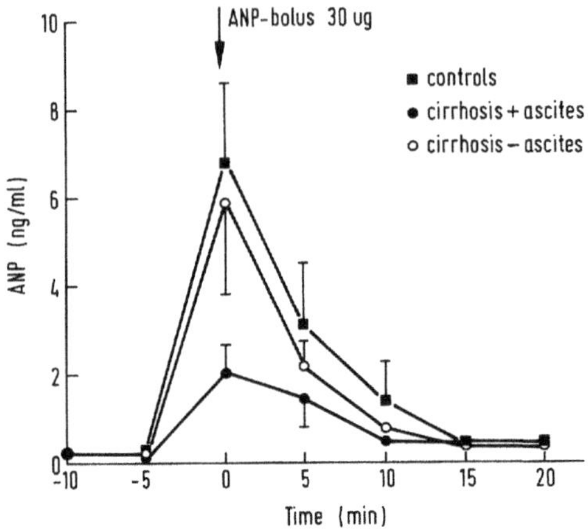

Fig. 4. ANP plasma levels following ANP bolus injection in control patients (n = 7) and in patients with liver cirrhosis (n = 6) before (cirrhosis + ascites) and after (cirrhosis – ascites) successful treatment of the ascites

patients with markedly impaired sodium excretion the diuretic and natriuretic effects of ANP were attenuated. The authors evaluated in their cohort of patients a significant ($r = 0.81$, $p < 0.001$) positive correlation between sodium excretion and the renal response to ANP. In our group of 19 patients we could not demonstrate such a correlation but demonstrated a weak inverse correlation between basal ANP plasma levels and the magnitude of the natriuretic response to an ANP bolus injection ($r = 0.64$, $p < 0.05$).

We have previously reported on the experimental use of ANP on a clinical basis in patients with liver cirrhosis and ascites [3]. The observation that only pulsatile administration of the peptide but not chronic infusion is leading to an increase in sodium excretion might indicate a receptor down regulation responsible for the impaired renal response to ANP in some of the cirrhotic patients. On this theoretical basis it might be expected that pulsatile treatment possibly resensitizes such a downregulated system. However, in six cirrhotic patients chronically treated with a regime of five nightly bolus injections (30 μg each) of ANP a wide scatter of responses was observed. In some patients sodium excretion and urinary output significantly increased while body weight decreased. In other patients these parameters did not change at all. No factors could be elucidated to date to clearly predict which of the patients are likely to profit by such therapeutic approach and which are not.

These studies suggest a highly variable renal response to ANP which might be coregulated by a number of factors. The available data support the hypothesis that the effect of the peptide is impaired on the renal level at certain stages of liver cirrhosis.

Conclusion

Experimental data as well as studies in humans demonstrated that ANP secretion is normal or even increased in cirrhosis as compared to controls. The metabolism of the hormone seems to be unaltered in cirrhosis. ANP is probably not primarily involved in the dysregulation of sodium and water homeostasis in patients with cirrhosis but rather secondarily altered. The intact responsiveness of ANP to volume stimulus in cirrhosis makes it probable that elevated ANP levels indicate an elevated plasma volume, thus supporting the overflow theory of ascites formation. The reduced natriuretic and diuretic effects of exogenous ANP in cirrhosis suggests an inhibition of ANP effects on the renal level.

References

1. Arendt RM, Gerbes AL, Ritter D, Stangl E (1986) Molecular weight heterogeneity of plasma ANF in cardiovascular disease. Klin Wochenschr 64 [Suppl VI]:97–102
2. Bonkowsky HL, Hartle DK, Mellen BG, Kutner M, Galambos JT (1988) Plasma concentrations of immunoreactive atrial natriuretic peptide in hospitalized cirrhotic and noncirrhotic patients: Evidence for a role of

deficient atrial natriuretic peptide in pathogenesis of cirrhotic ascites. Am J Gastroenterol 83:531–535

3. Brabant G, Jüppner H, Kirschner M, Böker K, Schmidt FW, Hesch RD (1986) Human atrial natriuretic peptide (ANP) for the treatment of patients with liver cirrhosis and ascites. Klin Wochenschr 64 [Suppl VI]: 108–111
4. Brabant G, Stegner H, Lueg H, Stolze D, Brunkhorst R, Schmidt FW, Hesch RD (1988) Effect of an ANP bolus injection on endocrine and renal regulation in patients with liver cirrhosis and ascites. Springer, Berlin Heidelberg New York (in press)
5. Brunkhorst R, Malcharzik CH, Roth A, Koch KM, Kühn KW (1987) Renal effects of atrial natriuretic peptide in rats with liver cirrhosis with and without Captopril pretreatment. International Congress of Nephrology, London 1987 (abstract)
6. Burghardt W, Wernze H, Diehl KL (1986) Atrial natriuretic peptide in hepatic cirrhosis: Relation to stage of disease, sympathoadrenal system and renin-aldosteron axis. Klin Wochenschr 64 [Suppl VI]: 103–107
7. Campbell PJ, Skorecki KL, Logan AG, Wong PY, Leung W, Greig P, Blendis LM (1987) Acute effects of peritoneosvenous shunting on plasma atrial natriuretic peptide in cirrhotic patients with massive refractory ascites. Am J Med 84:112–119
8. De Bold AJ (1986) Atrial natriuretic factor: An overview. Fed Proc 45:2081–2085
9. Epstein M (1985) Derangements of renal water handling in liver diesease. Gastroenterology 89:1415–1425
10. Epstein M, Loutzenhiser RD, Friedland E (1986) Increases in circulating atrial natriuretic factor during immersion induced central hypervolemia in normal humans. J Hypertens 4 [Suppl 2]:S93–S99
11. Fernandez-Cruz A, Marco J, Cuadrado LM, Gutkowska J, Rodriguez-Puyol D, Caramelo C, Lopez-Novoa JM (1985) Plasma levels of atrial natriuretic peptide in cirrhotic patients. Lancet II:1439–1440
12. Fyhrquist F, Tötterman KJ, Tikkanen I (1985) Infusion of atrial natriuretic peptide in liver cirrhosis with ascites. Lancet 7:1439
13. Gerbes AL, Arendt RM, Ritter D, Jungst D, Zahringer J, Paumgartner P (1986) Plasma atrial natriuretic factor in patients with cirrhosis. N Engl J Med 313:1609–1610
14. Gines P, Jimenez W, Arroyo V, Navasa M, Lopez C, Tito L, Serra A, Bosch J, Sanz G, Rivera F, Rodes J (1988) Atrial natriuretic factor in cirrhosis with ascites: Plasma levels, cardiac release and splachnic extraction. Hepatology 8:636–642
15. Itoh H, Nakaao K, Sugawara A, Saito Y, Mukoyama M, Morii N, Yamada T, Shiono S, Arai H, Hosoda K, Imura H (1988) Atrial natriuretic polypeptide (ANP) derived peptides in human plasma: Cosecretion of N-terminal ANP fragment and ANP. J Clin Endocrinol Metab 67:429–437
16. Jüppner H, Brabant G, Kapteina U, Kirschner M, Klein H, Hesch RD (1986) Direct radioimmunoassay for human atrial natriuretic peptide and its clinical evaluation. Biochem Biophys Res Commun 139: 1215–1223
17. Kawasaki H, Uemasu J, Maeda N, Hirayama C, Kobayashi T, Sakurai H (1987) Plasma levels of atrial natriuretic peptides in patients with chronic liver disease. Am J Gastroenterol 82:727–731
18. Levy M (1977) Sodium retention in dogs with cirrhosis and ascites. Efferent mechanisms. Am J Physiol 233:F586–F592
19. Liebermann FL, Denison EK, Reynolds TB (1970) The relationship of plasma volume, portal hypertension, ascites and renal sodium retention in cirrhosis: The overflow theory of ascites formation. Ann NY Acad Sci 170:202–212
20. Morgan T, Imada T, Inagami T (1986) Atrial natriuretic protein in the hepatorenal syndrome. Hepatology 6:1215 (abstract)
21. Nishiuchi T, Saito H, Yamasaki Y, Saito S (1986) Radioimmunoassay for atrial natriuretic peptide: method and results in normal subjects and in patients with various dieseases. Clin Chim Acta 159:45–57
22. Nozuki M, Mouri T, Itoi K, Takahashi K, Totsune K, Saito T (1986) Plasma concentration of atrial natriuretic peptide in various diseases. Tohoku J Exp Med 148:439–447
23. Olivera A, Gutkowska J, Rodriguez-Puyol D, Fernandez-Cruz A, Lopez-Novoa JM (1988) Atrial natriuretic peptide in rats with experimental cirrhosis of the liver without ascites. Endocrinology 122:840–846
24. Papper S (1958) The role of the kidney in Laennec's cirrhosis of the liver. Medicine (Baltimore) 37:299–316

Atrial Natriuretic Peptide and Chronic Renal Failure

W. Rascher and M. Bald,

Universitätsklinik für Kinder- und Jugendmedizin (GHS), Essen, FRG

Summary. Experimental and clinical studies are reviewed on the role of atrial natriuretic peptide in fluid volume and cardiovascular homeostasis in chronic renal failure. In patients with end-stage renal disease, atrial natriuretic peptide is elevated prior to hemodialysis and lowered by hemodialysis, hemofiltration or ultrafiltration. Volume overload is the most important stimulus for elevation of plasma ANP in chronic renal failure, and concomitant cardiac enlargement and arterial hypertension may play a role.

Plasma ANP does not contribute to long-term regulation of sodium homeostasis, but is released in an exaggerated manner in response to acute volume load in chronic renal failure. Plasma ANP is a useful index of volume overload in patients with chronic renal failure.

Key words: Atrial natriuretic peptide – Chronic renal failure – Continuous ambulatory peritoneal dialysis – Hemodialysis – Hemofiltration – Volume overload

Atrial natriuretic peptide (ANP) appears to play an important role in the regulation of fluid volume and arterial blood pressure [8, 15]. Since volume homeostasis is markedly altered in chronic renal failure (CRF), early investigations on the role of ANP as sodium and water sensitive circulating hormone system included patients with end-stage renal disease on intermittant hemodialysis [21]. The present communication summarizes briefly clinical and experimental studies of ANP in CRF, and demonstrates the clinical relevance of measurement of ANP as marker of fluid volume overload.

Plasma ANP and Volume Overload

After the first observation of elevated plasma ANP measurements in children with end-stage renal disease on hemodialysis [21], numerous other investigators reported subsequently similar findings [1, 2, 4, 5, 6, 9, 10, 14, 16, 17, 18, 22, 23, 25, 26, 27, 30]. Predialysis plasma ANP is significantly higher than those in a normal control goup and it decreases during hemodialysis or hemofiltration (Fig. 1). The majority of the patients on dialysis had post-dialysis plasma ANP levels that did not differ from a normal control group. However, a minority of them had still elevated levels that may represent

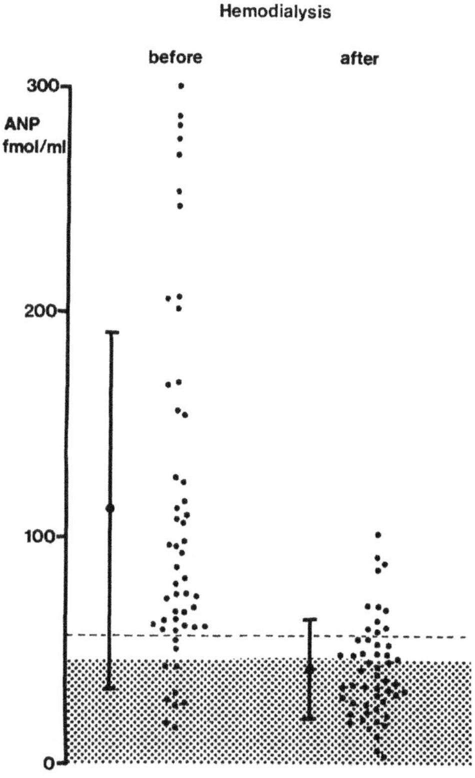

Fig. 1. Plasma concentration of atrial natriuretic peptide (ANP) before and after hemodialysis in children and adolescents with end stage renal disease. Hatched area represents x ± 2 SD of normal age-matched controls. Dotted line represents x + 3 SD of normal controls, the arbitrarily defined upper normal value

volume overload or cardiac involvement of their disease.

Since most patients undergoing hemodialysis accumulate sodium and water between dialysis sessions (in our own study about 5% of body weight), predialysis plasma ANP may be elevated due to volume overload. During hemodialysis or hemofiltration with fluid removal, plasma ANP decreases significantly. The most likely explanation of the changes during the dialysis session is that plasma ANP concentrations are volume-related and removal of fluid is associated with a fall of plasma ANP. This is corroborated by the close linear correlation between plasma ANP and right atrial pressure or pulmonary capillary wedge pressure in patients with renal replacement therapy [16, 22, 30]. In hemodialysed patients, these pressures correlated closely with the state of hydration [11]. Further studies using ultrafiltration, e.g. fluid removal without dialysis prior to hemodialysis [18, 20, 26] support further the role of ANP as volume related hormone in CRF. ANP falls rapidly without significant changes in plasma osmolality, urea and electrolytes [26] and paralleled changes in body weight [20, 26]. During reperfusion with normal saline of volume removed by ultrafiltration, plasma ANP concentration rises to similar or even higher levels compared to the pre-ultrafiltration state [18]. Pruszczynski et al. [18] calculated from this study that plasma ANP decreased 16–22 pg/ml for each 100 ml plasma water removed and increased 27–42 pg/ml for each 100 ml substitution fluid infused. Furthermore, plasma ANP is unchanged during isovolemic hemodialysis, i.e. dialysis without significant fluid removal or changes in body weight, because of high residual urinary output (Fig. 2).

In our studies the majority of children and adolescents treated by continuous ambulatory peritoneal dialysis (CAPD) achieved plasma ANP levels within the normal range which was calculated by the mean value 3 standard deviations of 96 control subjects aged 4 months to 16 years [19]. Twelve of our 32 pediatric patients on CAPD presented in Fig. 3 have been reported previously [20]. The date in children are in part at variance to that reported in adults on CAPD [5]. In adults mean plasma ANP was more than 4 times higher in patients on CAPD compared to control subjects. These authors demonstrated also that additional fluid volume retention in CAPD resulted in a further increase of plasma ANP in 8 patients.

Thus, plasma ANP is a volume-related hormone and the regulation (release and suppression) is well functioning in patients with CRF. Fluid volume overload is the most important stimulus for plasma ANP in CRF. However, other determinants of plasma ANP in CRF have to be discussed.

2. Plasma ANP and Glomerular Filtration Rate in CRF

Shenker et al. [23] reported a significant linear relationship between plasma ANP

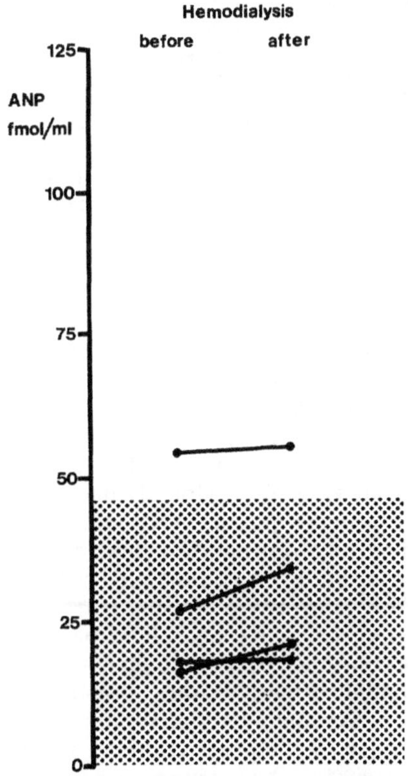

Fig. 2. Plasma concentration of atrial natriuretic peptide (ANP) before and after hemodialysis in 4 children and adolescents with endstage renal disease. Dialysis was performed without significant ultrafiltration and weight loss because of high residual urine output (isovolemic hemodialysis)

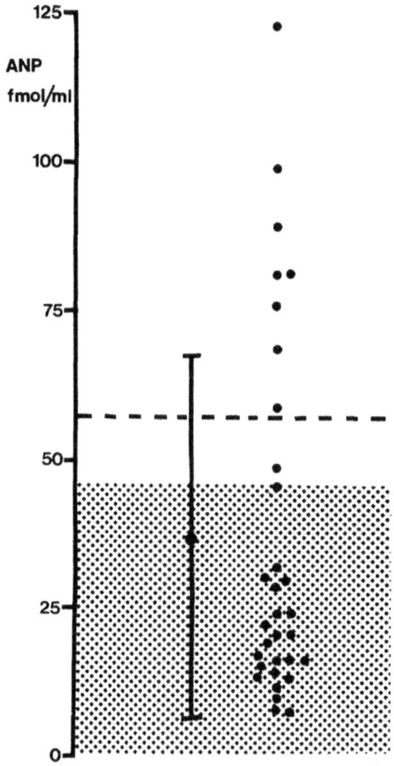

Fig. 3. Plasma concentration of atrial natriuretic peptide (ANP) in children and adolescents on continuous ambulatory peritoneal dialysis (CAPD). Symbols see Fig. 1

and blood urea nitrogen in patients suffering from CRF. Since patients with water retention and edema formation had higher plasma ANP concentrations, water overload appears to be the stimulus for ANP secretion. Predel et al. [17] found a linear correlation between plasma ANP and serum creatinine and plasma ANP and arterial blood pressure in 16 non-dialysed patients with CRF. Since blood pressure correlated with serum creatinine and blood pressure was not controlled by diuretic agents and/or other antihypertensive drugs, blood pressure elevation combined with sodium retention (urinary sodium excretion: 75 mmol/24 h) appeared to be the cause of ANP elevation. Similar findings were reported by other authors [9, 28]. Plasma ANP correlated with mean arterial blood pressure, but not with serum creatinine in non-dialysed patients. Plasma ANP was related to the cardio-thoracic ratio on chest X-ray films. In our own series of 12 children and adolescents with advanced chronic renal failure, we were unable to find a significant relationship between plasma ANP and clearances of inulin and paraminohippurate (Fig. 4). The patients had increased compensatory sodium excretion and blood pressure was controlled by diuretics and other antihypertensive agents.

3. Plasma ANP and Metabolism in CRF

The kidney may play an important role in the clearance of plasma ANP and impairment of renal function may account for elevated ANP in CRF. Luft et al. [12] observed that plasma half life of atriopeptin III is doubled and plasma clearance reduced in anephric rats compared to normal controls. During its passage to the kidneys about 50% of endogenous ANP disappears from the plasma [7, 29], indicating that the kidney is indeed an important ANP degrading organ. However, the observation of rapid decline of plasma ANP with plasma volume contraction during hemofiltration/ultrafiltration in uremic patients [21, 26] demonstrates that even at high levels of plasma ANP, a marked suppression of ANP can occure. This suggests that the regulation of ANP is intact and increased secretion rather than low catabolism is responsible for elevated plasma ANP in CRF.

Saxenhofer et al. [22] have calculated that only 12% of the total plasma ANP clearance in normal man can be attributed to a kidney based mechanism supporting that decreased metabolism does not contribute significantly to raised plasma ANP in CRF. These authors further could demonstrate that only a small fraction of plasma ANP was removed through the hemofilter or hemodialyser during blood purification. Of the ANP cleared only 30% appeared in the ultrafiltrate and 14% in the dialysate, assuming that ANP is rapidly metabolised or/and bound to the dialysis membrane, filters or plastic material.

4. ANP and Sodium Homeostasis in CRF

Elevated plasma ANP in CRF may play a role in promoting adaptive increase in

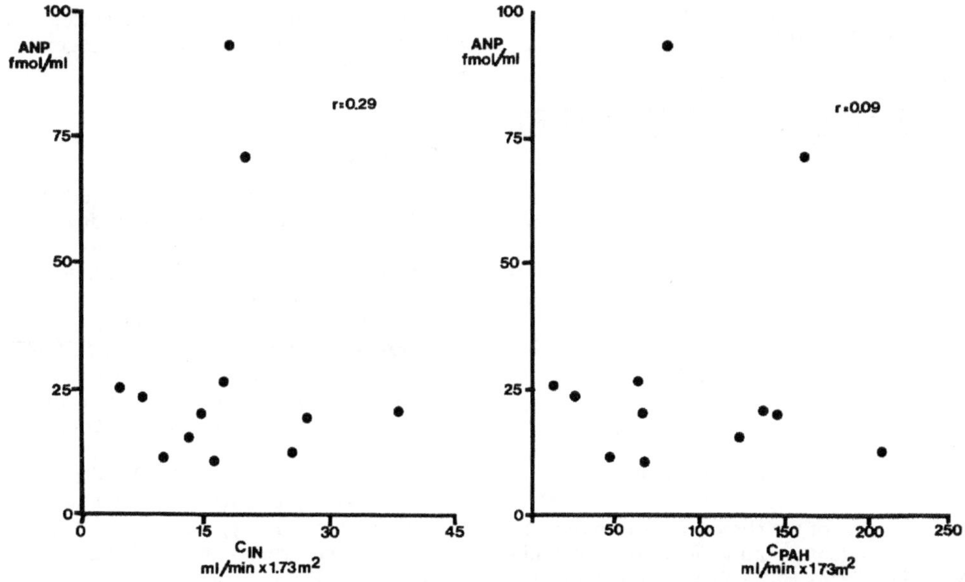

Fig. 4. Relationship between plasma concentration of atrial natriuretic peptide (ANP) and clearances of inulin (C_{IN}) or of paraminohippurate (C_{PAH}) in 12 children and adolescents with chronic renal failure

sodium excretion per nephron in CRF. Luft et al. [13] have shown that rats with CRF studied 3 to 4 weeks after subtotal nephrectomy had a wide range of fractional sodium excretion. Plasma ANP and atrial tissue content of ANP in sodium loaded rats were not related to differences in fractional sodium excretion. These results do not support the notion that ANP plays a role in the adaptation of remaining nephrons to a high sodium intake and thus, a long-term sodium homeostasis in CRF.

Lack of relationship between fractional sodium excretion and plasma ANP in children with CRF (Tulassay, Rascher and Schärer, unpublished observation) support this notion. However, Smith et al. [24] found that rats studied two days and two weeks after the total nephrectomy had indeed raised plasma levels of ANP when exposed to high sodium and water intake. Interestingly enough, plasma ANP was lower two weeks than two days after the nephrectomy, indicating that ANP response might be transient and not related to sodium intake per se, but to increased atrial pressure due to volume overload. Unfortunately, data on volume status (body weight) and the relation between plasma ANP and fractional or absolute sodium excretion were not reported in the study [24]. Cole et al. [3] reported an exaggerated diuretic and natriuretic response to acute infusion of atriopeptin III to rats with subtotal nephrectomy 4 weeks before the study.

Related findings were reported in clinical studies in patients with CRF. Acute volume expansion (saline infusion) induced a more pronounced stimulation of plasma ANP and increased fractional sodium excretion in patients with CRF compared to normal controls [4]. Analysis of covariance revealed that plasma ANP represented the main factor of changes in fractional sodium excretion after acute sodium and volume loading. This points to an important role of ANP in CRF to compensate for acute, short-termin sodium and volume overload.

5. Plasma ANP as Index of Volume Overload in Patients with CRF

Expansion of blood volume appears to be the most important stimulus for elevation of plasma ANP in patients with CRF. Concomitant cardiac enlargement and arterial hypertension may play a role. Thus, determination of plasma ANP is a clinical useful

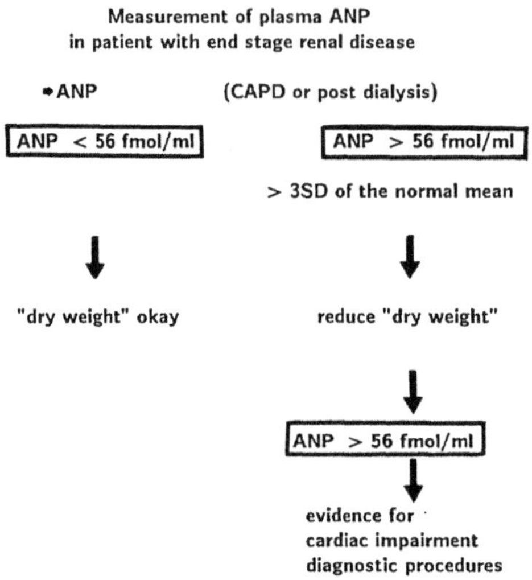

Fig. 5. Scheme of the clinical relevance of measurement of plasma atrial natriuretic peptide (ANP) in patients with end stage renal disease. Differential diagnosis of elevated plasma ANP in patients with renal replacement therapy

tool to detect fluid volume overload in patients with CRF, especially in those with renal replacement therapy [6, 20, 26].

Plasma ANP levels less than 56 fmol/ml in our assay, corresponding to less than 3 standard deviation of the mean value of control subjects [19] are arbitrarily defined as normal body fluid volume status. Higher plasma ANP concentrations in patients on CAPD, after hemodialysis or ultrafiltration may indicate volume overload or cardiac impairment (Fig. 5).

In line with the clinical examination (blood pressure, edema, dyspnoe, chest X-ray, and echocardiography) body weight should be reduced by increasing ultrafiltration in patients with raised ANP levels. In case of persisting high ANP plasma concentrations at the end of hemodialysis or hemofiltration despite weight reduction or if weight reduction is not tolerated, cardiac diagnostic procedures should be performed to detect the cause of underlying cardiac insufficiency.

In our hands, routine determination of plasma ANP helps to detect fluid volume overload in patients with chronic renal failure.

The studies of the authors were supported by a grant from the Deutsche Forschungsgemeinschaft (Ra 326/1-3)

References

1. Anderson JV, Raine AEG, Proudler A, Bloom SR (1980) Effect of haemodialysis on plasma concentrations of atrial natriuretic peptide in adult patients with chronic renal failure. J Endocr 110:193–196
2. Cannella G, Rodella A, Brunori G, Caggiotti M, Sandrini M, Maiorca R (1987) Plasma concentrations of atrial natriuretic peptide in relation to body fluid status in chronic uraemia. Nephrol Dial Transplant 2:158–160
3. Cole BR, Kuhnline MA, Needleman P (1985) Atriopeptin III – A potent natriuretic, diuretic, and hypotensive agent in rats with chronic renal failure. J Clin Invest 76:2413–2415
4. Czekalski S, Michel C, Dussaule JC, Touraine P, Mignon F, Ardaillou R (1988) Atrial natriuretic peptide and adaption of sodium urinary excretion in patients with chronic renal failure. Clin Sci 75:243–249
5. Deray G, Maistre G, Basset JY, Cacoub P, Carayon A, Anouar M, Baumelou A, Legrand JC, Ancri D, Jacobs C (1988) Plasma levels of atrial natriuretic peptide in chronically dialyzed patients. Kidney Int 34 [Suppl 25]:S86–S88
6. Eisenhauer T, Talartschik J, Scheler F (1986) Detection of fluid overload by plasma concentration of human atrial natriuretic peptide (h-ANP) in patients with renal failure. Klin Wochenschr 65 [Suppl VI]:68–72
7. Espiner EA, Nicholls MG, Yandle TG, Crozier IG, Cuneo RC, McCormick D, Ikram H (1986) Studies on the secretion, metabolism and action of atrial natriuretic peptide in man. J Hypertens 4 [Suppl 2]: S85–S91
8. Goetz KL (1988) Physiology and pathophysiology of atrial peptides. Am J Physiol 254:E1–E15
9. Hasegawa K, Matsushita Y, Inoue T, Morii H, Ishibashi M, Yamaji T (1986) Plasma levels of atrial natriuretic peptide in patients with chronic renal failure. J Clin Endocrinol Metab 63:819–822
10. Hodsman GP, Jackson B, Debrevi LM, Ogawa K, Johnston CI (1987) Atrial natriuretic factor in chronic renal failure: Studies in man and the rat. Clin Exp Pharmacol Physiol 14:247–251
11. Jahn H, Schohn D, Schmitt R (1981) Hemodynamic studies in chronic terminal

renal insufficiency – Effects of hemodialysis, hemofiltration and ultrafiltration procedures. Nephrologie 2:53–62
12. Luft FC, Lang RE, Aronoff GR, Ruskoaho H, Toth M, Ganten D, Sterzel RB, Unger T (1986) Atriopeptin III kinetics and pharmacodynamics in normal and anephric rats. J Pharmacol Exp Ther 236:416–418
13. Luft FC, Sterzel RB, Lang RE, Trabold EM, Veelken R, Ruskoaho H, Gao Y, Ganten D, Unger T (1986) Atrial natriuretic factor determinations and chronic sodium homeostasis. Kidney Int 29:1004–1010
14. Morris M, Cain M, Russell A, Elliott J, Chalmers J (1987) Direct radioimmunoassay of human plasma atrial natriuretic peptide in various normal and pathophysiological states: Increase in renal and cardiac failure during exercise. Clin Exp Hypertens A9: 703–718
15. Needleman PH, Greenwald (1986) Atriopeptin: A cardiac hormone intimately involved in fluid, electrolyte, and blood-pressure homeostasis. N Engl J Med 314: 828–834
16. Pacher R, Frass M, Hartter E, Woloszczuk W, Leithner C (1986) Continuous pump-driven hemofiltration associated with a decline in alpha-atrial natriuretic peptide. Crit Care Med 14:1010–1014
17. Predel HG, Bäcker A, Kipnowski J, Düsing R, Kramer HJ (1987) Relationship of plasma concentrations of human atrial natriuretic peptide to renal function and blood pressure in patients with progressive chronic renal failure. Klin Wochenshcr 65 [Suppl VIII]: 127–132
18. Pruszczynski W, Viron B, Gzekalski S, Mignon F, Ardaillou R (1987) Role of cardiac parasympathetic dysfunction in atrial natriuretic peptide response to volume changes in patients with chronic renal failure. Mineral Electrolyte Metab 13:333–339
19. Rascher W, Bald M, Kreis J, Tulassay T, Heinrich U, Schärer K (1987) Atrial natriuretic peptide in infants and children. Hormone Res 28:58–63
20. Rascher W, Bald M, Kröner F, Tulassay T, Müller-Wiefel DE (1988) Klinische Wertigkeit der Messung des atrialen natriuretischen Peptids im Plasma von Kindern mit chronischer Niereninsuffizienz. Z Kardiol 7 [Suppl 2]: 61–64
21. Rascher W, Tulassay T, Lang RE (1985) Atrial natriuretic peptide in plasma of volume-overloaded children with chronic renal failure. Lancet II:303–305
22. Saxenhofer H, Gnädinger MP, Weidmann P, Shaw S, Schohn D, Hess C, Uehlinger DE, Jahn H (1987) Plasma levels and dialysance of atrial natriuretic peptide in terminal renal failure. Kidney Int 32:554–561
23. Shenker Y, Port FK, Swartz RD, Gross MD, Grekin RJ (1987) Atrial natriuretic hormone secretion in patients with renal failure. Life Sci 41:1635–1644
24. Smith S, Anderson S, Ballermann BJ, Brenner BM (1986) Role of atrial natriuretic peptide in adaption of sodium excretion with reduced renal mass. J Clin Invest 77: 1395–1398
25. Talartschik J, Eisenhauer T, Voth E, Sold G, Scheler F (1988) Ist der Plasma-ANP-Spiegel ein Index für die Volumenexpansion bei Dialysepatienten? Z Kardiol 77 [Suppl 2]: 72–77
26. Wilkins MR, Wood JA, Adu D, Lote CJ, Kendall MJ, Michael J (1986) Change in plasma immunoreactive atrial natriuretic peptide during sequential ultrafiltration and haemodialysis. Clin Sci 71:157–160
27. Yamamoto Y, Higa T, Kitamura K, Tanaka K, Kangawa K, Matsuo H (1985) Plasma concentration of atrial natriuretic polypeptide in chronic hemodialysis patients. Regulatory Peptides 4 [Suppl]:110–112
28. Yamamoto Y, Higa T, Kitamura K, Tanaka K, Kangawa K, Matsuo H (1987) Plasma concentration of human atrial natriuretic polypeptide in patients with impaired renal function. Clin Nephrol 27:84–86
29. Yandle TG, Richards AM, Nicholls MG, Cuneo R, Espiner EA, Livesey JH (1986) Metabolic clearance rate and plasma half life of alpha-human atrial natriuretic peptide in man. Life Sci 38:1827–1833
30. Zoccali C, Ciccarelli M, Mallamaci F, Delfino D, Salnitro F, Parlongo S, Maggiore Q (1986) Effect of ultrafiltration on plasma concentrations of atrial natriuretic peptide in haemodialysis patients. Nephrol Dial Transplant 1:188–191

Pharmacological Modification of the ANP System

C. Hirth, J.-P. Stasch, D. Neuser and S. Kazda

Bayer AG, Institut für Pharmakologie, Wuppertal, FRG

Summary. The search for drugs interacting with the ANP system to give favourable therapeutic effects has concentrated on the release and the metabolism of ANP. Regarding the release of ANP direct effects have to be distinguished from indirect ones. Both drug induced increases and decreases of ANP plasma levels may be indirectly mediated: Increased ANP plasma levels are noted after sodium retaining antihypertensives such as reserpine and minoxidil. On the other hand, the pathological high ANP plasma levels of SHR are normalized in parallel to the amelioration of cardiac hypertrophy by the natriuretic calcium antagonist nitrendipine. The mechanism for β-blocker-induced increase in plasma ANP is not clear as yet.

Direct effects on ANP release can be demonstrated using in vitro assays of isolated atria. An increase of ANP has been reported for agents increasing the intracellular calcium concentration such as the calcium agonist BAY K 8644, the newly discovered endogenous vasoconstrictor endothelin or the protein kinase C activator TPA. These effects can be antagonized by calcium antagonists, but calcium antagonists have no effect on baseline ANP release, and a reduction in intracellular or extracellular calcium has also been reported to increase ANP release in vitro.

A direct stimulatory effect on ANP release of isolated rat atria was found with the endogenous opioid peptide dynorphin. In contrast, the increase in ANP plasma levels after high dose of morphine seems to be mediated by the central nervous system.

For natriuretic drugs antagonization of ANP by monoclonal antibodies is another way to detect mechanisms of action involving endogenous ANP. Although the effects of exogenous and endogenous ANP were effectively blocked by the antibody in vivo, no diminution of the natriuretic effects of calcium antagonists or clonidine in rats could be observed.

Research in the metabolism of ANP has led to the discovery that enkephalinase inhibitors prolong the half life of ANP and enhance the effects of ANP. The therapeutic relevance of this mechanism has to be evaluated.

Key words: ANP – Pharmacology – reserpine – minoxidil – clonidine – nitrendipine – BAY N 1468

ANP is an attractive target for pharmacological interventions as it combines the effects of vasodilatation, natriuresis and suppression of the renin-aldosterone system. Drugs that mimick or enhance the effect of ANP might be useful in the treatment of hypertension, cardiac failure and other diseases associated with increased circulating volume. Theoretically, pharmacological interventions can be made at different levels: At the level of ANP release, or ANP metabolism or ANP receptor or even intracellularly involving the second messenger cGMP.

Effects on the release of ANP have been studied with various drugs in vivo and in vitro. Morphine was the first drug recognized to increase ANP plasma levels. In rats high doses of morphine increase plasma ANP as was shown by Gutkowska et al. [8], and this effect is blocked by naloxone. Naloxone alone also decreases basal ANP plasma levels. When morphine is administered centrally, far lower doses are required to give the same increase in ANP [3]. The effect of morphine on ANP release thus seems to be centrally mediated. In keeping with these results we also found no stimulatory effect of morphine on ANP-release of isolated atria [26]. The μ opioid agonist fentanyl was reported by Vollmar et al. [30] to act via a mechanism similar to morphine.

The ϰ opioid agonist dynorphin has been reported to increase ANP plasma levels after i.v. administration of high doses (162 nmol/kg i.v.) in rats [31].

In isolated rat atria dynorphin A (1–13) concentrations in the micromolar range cause a dose-dependent increase in ANP release (baseline: 240 ± 20 pg/ml, min; 8×10^{-7} mol/l dynorphin: 569 ± 224; 8×10^{-6} mol/l dynorphin: 1731 ± 155 pg/ml, min). This increase can be totally blocked by naloxone. 2×10^{-7} mol/l dynorphin is without effect on ANP secretion in vitro. This may explain the lack of effect on plasma ANP levels observed with lower dynorphin doses (23 nmol/kg i.v., Crum and Brown [3]). Basal plasma levels of endogenous dynorphine as determined by radioimmunoassay were 33 ± 1.7 pg/ml (n = 9) in conscious normotensive rats (Stasch and Hirth, unpublished results). They were unchanged (36 ± 2.3 pg/ml, n = 9) five minutes after acute volume expansion (20 ml/kg i.v. saline). Thus it seems very unlikely that the high concentrations of dynorphin needed for stimulation of ANP release are reached in the circulation. However, endogenous dynorphin is also localized in the heart [6], and local increases in dynorphin concentration might influence ANP release. Dynorphin is a ϰ-opioid agonist, and ϰ agonists are shown to enhance diuresis [15]. However, this increase in urine volume is accompanied by a decrease in urinary sodium concentration [13]. This pattern of effects cannot be attributed to ANP which causes a marked increase in urinary sodium concentration. In summary, the opioids give interesting hints to the regulation of ANP release but the picture is puzzling still and no therapeutical application of the ANP system has emerged as yet.

It was also tested whether some of the known antihypertensive drugs exert at least part of their effect via the ANP system.

We found a substantial increase in plasma ANP in strongly reserpinized rats (Fig. 1). However, this increase was associated with severe sodium retention and thus seems to be a secondary effect. Reserpine has numerous pharmacological actions and in order to have less side effects we turned to the arteriolar vasodilatator minoxidil. In fed rats subchronically treated with minoxidil sodium excretion is diminished during the first day and normalizes afterwards (Fig. 2). However, decreased hematocrit indicates sustained volume expansion and ANP levels are substantially increased with respect to controls on the third day of minoxidil treatment (Fig. 2). We wondered whether the normalization of sodium excretion is brought about by ANP. We therefore repeated the experiments with two groups of minoxidil and two groups of control rats (Fig. 3A). On the first day sodium excretion was reduced in the minoxidil group. On the second day the rats received an oral sodium loading and were fasted over night. These manoeuvers prolong the antinatriuretic action of minoxidil. Sodium excretion of the minoxidil treated rats normalized on the third day (Fig. 3B). However, this normalization was not brought about by ANP, as a

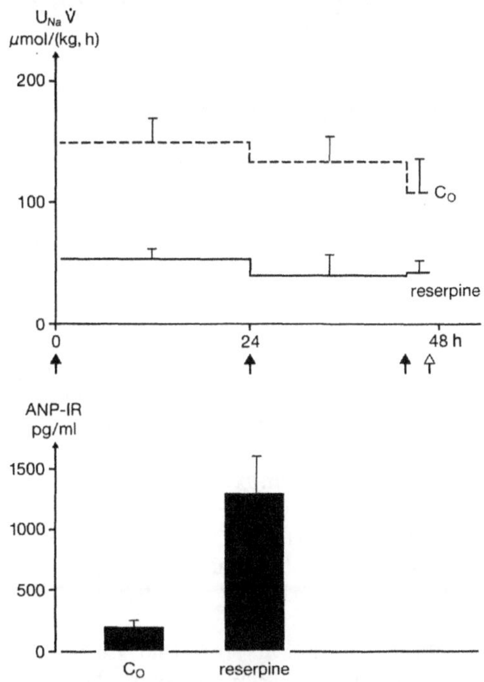

Fig. 1. *Top:* Sodium excretion ($U_{Na}\dot{V}$) of conscious rats in metabolic cages with free acess to food and drinking water. Solid line: treatment with 1.5 mg/kg i.p. reserpine at the times indicated by solid arrows. Broken lines: corresponding control. *Bottom:* Plasma ANP immunoreactivity (ANP-IR) of the same rats determined at the time indicated by the open arrow, n = 10 for each group

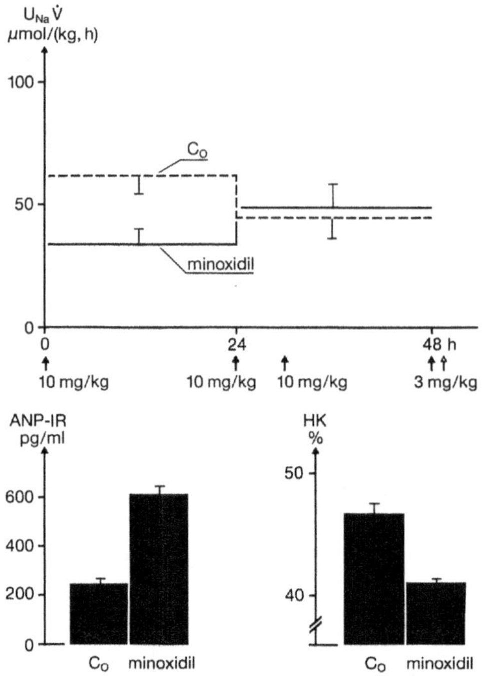

Fig. 2. *Top:* Sodium excretion ($U_{Na}\dot{V}$) of conscious rats in metabolic cages with free acess to food and drinking water. Solid line: oral treatment with minoxidil, times and dosages indicated by solid arrows. Broken line: corresponding control. *Bottom:* Plasma ANP immunoreactivity (ANP-IR) and hematocrit (HK) determined 90 min (open arrow) after the last p.o. administration, n = 10 for each group

monoclonal antibody that acts as a long-lasting ANP antagonist and was injected on the third day did not change sodium excretion (Fig. 3B) [12].

The effect of minoxidil on ANP can also be shown in acute experiments: When oral sodium loading is given, minoxidil produces a pronounced antinatriuresis and increased ANP levels can be measured after two hours (Table 1).

These experiments show that drug effects on ANP plasma levels have to be interpreted cautiously because the ANP system responds to alterations in volume status. Especially when ANP is activated, drug effects may be different than under normal conditions. It has been reported by many authors by now that ANP plasma levels are increased in spontaneously hypertensive rats (SHR) in comparison to the normotensive control strain of Wistar Kyoto rats (WKY). We made a long term treatment of SHR and WKY with nitrendipine and minoxidil for 11 weeks [25]. The antihypertensive effects of both drugs were similar, but the minoxidil treated rats gained more weight. When the rats were sacrificed at the end of the treatment period, the cardiac hypertrophy of SHR was aggravated by minoxidil and diminished by nitrendipine. In parallel, the high ANP plasma levels were further increased by minoxidil and almost normalized by nitrendipine. However, nitrendipine is not a drug that decreases ANP plasma levels per se as in normotensive WKY nitrendipine has no effect on ANP plasma levels, while minoxidil here again increases relative heart weight and ANP plasma levels.

Drug induced elevation of ANP plasma levels is not necessarily a benefit, it may also indicate unfavourable cardiac side effects.

In the case of sodium retention the mechanism is immediately clear, but sometimes it is hard to determine whether a drug exerts its effect on the ANP system by hemodynamic changes. For example, β-blockers are reported to increase ANP plasma levels: The β-blocker metroprolol was shown to cause a slight (50%) increase in plasma ANP levels after acute administration [18] in conscious hypertensive rats. This increase might account for the concomitant transient natriuresis. We found a doubling of ANP plasma levels by one week of treatment with propranolol in young spontaneously hypertensive rats (controls: 161 ± 15 pg/ml, propranolol: 336 ± 70 pg/ml, n = 8–9) (Hirth and Stasch, unpublished results). This effect of β-blockers was also demonstrated in humans: Thamsborg et al. [28] found an increase in ANP plasma levels of healthy volunteers with atenolol both at rest and during exercise. This β-blocker also increases ANP plasma levels in hypertensive patients [17]. It is suggested that hemodynamic changes are responsible for the effect of β-blockers but right atrial or pulmonary arterial pressure were not measured in parallel to ANP.

Good candidates for ANP releasing drugs should be those that are both antihypertensive and natriuretic. Contrasting to the situation in humans clonidine is strongly nat-

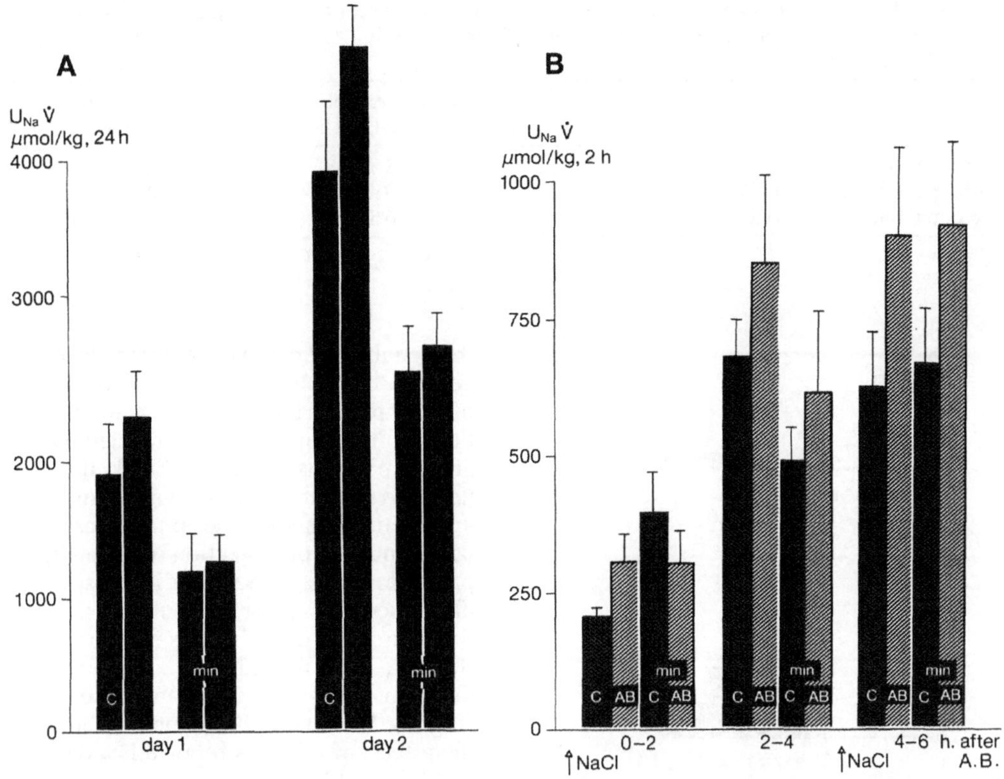

Fig. 3. A, B. Sodium excretion ($U_{Na}\dot{V}$) of conscious rats administered minoxidil (min, 3 mg/kg p.o.) or vehicle (c) twice daily. **A** first day: food and drinking water ad lib. second day: fasting, oral saline (20 ml/kg) loading, water ad lib. **B** third day: injection of the monoclonal antibody (AB, striped bas) or control solution with equal protein concentration (C). Oral saline loading both immediately and 4 h after injection

riuretic in the rat and it has been reported by Baranowska et al. [1] to increase ANP plasma levels after intravenous administration. However, the dose employed (50 μg) causes a sharp transient increase in blood pressure that is likely to promote ANP release. We therefore administered clonidine p.o. and tried to block the resulting natriuresis by administration of a monoclonal antibody against ANP. The clonidine induced natriuresis was not blocked (Table 2).

The antibody employed in these studies is an effective antagonist of exogenous ANP and endogenous ANP release by volume expansion [11]. On the other hand, it does not prevent the natriuresis induced by diuretics: furosemid is still active after antibody pretreatment [11]. The effect of muzolimine, another high ceiling diuretic, was also not

Table 1. Sodium excretion and ANP plasma levels determined 0–2 h and 2 h, respectively, after 3 mg/kg p.o. minoxidil or vehicle administered together with an oral sodium load (30 ml/kg, 0.9% NaCl) ($\bar{x} \pm$ SEM of 10 rats)

	sodium excretion μmol/kg, 2 h	plasma ANP pg/ml
minoxidil	241 ± 52	478 ± 34
control	793 ± 82	354 ± 19

Table 2. Effect of clonidine (0.1 mg/kg p.o. in tylose) and tylose control on sodium excretion and urine volume in conscious rats pretreated with monoclonal antibody (AB) or control mouse IgG (IgCo), n = 7 in each group

	sodium excretion µmol/kg, 2 h	urine volume ml/kg, 2 h
group I tylose control + IgCo	373 ± 98	12.7 ± 1.4
group II clonidine + IgCo	2960 ± 238	48.5 ± 2.1
group III clonidine + AB	2496 ± 124	47.2 ± 2.2
	n.s. vs. group II	

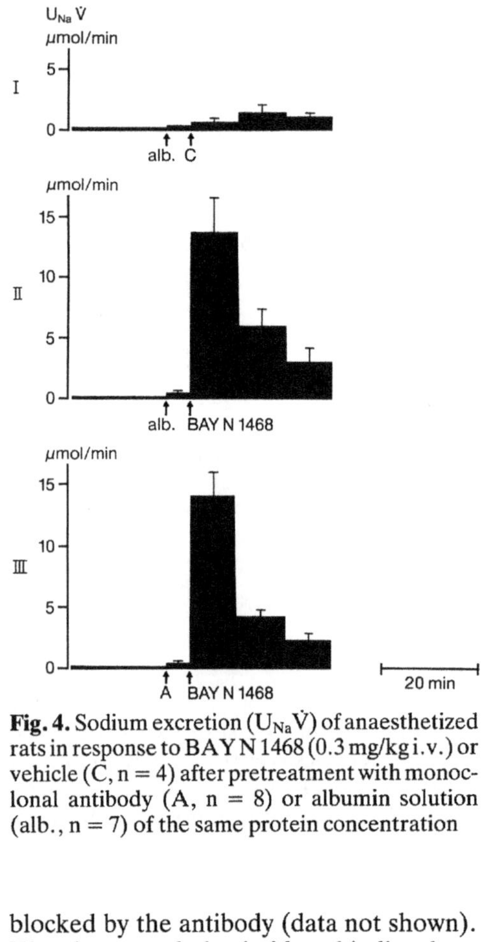

Fig. 4. Sodium excretion ($U_{Na}\dot{V}$) of anaesthetized rats in response to BAY N 1468 (0.3 mg/kg i.v.) or vehicle (C, n = 4) after pretreatment with monoclonal antibody (A, n = 8) or albumin solution (alb., n = 7) of the same protein concentration

blocked by the antibody (data not shown). We also tested the imidazothiadiazol-acrylamide BAY N 1468 (Fig. 4). Compounds of this class resemble ANP in their renal action as they increase GFR and renal blood flow [23]. But despite this similarity in the renal effect the natriuretic effect of BAY N 1468 is not mediated by ANP.

Of course the natriuretic effect of calcium antagonists prompted the question whether this renal effect could be mediated by endogenous ANP release. We found no increase of ANP plasma levels after oral administration of nitrendipine and other calcium antagonists. We also tried to block the pronounced natriuretic effect of nitrendipine in anesthetized rats by the monoclonal antibody: Intravenous injection of nitrendipine produces a dose-dependent increase in sodium excretion. Pretreatment with the antibody does not diminish this response, thus showing that the calcium antagonist induced natriuresis is independent of ANP (Fig. 5). However, nifedipine may enhance the effects of ANP, as reported by Seino et al. [21] in rabbits.

In humans reports on the effects of calcium antagonists on the ANP system are conflicting: On one hand, verapamil diminishes the increase of ANP plasma levels brought about by atrial pacing as reported by Haufe et al. [9]. The effects on ANP were paralleled by effects on cGMP. On the other hand, slight (20%) increases of ANP plasma levels have been reported after nifedipine sublingually by Rapelli et al. [19] and Shima et al. [22]. Cyclic GMP was not determined in these studies. Obviously the effect of calcium antagonists on the secretion of ANP is difficult to determine in humans after acute administration since ANP secretion is increased by tachycardia and since the ANP response is very quick and phasic.

In order to investigate the effect of drugs affecting the calcium homeostasis, it is perhaps better to start with an in vitro assay: The ANP release from isolated rat atria. The calcium agonist BAY K 8644 promotes the secretion of ANP [20]. BAY K 8644 is a racemat consisting of a calcium agonistic and a calcium antagonistic enantiomer. The promotion of ANP secretion is brougth

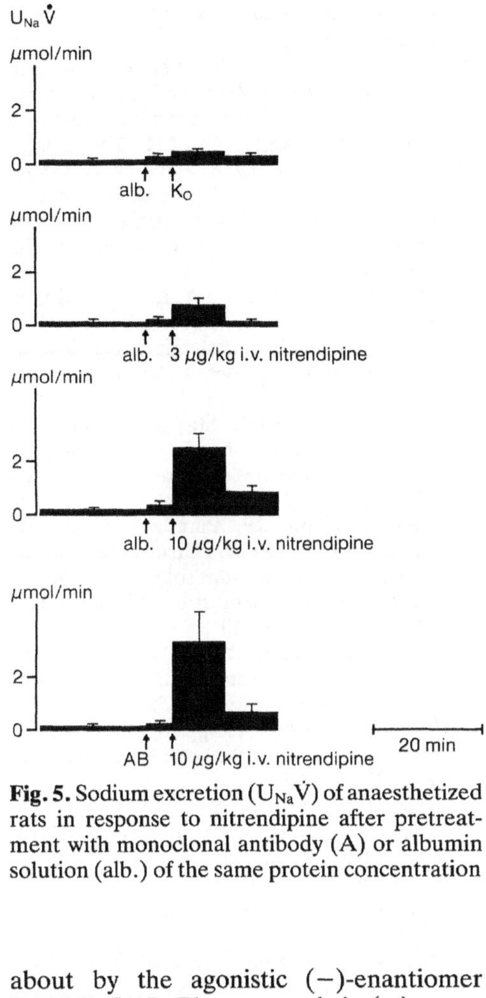

Fig. 5. Sodium excretion ($U_{Na}\dot{V}$) of anaesthetized rats in response to nitrendipine after pretreatment with monoclonal antibody (A) or albumin solution (alb.) of the same protein concentration

about by the agonistic (−)-enantiomer BAY R 5417. The antagonistic (+)-enantiomer BAY R 4407 has little effect on ANP secretion in vitro (H. Grote et al., unpublished results). This is also true for other calcium antagonists in our in vitro system. The newly discovered endogenous peptide endothelin that acts in many aspects like a calcium agonist also promotes the secretion of ANP as was shown by Fukuda et al. [5] in neonatal rat atria cardiocytes. The calcium antagonist nicardipine attenuates the effect of endothelin, but has no effect on ANP secretion under basal conditions. The protein kinase C activator TPA also has a positive effect on ANP secretion that adds to the effect of endothelin. TPA also potentiates the effect of the calcium agonist BAY K 8644 as was shown by Ruskoaho et al. [20]. These data suggest that intracellular calcium promotes the secretion of ANP. On the other hand, de Bold [2] observed an increase in ANP secretion from isolated atria after removal of extracellular calcium in EGTA containing perfusion fluid. Recently, Greenwald et al. [7] reported an increase of stimulated ANP secretion in isolated myocytes by the intracellular calcium chelator BAPTA. These investigations suggest that the dependence of ANP secretion on intracellular calcium concentration follows a bell-shaped curve. The in vitro system can thus help us to discriminate between direct and indirectly mediated drug effects on ANP release but the intracellular factors influencing ANP release are still unknown.

An in vitro incubation of isolated atria was combined with an ANP bioassay by Veress et al. [29]. In this assay, ANP secretion is promoted by angiotensin II and vasopressin. The effects were pronounced especially in the case of angiotensin II, but the physiological significance of this effects remains unknown since Lachance and Garcia [14] found an in vivo effect of angiotensin II only with pressor doses.

Physiological data on the metabolism of ANP are still incomplete in important points: Internalization of the receptor-bound protein is discussed as a main mechanism for inactivation. The role of the so called clearance receptor that binds ANP but is not coupled to guanylate cyclase is unknown as yet. However, it has also been recognized that a neutral metallopeptidase in kidney brush border membranes participates in ANP metabolism: This endopeptidase 24.11 cleaves the cysteine-phenylalanine bond within the ring structure and can be inhibited by known enkephalinase inhibitors such as thiorphan and phosphoramidone [27, 24]. This enzyme is regarded as the major factor degrading ANP in the kidney [24]. It has to be clarified whether enkephalinase inhibitors increase ANP plasma levels in humans, especially in patients with heart failure or severe hypertension.

Non-peptide drugs binding to the receptor that mediates the biological actions of ANP have not been found as yet, but the long known antikaliuric diuretic amiloride (for review see [4]) increases the sensitivity of guanylate cyclase to atrial natriuretic factor [10]. Amiloide potentiates ANP binding to the receptor even in purified adrenal zona glomerulosa receptors suggesting the presence of an allosteric binding site for amiloride on the receptor protein [16]. It is not clear as yet how the interaction with the ANP receptor might be related to the inhibitory effect of amiloride on Na^+/H^+ exchange and epithelial Na^+ channels.

Summing up the data on pharmacological effects on the ANP system provides no clear picture but rather a patchwork of effects and hypotheses. But such a patchwork also represents a challenge and a source of new ideas for the pharmacologist, and we may expect interesting new results to emerge in the next few years.

References

1. Baranowska B, Gutkowska J, Talbot P, Genest J, Cantin M (1987) Plasma immunoreactive atrial natriuretic factor is inhibited by selective blockade of $alpha_2$ adrenergic receptors in conscious Sprague-Dawley rats. Neurosc Lett 76:119–123
2. de Bold A (1987) Functional morphology of the endocrine component of the heart. In: Brenner M, Laragh JH (eds) Biologically active atrial peptides, vol 1. American Society of Hypertension Symposium Series, Raven Press, New York
3. Crum RL, Brown MR (1988) Effects of morphine and opioid peptides on plasma levels of atrial natriuretic peptides. Life Sci 43:851–858
4. Frelin C, Vigne P, Barbry P, Lazdunski M (1987) Molecular properties of amiloride action and of its Na^+ transporting targets. Kidney Int 32:785–793
5. Fukuda Y, Hirata Y, Yoshimi H, Kojima T, Kobayashi Y, Yanagisawa M, Masaki T (1988) Endothelin is a potent secretagogue for atrial natriuretic peptide in cultured rat atrial myocytes. Biochem Biophys Res Commun 155:167–172
6. Goldstein A (1983) Biology and chemistry of the dynorphin peptides. In: Meienhofer J, Udenfried S (eds) The peptides: analysis synthesis biology, vol 7. Academic Press, New York
7. Greenwald JE, Apkon M, Sides SD, Needleman P (1988) Cellular mechanisms regulating atriopeptin release. J Cell Biochem [Suppl] 12A:4
8. Gutkowska J, Racz K, Garcia R, Thibault G, Kuchel O, Genest J, Cantin M (1986) The morphine effect on plasma ANF. Eur J Pharmacol 131:91–94
9. Haufe MC, Gerzer R, Weil J, Ernst JG, Theisen K (1988) Verapamil impairs secretion of stimulated atrial natriuretic factor in humans. J Am Coll Cardiol 11:1199–1203
10. Heim JM, Ivanova K, Gerzer R (1988) Amiloride increases the sensitivity of particulate guanylate cyclase to atrial natriuretic factor. Biochem Biophys Res Commun 152: 1263–1268
11. Hirn C, Stasch JP, John A, Kazda S, Morich F, Neuser D, Wohlfeil S (1986) The renal response to acute hypervolemia is caused by atrial natriuretic peptides. J Cardiovasc Pharmacol 8:268–275
12. Hirn C, Kauczor HK, Stasch JP, Wohlfeil S (1988) The release of atrial natriuretic peptides and its role in volume regulation. J Cell Biochem [Suppl] 12A:8
13. Huidiboro-Toro JP, Parada S (1985) K-opiates and urination: Pharmacological evidence for an endogenous role of the K opiate receptor in fluid and electrolyte balance. Eur J Pharmacol 107:1–10
14. Lachance D, Garcia R (1988) Atrial natriuretic factor release by angiotensin II in the conscious rat. Hypertension 11:502–508
15. Leander JD (1983) A kappa opioid effect: Increased urination in the rat. J Pharmacol Exp Ther 224:89–94
16. Meloche S, McMcoll N, Lin B, Ong H, De Lean A (1988) Atrial natriuretic factor R_1 receptor from Bovine adrenal zona glomerulosa: Purification, characterization and modulation by amiloide. Biochemistry 27: 8151–8158
17. Nakaoka H, Kitahara Y, Amano M, Imataka K, Fujii J, Ishibashi M, Yamaji T (1987) Effect of β-adrenergic receptor blockade on atrial natriuretic peptide in essential hypertension. Hypertension 10:221–225
18. Pettersson K, Anderson J, Sjölander M, Bloom SR (1987) Atrial natriuretic peptide and the natriuresis due to acute β-blockade in conscious hypertensive rats. Clin Exp Ther Pract A9:95–107
19. Rapelli A, Dessi-Fulgheri P, Madeddu P, Glorioso N (1987) Studies on the natriuretic effect of nifedipine in hypertensive patients: Increase in levels of plasma atrial natriuretic factor without participation of the renal kallikrein-kinin system. J Hypertension 5: S61–S65
20. Ruskoaho H, Toth M, Ganten D, Unger T, Lang RE (1986) The phorbol ester induced atrial natriuretic peptide secretion is stimulated by forskolin and BAY K 8644 and inhibited by 8 Bromo-cyclic-GMP. Biochem Biophys Res Commun 139:266–274

21. Seino M, Abe K, Nushiro N, Yoshinaga K (1988) Nifedipine enhances the vasodepressor and natriuretic effects of atrial natriuretic peptide. Hypertension 11:34–40
22. Shima J, Ogihara T, Hara H, Iinuma K, Kumahara Y (1987) Effects of calcium antagonists on the secretion of atrial natriuretic peptide in normal volunteers. Curr Therap Res 42:115–123
23. Sigrist G, Fuchs B, Greven J (1985) Characterization of the renal effects of an imidazothiadiazol-acrylamide derivative in rats. Naunyn-Schmiedeberg's Arch Pharmacol 330:R31
24. Sonnenberg JL, Sakane Y, Jeng AY, Koehn JA, Ansell JA, Wennogle LP, Ghai RD (1988) Identification of protease 3.4.24.11 as the major atrial natriuretic factor degrading enzyme in rat kidney. Peptides 9:173–180
25. Stasch JP, Kazda S, Hirn C (1987) The different effects of a calcium antagonist and a sodium retaining vasodilatator on blood pressure, cardiac hypertrophy and atrial natriuretic peptides in SHR. J Hypertens 5: S211–S213
26. Stasch JP, Grote H, Kazda S, Hirn C (1989) Dynorphin stimulates release of ANP from isolated rat atria. Eur J Pharmacol (submitted)
27. Stephenson SL, Kenny AJ (1987) The hydrolysis of alpha-human atrial natriuretic peptide by pig kidney microvillar membranes is initiated by endopeptidase 24.11. Biochem J 243:183–187
28. Thamsborg G, Sykulski R, Larsen J, Storm T, Keller N (1987) Effect of β_1 adrenoceptor blockade on plasma levels of atrial natriuretic peptide during exercise in normal man. Clin Physiol 7:313–318
29. Veress AT, Milojevic S, Yip C, Flynn TG, Sonnenberg H (1988) In vitro secretion of atrial natriuretic factor: receptor-mediated release of prohormone. Am J Physiol 254: R809–814
30. Vollmar AM, Arendt RM, Schulz R (1987) The effect of opioids on rat plasma atrial natriuretic peptide. Eur J Pharmacol 143: 315–321
31. Xie CW, Yin LY, Xie XZ, Gao XM, Xia ZQ, Chang JK, Tang J (1988) A dynorphin peptide induces hypotension by stimulating the release of atrial natriuretic peptide from rat atrium. Life Sci 42:1117

The Heart as a Target Organ

Thyroid Hormones and the Heart

H.-G. Zimmer

Physiologisches Institut der Universität München, FRG

Summary. Recent research has revealed some new and surprising aspects of thyroid hormone action. 1. Many of the marked effects of thyroid hormones can be explained by nuclear binding, alteration in gene expression, increaed mRNA formation and subsequent enhancement of protein synthesis. 2. Several enzymes of carbohydrate and fatty acid metabolism are stimulated. However, those involved in the oxidative pentose phosphate pathway, glucose-6-phosphate dehydrogenase and 6-phosphogluconate dehydrogenase, are not altered in the rat heart by 3,3′,5-triiodo-L-thyronine. 3. The positive chronotropic and inotropic effects of 3,3′,5-triiodo-L-thyronine are mediated by catecholamines via an increased number of β-adrenergic receptors, they can be abolished by β-adrenergic blockade with metoprolol. 4. This β-receptor blocker, however, does not affect the 3,3′,5-triiodo-L-thyronine induced increase in cardiac output, the stimulation of myocardial metabolism and the development of cardiac hypertrophy. Thus, these alterations occur independently of catecholamines. 5. The hypertrophic response seems not to be exclusively the result of direct stimulation of myocardial metabolism, but also the consequence of an additional and indirect factor such as increased hemodynamic load.

Key words: Cardiac hypertrophy – Catecholamines – β-Receptor blockers – Heart function in rats – Myocardial Metabolism – 3,3′,5-Triiodo-L-thyronine

Introduction

Thyroid hormones play an important role in many biological functions. They are involved in growth and development, in stimulation of metabolism and thermogenesis, and they have a permissive effect on the action of other hormones. They are produced in and secreted by the thyroid gland (Fig. 1). The main products

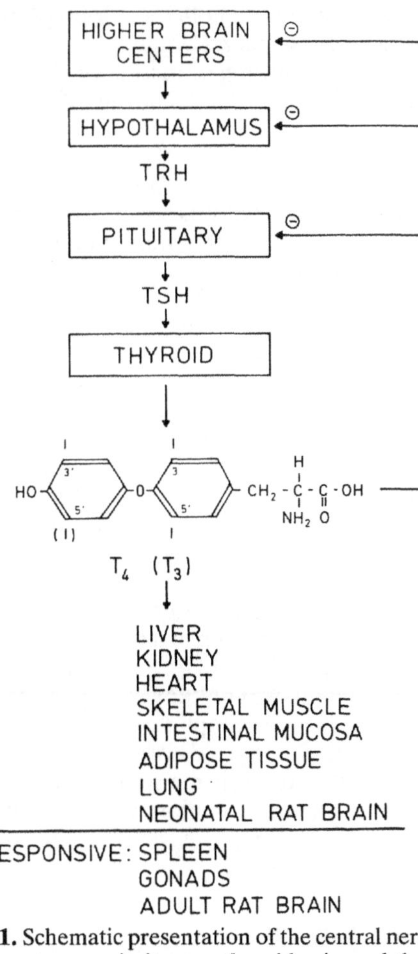

Fig. 1. Schematic presentation of the central nervous system – pituitary – thyroid axis, and the long loop feedback system as well as the target organs for thyroid hormones

are thyroxine (T_4) and 3,3′,5-triiodo-L-thyronine (T_3). 15% of the circulating T_3 come from direct thyroid secretion, 85% are the product of conversion from T_4 in peripheral tissues. T_3 is the major physiologically active hormone. The secretion is regulated by thyroid stimulating hormone (TSH) or thyrotropin from the pituitary gland which in turn is controlled by thyrotropin releasing hormone (THR) of hypothalamic origin. Thyroid hormones exert a feedback inhibition at the pituitary and hypothalamic levels and even at higher brain centers (Fig. 1). This is the so-called long loop feedback system. There are various target organs listed in Fig. 1 with the notable exception of spleen, the gonads and the adult brain, at least in the rat. In this article, the main emphasis will be placed on the heart as a target organ.

Hyper- and hypofunction of the thyroid gland have marked clinical effects. The symptoms of hyperthyroidism are known as Graves' or Basedow's disease since the middle of the last century. This disease was considered to be "of unknown origin, characterized by exophthalmos, enlargement of the thyroid, and function disturbance of the vascular system. Cardiac and vascular symptoms are usually first to develop and the patient complains of palpitation with breathlessness. The pulse-rate at first may not be more than 95 or 100, but when the disease is established may reach 140 or 160. Any emotional excitement sets the heart beating with great intensity. In the long-standing cases the heart may be hyperthrophied and the sounds very intense" [14].

This classical description of clinical symptoms was given at a time when therapy was not possible and the pathophysiological background was unknown. In view of these symptoms, three topics will be discussed: 1. The action of thyroid hormones at the cellular level resulting in metabolic effects, 2. the effects on heart function, and 3. the mechanisms underlying the development of cardiac hypertrophy.

Metabolic Effects

A large body of evidence obtained in recent research supports the concept that T_3 binds to a receptor localized at the DNA of the cell nucleus [13]. The receptor is a chromatin-associated protein with a molecular weight of 50 000 to 55 000. Unlike steroid hormones, a cytoplasmic form of a T_3-receptor has not been identified or characterized. It is interesting that the thyroid hormone receptor protein is similar to the one encoded by the c-erb-A-oncogene which also binds T_3 specifically [21]. Thyroid hormone appears to promote the growth and metastatic potential of certain types of neoplasias demonstrating an enhancement of tumor progression. In addition, the transformation of cultured cells by radiation or adenovirus infection is facilitated by thyroid hormone [3]. After binding, thyroid hormones mediate a rapid and selective activation of gene expression and increase the transcription processes resulting in enhanced mRNA formation (Fig. 2). After translation, protein synthesis is stimulated [2, 19, 27] which results in altered cell function (Fig. 2).

It is well established that T_3 rapidly increases the transcription of the growth hormone gene in the pituitary [10] which is then involved in growth and development. Furthermore, it has been shown that the number of β-adrenergic receptors in cardiac membranes derived from hyperthyroid animals is increased thus leading to an enhanced sensitivity of the heart to catecholamines [8, 22]. T_3 also augments the Na^+/K^+-transport via activation of the ATP-dependent Na^+/K^+-ATPase which functions as a pump [5]. Consequent changes in the ATP/ADP ratio stimulate mitochondrial respiratory rates resulting in increased oxygen consumption, stimulation of metabolism and enhanced thermogenesis (Fig. 2).

The T_3-induced increase in protein synthesis also concerns several enzymes which may remain in the cytoplasm or will be transported into the mitochondria such as α-glycerophosphate dehydrogenase. Increase of the activity of many enzymes contributes to stimulation of metabolism and is in some cases associated with the development of cardiac hypertrophy, although it may not always be essential for the hypertrophic response [1, 15, 16]. T_3 may also increase the transcription and translation of

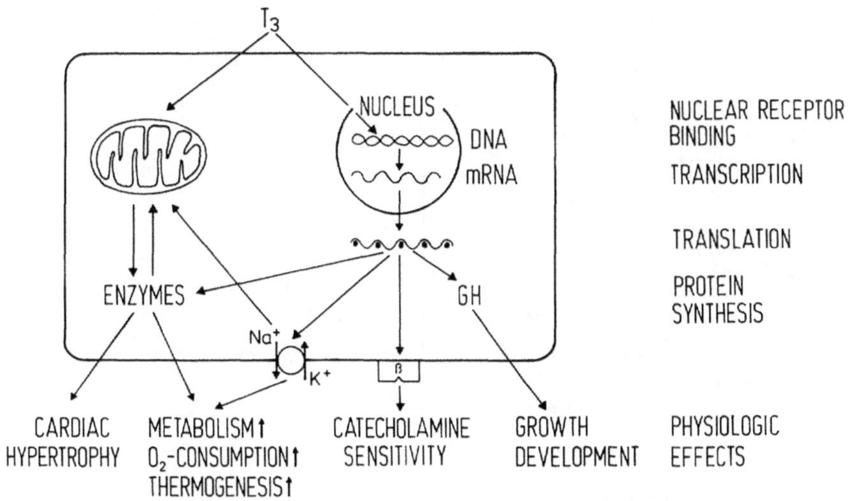

Fig. 2. Action of 3,3′,5-triiodo-L-thyronine at the cellular level, and the physiologic effects

several mitochondrial proteins [12, 17] such as cytochrome oxidase. It has been shown for the heart that glycolysis is enhanced, in particular, the activity of phosphofructokinase [18], a key enzyme in this pathway. Likewise, the activity of some enzymes of the Krebs cycle such as citrate synthase and malate dehydrogenase, has been found to be enhanced [20]. In this way, ATP can be produced both via glycolysis and via oxidative phosphorylation that is necessary for the increased activity of Na^+/K^+-ATPase. Of particular concern is the question whether in the heart the activity of enzymes involved in fatty acid metabolism may also be increased. It has been shown for the liver that the activity of four lipogenic enzymes is increased in response to T_3, and that this response is even more pronounced when a high carbohydrate diet is fed to the animals [9]. These enzymes were fatty acid synthase, malic enzyme, glucose-6-phosphate dehydrogenase and 6-phosphogluconate dehydrogenase. A common feature of the last three is that in the reactions catalyzed by the respective enzymes NADPH is produced which can be used for fatty acid synthesis. In our own studies, particular attention was directed to the activity of glucose-6-phosphate dehydrogenase and 6-phosphogluconate dehydrogenase in the myocardium. These are enzymes of the oxidative pentose phosphate pathway (Fig. 3).

This pathway is a link between carbohydrate metabolism on the one hand and pyrimidine and purine nucleotide metabolism on the other hand. It serves mainly two functions: It provides 5-phosphoribosyl-1-pyrophosphate for the synthesis of pyrimidine and purine nucleotides. Moreover, reducing equivalents in the form of NADPH are generated in the reactions catalyzed by glucose-6-phosphate dehydrogenase and 6-phosphogluconate dehydrogenase. NADPH can be used both for fatty acid synthesis and for detoxification processes in which glutathione is involved (Fig. 3). The flow through the oxidative pentose phosphate pathway is regulated by the first enzyme, glucose-6-phosphate dehydrogenase. Comparative studies have revealed that the activity of this enzyme, the available pool of 5-phosphoribosyl-1-pyrophosphate and the rate of adenine nucleotide biosynthesis are all very low in the rat heart. This seems to be true also for human hearts [29]. It was therefore examined whether thyroid hormone can influence the oxidative pentose phosphate pathway. Time course studies on the effect of daily T_3 administrations in cyclic AMP (cAMP), on the glucose-6-phosphate dehydrogenase and 6-phosphogluconate dehydrogenase activities, as well as on adenine nucleotide and protein synthesis showed (Fig. 4) that there was a moderate, but sustained increase in

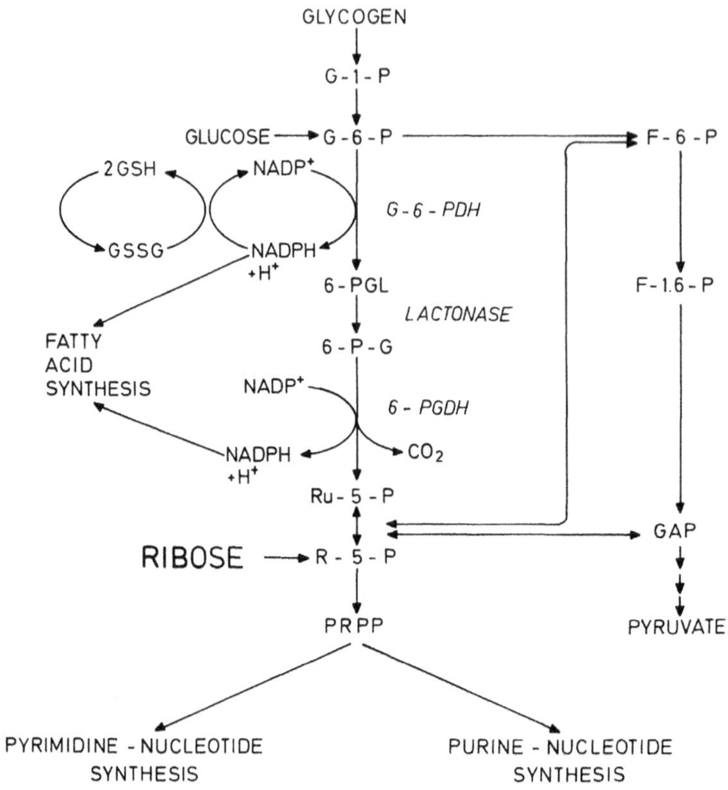

Fig. 3. Simplified scheme of the oxidative pentose phosphate pathway as a link between carbohydrate metabolism and the synthesis of pyrimidine and purine nucleotides. Glycolysis is indicated on the right hand side of the scheme. The connections between glycolysis and the endproducts of the oxidative pentose phosphate pathway via the transaldolase and transketolase reactions of the nonoxidative segment are symbolized by two arrows. *Abbreviations:* G-1-P: Glucose-1-phosphate; G-6-P: Glucose-6-phosphate; F-6-P: Fructose-6-phosphate; F-1,6-P: Fructose-1,6-phosphate; GAP: Glyceraldehyde-3-phosphate; 6-PGL: 6-Phosphogluconolactone; 6-PG: 6-Phosphogluconate; Ru-5-P: Ribulose-5-phosphate; R-5-P: Ribose-5-phosphate; PRPP: 5-Phosphoribosyl-1-pyrophosphate; G-6-PDH: Glucose-6-phosphate dehydrogenase; 6-PGDH: 6-Phosphogluconate dehydrogenase; GSSG: Oxidized glutathione; GSH: Reduced glutathione; $NADP^+$: Nicotinamide adenine dinucleotide phosphate; NADPH: Reduced form of $NADP^+$

the level of cardiac cAMP indicating a prolonged stimulation of glycogenolysis. There was also an enhancement of adenine nucleotide and protein synthesis. In contrast, the activities of glucose-6-phosphate dehydrogenase and 6-phosphogluconate dehydrogenase did not change at all (Fig. 4). From these results it can be concluded that the non-oxidative pentose phosphate pathway (Fig. 3) is enhanced under the influence of T_3 thereby leading to an elevation of the 5-phosphoribosyl-1-pyrophosphate pool and to the stimulation of nucleotide synthesis. It is interesting that these two metabolic parameters were also elevated specifically by ribose which bypasses the critical step in the oxidative pentose phosphate pathway. It was shown in previous studies that ribose stimulated adenine nucleotide biosynthesis in some pathophysiologic stituations to such an extent that the decline in ATP was greatly attenuated or even completely prevented [26, 28]. Ribose thus compensates for the limited capacity of the oxidative pentose phosphate pathway and thereby becomes cardioprotective. That T_3 is unable to stimulate the enzymes of this pathway is in contrast to its effects on the rat liver [9]. This

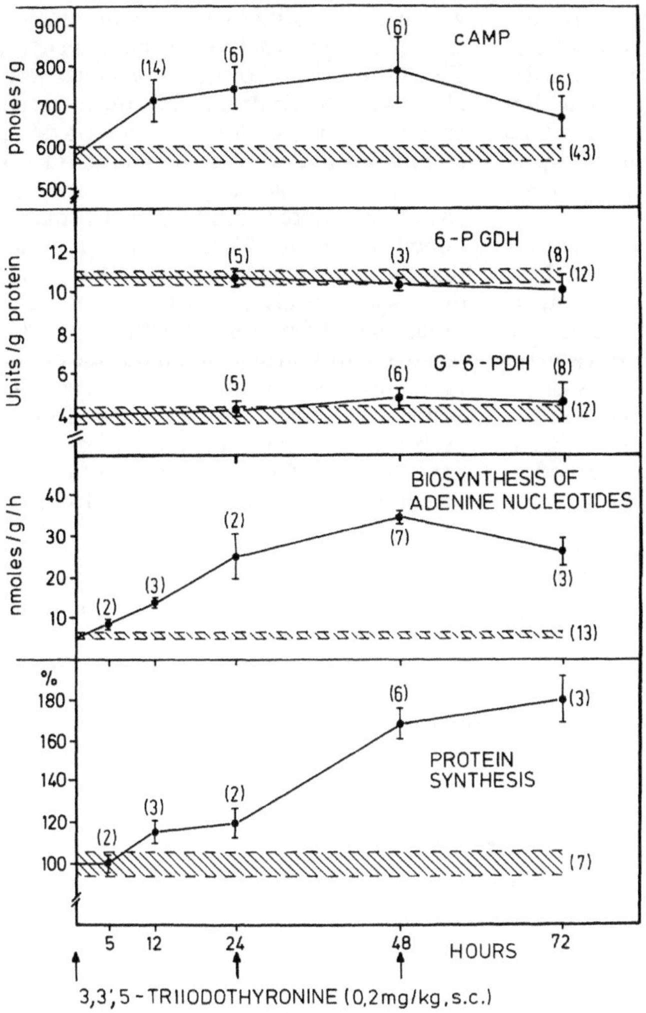

Fig. 4. Effect of daily s.c. injections of 3,3′,5-triiodo-L-thyronine (0.2 mg/kg) on the level of 3′,5′-cyclic AMP, on the activities of glucose-6-phosphate dehydrogenase (G-6-PDH) and of 6-phosphogluconate dehydrogenase (6-PGDH), and on adenine nucleotide and protein synthesis in rat hearts. Mean values ± SEM; number of experiments in parentheses

lack of hormone adaptation and inadequate metabolic reaction may help explain the susceptibility of the heart to various disease processes.

Effects on Heart Function

A particular enzyme that plays an important role in heart muscle and that does react very sensibly to thyroid hormone is myosin. In the heart of rats and rabbits there are three myosin isoenzymes, named V_1, V_2 and V_3 which differ in electrophoretic mobility in pyrophosphate gels and in the myosin AT-Pase activity, V_1 having the highest activity [4, 11, 16]. Hyperthyroidism leads to gene expression of the V_1 isoenzyme, and hypothyroidism induced by propylthiouracil produces exclusively the V_3 isomyosin [16]. Also during development, there are marked changes in the isomyosin pattern. In the neonatal rat, all three isoenzymes are present. In the first 4 to 5 weeks during postnatal development, the isoenzymes are shifted toward V_1 [4], and this shift goes parallel to the increase in the serum free T_3 levels. Thereafter, the T_3 level decreases, and this is followed by a corresponding shift towards V_3. However, the V_1 isoenzyme with the highest ATPase activity still predominates. Accordingly, the rat heart is a fast myocardium (Fig. 5).

Heart rate in normal, anesthetized rats is quite high as is LV dp/dt_{max}. In these studies, the hemodynamic measurements were obtained by left heart catheterization with the Millar ultraminiature catheter pressure transducer [25]. When T_3 was administered, heart rate increased markedly, and LV dp/dt_{max} was about twice as high as in the control. LVSP increased only moderately (Fig. 5). The crucial question was whether this positive chronotropic and inotropic effect was exclusively the result of the T_3 action or whether catecholamines were also involved. To decide this, the β_1-receptor blocker metoprolol was applied in rats as continuous i.v. infusion for 3 days, since at this time the hemodynamic parameters stimulated under the influence of T_3 had attained a plateau. These studies revealed that the increase in heart rate and in LV dp/dt_{max} was entirely prevented when metoprolol was administered [30]. Thus, the positive chronotropic and inotropic effects of T_3 obviously are mediated by catecholamines. This effect can be explained on the basis of radioligand binding studies which have shown that the number of β-adrenergic receptors in cardiac membranes from hy-

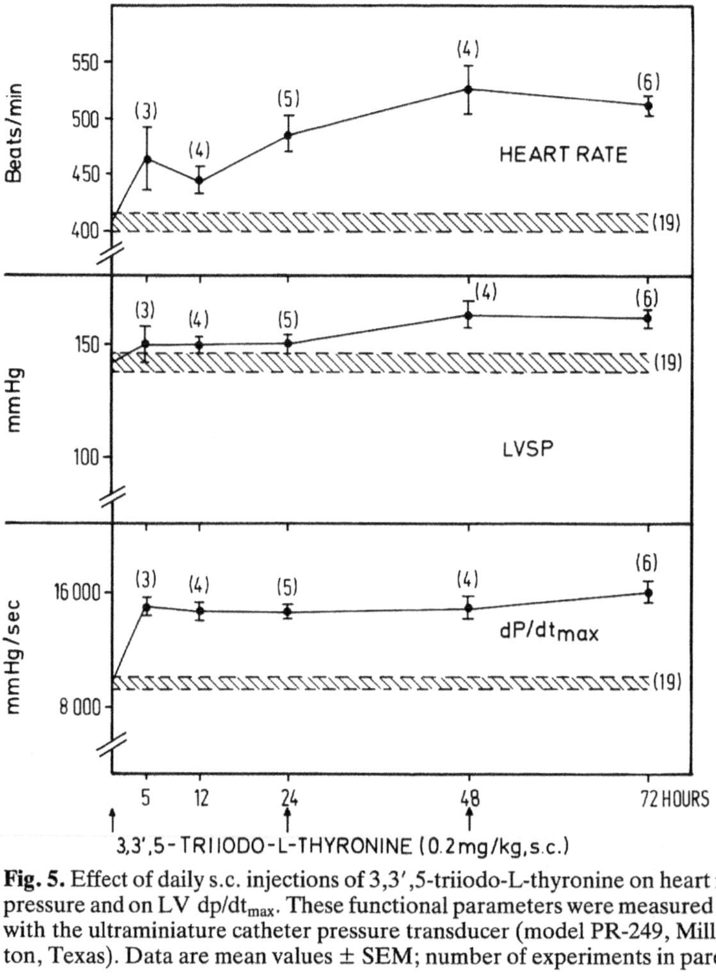

Fig. 5. Effect of daily s.c. injections of 3,3',5-triiodo-L-thyronine on heart rate, left ventricular systolic pressure and on LV dp/dt_{max}. These functional parameters were measured by left heart catheterization with the ultraminiature catheter pressure transducer (model PR-249, Millar Instruments, Inc., Houston, Texas). Data are mean values ± SEM; number of experiments in parentheses

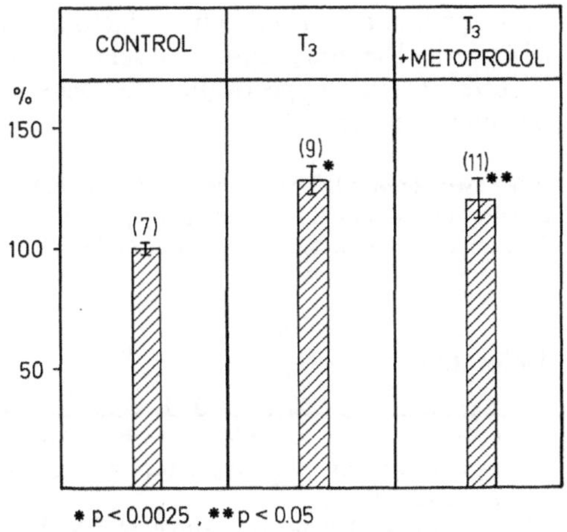

Fig. 6. Content of cardiac 3′,5′-cyclic AMP in rats treated with 3,3′,5-triiodo-L-thyronine (0.2 mg/kg, s.c. daily) for 3 days, and the effect of continous i.v. infusion of the β-adrenergic blocker metoprolol (1 mg/kg/h). Data are mean values ± SEM; number of experiments in parentheses. Increases given as percent of controls (= 100%)

perthyroid animals was increased roughly twofold [22]. This leads to an increased sensitivity of the heart to catecholamines. As a consequence, the positive chronotropic and inotropic effects can be abolished by β-receptor blockers. On the basis of these results, the question was asked whether the increase in oxygen consumption and in metabolism that occurs under the influence of T_3 may also be affected by β-receptor blockade and whether cardiac hypertrophy may still develop.

Development of Cardiac Hypertrophy

Previous studies had already shown that thyroid hormones increase adenylate cyclase activity. This effect could not be affected by the β-receptor blocker propranolol, although this blocker abolished the norepinephrine-induced activation of the enzyme [7]. These results indicated that this effect of thyroid hormones is not mediated by the β-adrenergic receptor. In our own studies, the T_3-elicited elevation of myocardial cAMP was not altered by metoprolol (Fig. 6). Likewise, the stimulation of adenine nucleotide and protein synthesis induced by T_3 was not changed when metoprolol was administered which by itself had no effect (Fig. 7). As a consequence, the development of cardiac hypertrophy measured as the increase in heart weight was not affected by metoprolol [30]. In addition, time course studies were carried out in

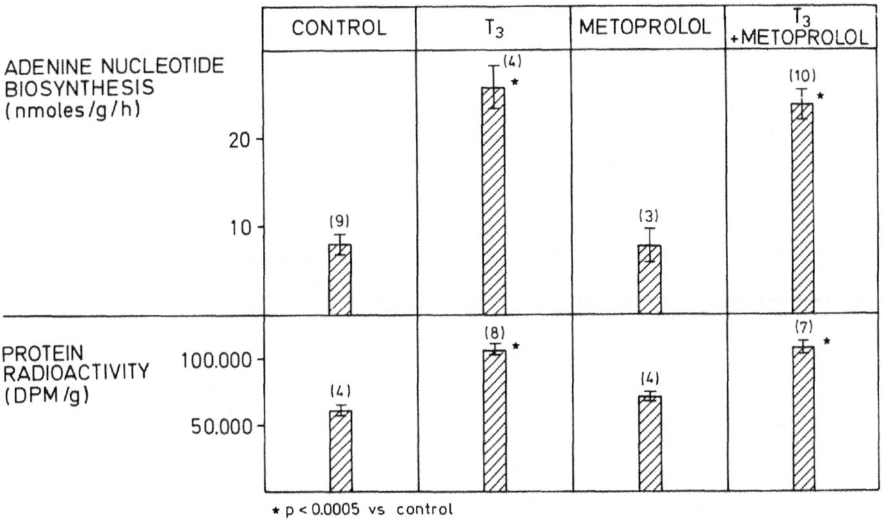

Fig. 7. Changes in cardiac adenine nucleotide biosynthesis and in the radioactivity of myocardial proteins due to incorporation of 1-^{14}C-glycine in rats after 3 days of treatment with 3,3′,5-triiodo-L-thyronine (0.2 mg/kg, s.c. daily) and with metoprolol (1 mg/kg/h, continuous i.v. infusion) alone and in combination. Mean values ± SEM; number of experiments in parentheses

which it was demonstrated that T_3 induced an increase in cardiac output. This was more pronounced after 48 and 72 hours than after 18 hours. Metoprolol first antagonized the T_3-induced increase in cardiac output, but after 48 and 72 hours, cardiac output was as high as in the group treated with T_3 alone [24]. Since heart rate was normal in animals simultaneously treated with T_3 and metoprolol, this increased cardiac output must be maintained by an increase in stroke volume. Also in patients with hyperthyroidism, the β-receptor blocker nethalide did not significantly change the increase in oxygen consumption and in cardiac output [23].

From all these results it appears that under the influence of thyroid hormones there is an increased number of cardiac β-adrenergic receptors. It is for this reason that the resulting increase in heart rate and in LV dP/dt_{max} can be abolished entirely by β-receptor blockade (Fig. 2). T_3, however, also binds to nuclear receptors, leads via increased mRNA formation to stimulation of RNA, nucleotide and protein synthesis and to cardiac hypertrophy. On the other hand, oxygen consumption is enhanced in general leading to volume overload, and this also contributes to cardiac hypertrophy. These actions of T_3 cannot be affected by β-receptor blockers. Therefore, cardiac metabolism and volume overload are still enhanced, and hypertrophy develops. On the basis of our own results we cannot determine the contribution which volume overload on the one hand and stimulation of cardiac metabolism on the other hand have in the initiation and maintenance of cardiac hypertrophy. However, recent results of another research group suggest that volume overload may play a decisive role. In these experiments, hearts from hypothyroid donors were transplanted into the abdominal cavity of hypothyroid recipient rats. Administration of thyroid hormone induced a comparable increase in heart function and in the isoenzyme shift of myosin from V_3 to V_1 in both the recipient and the transplanted heart. However, the transplanted heart, in contrast to the recipient heart, did not develop hypertrophy, but underwent atrophy [6]. Thus, direct stimulation of cardiac metabolism by T_3 seems not to be a sufficient trigger for cardiac hypertrophy. Obviously, an additional and indirect factor such as increased hemodynamic load seems to be required for the hypertrophic response to become effective.

Acknowledgement: The results referred to in this article were obtained in studies supported by the Deutsche Forschungsgemeinschaft (Zi 199/4–5).

References

1. Bartolome J, Huguenard J, Slotkin TA (1980) Role of ornithine decarboxylase in cardiac growth and hypertrophy. Science 210:793–794
2. Crie JS, Wakeland JR, Mayhew BA, Wildenthal K (1983) Direct anabolic effects of thyroid hormone on isolated mouse heart. Am J Physiol 245:C328–C333
3. Fisher PB, Guernsey DL, Weinstein IB, Edelman IS (1983) Modulation of adenovirus transformation by thyroid hormone. Proc Natl Acad Sci USA 80:196–200
4. Hoh JFY, McGrath PA, Hale PT (1977) Electrophoretic analysis of multiple forms of rat cardiac myosin: Effects of hypothysectomy and thyroxine replacement. J Mol Cell Cardiol 10:1053–1076
5. Ismail-Beigi F, Bissell DM, Edelman IS (1979) Thyroid thermogenesis in adult rat hepatocytes in primary monolayer culture. Direct action of thyroid hormone in vitro. J Gen Physiol 73:369–383
6. Korecky B, Zak R, Schwartz K, Aschenbrenner V (1987) Role of thyroid hormone in regulation of isomyosin composition, contractility, and size of heterotopically isotransplanted rat heart. Circ Res 60:824–830
7. Levey GS, Epstein SE (1969) Myocardial adenyl cyclase: Activation by thyroid hormones and evidence for two adenyl cyclase systems. J Clin Invest 48:1663–1669
8. Limas C, Limas CJ (1987) Influence of thyroid status on intracellular distribution of cardiac adrenoceptors. Circ Res 61:824–828
9. Mariash CN, Kaiser FE, Schwartz HL, Towle HC, Oppenheimer JH (1980) Synergism of thyroid hormone and high carbohydrate diet in the induction of lipogenic enzymes in the rat. Mechanisms and implications. J Clin Invest 65:1126–1134
10. Martial JA, Baxter JD, Goodman HM, Seeburg PH (1977) Regulation of growth hormone messenger RNA by thyroid and glucocorticoid hormones. Proc Natl Acad Sci USA 74:1816–1820
11. Martin AF, Pagani ED, Solaro RJ (1982) Thyroxine-induced redistribution of isoen-

zymes of rabbit ventricular myosin. Circ Res 50:117–124
12. Nelson BD, Joste V, Wielburski A, Rosenqvist U (1980) The effects of tri-iodothyronine on the synthesis of mitochondrial proteins in isolated rat hepatocytes. Biochim Biophys Acta 608:422–426
13. Oppenheimer JH (1979) Thyroid hormone action at the cellular level. Science 203: 971–979
14. Osler W (1892) The principles and practice of medicine. New York, 712–713
15. Pegg AE, Hibasami H (1980) Polyamine metabolism during cardiac hypertrophy. Am J Physiol 239:E372–E378
16. Rupp H (1982) Polymorphic myosin as the common determinant of myofibrillar AT-Pase in different heaemodynamic and thyroid states. Basic Res Cardiol 77:34–46
17. Schimmelpfennig K, Sauerberg M, Neubert D (1970) Stimulation of mitochonrial RNA synthesis by thyroid hormone. FEBS Letters 10:269–272
18. Seymour A-ML, Eldar H, Radda GK (1988) Hyperthyroidism results in increased glycolytic capacity in the rat heart. J Mol Cell Cardiol 20 [Suppl V]:47
19. Siehl D, Chua BHL, Lautensack-Belser N, Morgan HE (1985) Faster protein and ribosome synthesis in thyroxine-induced hypertrophy of rat heart. Am J Physiol 248: C309–C319
20. Tanaka T, Morita H, Koide H, Kawamura K, Takatsu T (1985) Biochemical and morphological study of cardiac hypertrophy. Effects of thyroxine on enzyme activities in the rat. Basic Res Cardiol 80:165–174
21. Weinberger C, Thompson CC, Ong ES, Lebo R, Gruol DJ, Evans RM (1986) The c-erb-A gene encodes a thyroid hormone receptor. Nature 324:641–646
22. Williams LT, Lefkowitz RJ, Watanabe AM, Hathaway DR, Besch HR (1977) Thyroid hormone regulation of β-adrenergic receptor number. J Biol Chem 252:2787–2789
23. Wilson WR, Theilen EO, Fletcher FW (1964) Pharmacodynamic effects of beta-adrenergic receptor blockade in patients with hyperthyroidism. J Clin Invest 43: 1697–1703
24. Zierhut W, Zimmer H-G (1987) Time course of triiodothyronine-induced hemodynamic changes and the effect of metoprolol. Pflügers Arch 408 [Suppl 1]:R13
25. Zimmer H-G (1983) Measurement of left ventricular hemodynamic parameters in closed-chest rats under control and various pathophysiologic conditions. Basic Res Cardiol 78:77–84
26. Zimmer H-G (1983) Normalization of depressed heart function in rats by ribose. Science 220:81–82
27. Zimmer H-G, Gerlach E (1980) Early metabolic alterations during the development of experimentally induced cardiac hypertrophy. Arzneim-Forsch/Drug Res 30 (II) 11a:2001–2007
28. Zimmer H-G, Ibel H (1984) Ribose accelerates the repletion of the ATP pool during recovery from reversible ischemia of the rat myocardium. J Mol Cell Cardiol 16:863–866
29. Zimmer H-G, Ibel H, Suchner U, Schad H (1984) Ribose intervention in the cardiac pentose phosphate pathway is not species-specific. Science 223:712–714
30. Zimmer H-G, Peffer H (1986) Metabolic aspects of the development of experimental cardiac hypertrophy. Basic Res Cardiol 81 [Suppl 1]:127–137

Molecular Biology of Tissue Renin

J. Peters, K. Lindpaintner and D. Ganten

German Institute for High Blood Pressure Research and Department of Pharmacology, University of Heidelberg, FRG

Summary. The actions of converting enzyme (CE) inhibitors at the tissue level (brain, heart, blood vessels) and their interferences with the autonomic nervous system through central and peripheral actions may under certain conditions be more important than inhibition of the hormonal circulating plasma ANG II. Recent clinical and experimental studies and new insights in the molecular biology of the renin-angiotensin system (RAS), especially gene expression of renin and angiotensinogen in tissues of the cardiovascular system support this view. These findings have consequences not only for the understanding of pharmacokinetics and pharmacodynamics of CE inhibitors but also for their practical therapeutic use.
Key words: Converting enzyme – Converting enzyme inhibitors – Angiotensin – Renin- angiotensin system – Brain – Heart – Blood vessels

Introduction

The renin-angiotensin system (RAS) is one of the key modulators of cardiovascular homeostasis. Over the past two decades the development of potent inhibitors of the renin-angiotensin axis, such as renin- or converting enzyme (CE) inhibitors and angiotensin II antagonists, has fostered a rapid expansion of our understanding of its physiological significance. Recently, it has gained additional interest due to the discovery of local tissue renin-angiotensin systems. Studies in hypertensive patients had shown a poor correlation between hypotensive effect of CE inhibitors and plasma renin activity. Thus, changes in the activity of renin-angiotensin systems residing locally in tissues important for blood pressure regulation were invoked to explain this finding. Additional support for the existence and physiological significance of tissue renin angiotensin systems came from studies in rats, where blood pressure was found to correlate better with renin activity in the vascular wall than with plasma renin activity [1, 2]. Also, mineralcorticoid concentrations and their modulation by nephrectomy, potassium loading or sodium depletion correlate better with renin activity in the rat adrenal gland than in plasma [3–5].

The existence of such intrinsic renin-angiotensin systems, which may act independently of the plasma RAS in an autocrine or paracrine fashion, has now also been confirmed by a number of recent studies demonstrating unequivocally expression of the genes for renin and angiotensinogen in a variety of tissues (e.g. brain, adrenal gland, heart, arterial wall, testis, ovary and kidney [6, 7]).

In this review we shall summarize some of the recent findings concerning tissue renin-angiotensin system and their possible functions in tissues relevant for cardiovascular regulation.

The Brain Renin-Angiotensin System

A crucial step in confirming the existence of an endogenous renin-angiotensin system in the brain was the demonstration of local presence and synthesis of renin and angiotensinogen and their respective messenger RNAs in the brain. The renin gene has been cloned and characterized and found to consist of 9 exons and 8 introns in mouse and rat and of 10 exons and 9 introns in humans. Using radiolabelled synthetic cRNA as a hybridization probe in an in situ-hybridization assay system, we were able to demonstrate the presence of renin mRNA in the lateral hypothalamus and the medulla oblongata of rats. Using the same methodology, renin mRNA was also demonstrated in the afferent ateriole of the glomerulum in the kidney, consistent with the results of earlier studies.

Using a different approach, we also documented the presence of renin mRNA in the brain by Northern blotting. This method encompasses electrophoretic fractionation of total extracted RNA on agarose gels and transfer to nitrocellulose membranes, which were subsequently hybridized against radiolabelled renin cRNA under stringent conditions. Thus, the presence of a 1.6 kilobase renin mRNA in brain extracts was confirmed, identical in appearence to kidney renin mRNA. These experiments showed that the renin gene is expressed in the brain, strongly supporting local renin synthesis in the CNS [8–12].

The genomic DNA and cDNA of the high molecular weight precursor of ANG I and ANG II, angiotensinogen, has also been cloned. Therefore, in a similar way, we were able to test the presence of angiotensinogen mRNA in the brain by using a radiolabelled synthetic cRNA [13–15]. In Northern blot experiments, large amounts of angiotensinogen mRNA were demonstrated in brain tissue, in addition to the liver, the classical site of synthesis. Angiotensinogen mRNA was also found in cardiac atria, ventricles, the adrenal gland and the kidney. In situ-hybridization experiments localized angiotensinogen-mRNA to the paraventricular nucleus; this is an area where ANG II has previously been shown to be present in high concentrations. Thus, the present data on renin and angiotensinogen gene expression in the brain complement and confirm earlier results obtained by immunhistochemistry and lend additional strong support to the concept of locally integrated RAS in the CNS [9–11].

In collaboration with Fuxe, Lind, and others, we have done extensive mapping of central ANG II pathways by immunocytochemistry [see 16–18]. There is a dense network in the lateral hypothalamus, the subfornical organ, the medial preoptic area, the paraventricular nucleus with projections into the pituitary and the spinal cord. Many of these areas are important cardiovascular centers. To be of functional significance, they have to contain specific angiotensin receptors. Indeed, receptor binding studies by several authors show a high density of angiotensin binding sites in the subfornical organ, nucleus paraventricularis and periventricularis of the hypothalamus, nucleus supra-chiasmaticus, lateral optical tract, and also in the amygdala.

A further test concerning the biological relevance was the stimulation of the subfornical organ by local application of ANG II using microiontophoresis. Angiotensin resulted in increased spiking activity of the neurons, which could be specifically blocked by the angiotensin receptor antagonist, saralasin. This stimulation also resulted in an increase in blood pressure. Intracerebroventricularly (icv) given ANG II causes a much more prolonged increase of blood pressure than peripheral application of angiotensin II. It is noteworthy that the angiotensin receptor antagonist alone reduced spontaneous firing of the neurons [see 10, 19, 20].

In summary, the essential components of the renin-angiotensin system have been identified in brain tissue: angiotensinogen, renin, ANG II, and angiotensin binding sites. Furthermore, central angiotensin receptor stimulation results in blood pressure increases. It is thus highly likely that an intrinsic functional renin-angiotensin system exists in the brain. Measurements of renin and angiotensin support the notion that this system is stimulated in genetically hypertensive animals [21, 22].

The key experiment to test the system's contribution to the elevation of blood pressure is an examination of the inhibition of endogenous angiotensin synthesis in the brain. Unique for neuropeptides, this can be done at all levels of peptide synthesis and action by the inhibition of renin, converting enzyme and by angiotensin receptor blockade. Inhibition of renin with pepstatin resulted in retardation of blood pressure development. In the same spontaneously hypertensive rats the hypotensive effects of central inhibition of angiotensin receptors decreased blood pressure even more markedly after nephrectomy when a counterbalancing action of circulating angiotensin was excluded [23–28].

Intracerebroventricular (icv) application of different CE inhibitors lowered blood pressure in SHRSP [27, 29–31] as well as in renal hypertensive rats [32] and in DOCA-salt hypertensive rats [33], suggesting the brain as a site of action of CE inhibitors.

However, there is still controversity as to whether these drugs gain access to the central nervous system (CNS) upon systemic administration. While some earlier studies suggested that the CE inhibitor, captopril, does not penetrate the blood-brain barrier following acute systemic application [34–36], other groups have reported on an inhibition of CE in brain tissue homogenates after systemic treatment with CE inhibitors [37–40]. Results obtained from experiments using brain tissue homogenates must be interpreted with caution, because this method does not allow differentiation between CE activity derived from neuronal and vascular structures. Therefore, it is difficult to decide whether the marked inhibition seen in some brain areas after oral CE inhibitor treatment is due to an inhibition of neuronal CE activity, whether it reflects CE inhibition in the vascular wall of cerebral blood vessels, or if it perhaps reflects changes in CE activity of plasma that may also contaminate the preparation. A better approach for studying the possible access of orally applied CE inhibitors to the CNS is the measurement of CE inhibition in the cerebrospinal fluid (CSF), because interferences with blood plasma and brain vasculature can be ruled out by appropriate sampling techniques.

Indirect evidence for an inhibition of CE in CSF following systemic CE inhibitor administration was suggested by in-vivo studies demonstrating that the dipsogenic and pressor effects of icv injected renin or angiotensin I (ANG I) were decreased following a single oral dose of captopril [24, 28]. More recently, Gepetti et al. [41] showed a substantial inhibition of CE in the CSF after acute oral captopril treatment in man.

The Renin-Angiotensin System in the Adrenal Gland

All components of the RAS's catalytic cascade, angiotensinogen, renin, angiotensin I, angiotensin II, and converting enzyme have been demonstrated in the adrenal gland. Similarly, presence of the messenger RNAs for angiotensinogen and renin has been confirmed in the rat and mouse adrenal gland; moreover, expression of this local system has been shown to respond to maneuvers influencing steroid synthesis and release [42–51]. Angiotensin II receptors are present in all zones of the adrenal gland. Angiotensin II is known to stimulate aldosterone, corticosterone, or other steroids as well as the release of catecholamines from the adrenal medulla [52, 53].

About 90% of the renin activity as well as the majority of renin mRNA has been localized to the rat zona glomerulosa by immunocytochemistry and by in situ-hybridization techniques. The site of storage of the adrenal zona glomerulosa renin has been recently localized to dense "secretory" granules by density gradient centrifugation techniques [54]. 73% of adrenal angiotensin II is concentrated in the zona glomerulosa; likewise, angiotensin converting enzyme also appears to be present mainly in the outer part of the adrenal gland [3, 4, 53, 55].

Angiotensin II concentrations in cultured adrenal cells are decreased in the presence of captopril [56], supporting the concept of local generation of angiotensin II.

It has been suggested that the preferential localization of renin in the zona glomerulosa indicates that it plays a role in the regulation of aldosterone secretion. This hypothesis is supported by a number of recent findings: Renin activity in the zona glomerulosa is markedly enhanced by maneuvers which stimulate aldosterone secretion (nephrectomy, sodium deplection and potassium loading). Conversely, a high-sodium diet, which suppresses aldosterone secretion, also decreases zona-glomerulosa renin activity. By comparison, similar changes do not occur in the inner cortical layers (zona fasciculata and reticularis), and in the medulla [3, 4]. Importantly, these experiments demonstrated a dissociation between plasma- and adrenal renin activity, indicating that plasma and adrenal RAS are regulated independently of each other. Hence, high potasium diet lowers plasma renin activity while stimulating adrenal renin activity. Similarly, an independent regulation of plasma and adrenal RAS is illustrated by unchanged adrenal ANG II levels after nephrectomy, when plasma ANG II is undetectable. Comparative studies have established a positive correlation between zona glomerulosa renin activity and plasma aldosterone concentration [3, 4]. Moreover, this correlation has been found to be closer than the correlation between plasma renin activity and aldosterone.

Additional evidence for a role of renin in aldosterone regulation comes from experiments which demonstrated that potassium induced increases in aldosterone can be blocked in vivo and in vitro by captopril. This points to an interaction of potassium and angiotensin II in aldosterone regulation [53]. In this respect, it is interesting to note that in rats potassium loading (0.5% KCl in drinking water for 2 weeks) leads to a fixed elevation of aldosterone plasma levels, although potassium levels are only temporarily elevated. This effect might be mediated by the adrenal RAS, since adrenal renin also remains elevated.

In addition to modulating steroid hormone synthesis, angiotensin II may also regulate cell growth in the adrenal gland. Angiotensin II is a potent mitogen for bovine adrenocortical cells and it stimulates fibroblasts growth. This effect is specifically mediated through angiotensin II receptors and can be blocked by competetive angiotensin II receptor antagonists [56, 67]. These mitogenic effects are of particular interest in view of the fact that the mas-oncogene [58] has been reported to encode a protein functionally identical to an angiotensin receptor and that adrenal tumor tissue (aldosterone producing Conn's tumor) contains abnormally high renin activities [51]. Angiotensin II has also been shown to stimulate or trigger angiogenesis very efficiently [59], especially in situations of regeneration in endocrine glands [60]. Of note, angiotensin II stimulates prostaglandins, which in turn also have angiogenic effects.

These effects are probably not specific for the adrenal gland; rather, they may represent a more general effect of tissue RASs. Angiotensin II binding sites have been detected in liver chromatin [61], and angiotensin II has been found to increase RNA synthesis in hepatocytes (RNA) or hepatocytes nuclei (hnRNA) in vitro [62]. This has given rise to the concept that ANG II acts as a stimulant for transcriptional activity.

A possible participation of the adrenal RAS in the reguation of catecholamine metabolism or release has been proposed based on the demonstration of angiotensin II receptors in the adrenal medulla. Angiotensin II has been shown to stimulate the release of adrenal catecholamines [52, 53]. In this context it is of interest that paracrine interactions between the cortex and the medulla of the adrenal gland have been demonstrated, perhaps facilitated by the presence of interconnecting blood vessels [63, 64].

Several studies indicate the importance of the adrenal gland and of mineralcorticoids for the pathogenesis of hypertension in spontaneously hypertensive rats (SHR). Thus, the adrenal glands of SHR appear to be hyperplastic [65, 66] and the steroidogenic responsiveness of SHR adrenals to ACTH and potassium is increased. Elevated plasma levels of corticosterone and aldosterone in SHR compared to normotensive controls have been found by some, while others failed to show such differences [67]. Adrenalectomy prevents the development of hypertension in SHR, while substitution of low dose aldosterone in adrenalectomized animals restores the normally seen development of hypertension.

The Heart as a Target for CE Inhibitors

We have recently been successful in identifying and quantitating renin and angiotensinogen mRNA in the heart, confirming previous reports [12, 15, 68–75]. Indirect evidence for the intracardiac activation of angiotensin I to angiotensin II by CE was first presented by Needleman et al. [76] and Nakashima et al. [77], who used bioassay systems to show activation of exogenously infused angiotensin I after passage through the coronary circulation. The implicated presence of angiotensin converting enzyme in the heart was recently confirmed by biochemical measurements [37].

Angiotensin II has a pronounced vasoconstrictor effect on coronary arteries [78], and exogenously administered angiotensin II is a potent inotropic agent. Dose-dependent direct positive inotropic effects of angiotensin II were shown in isolated atria and papillary muscle strips of rabbits [79], dogs [80], cats [81, 82], and guinea pigs [78]. Different investigators have found that the magnitude of this response ranged from very small [80] to equipotent with the maximal response to sympathetic nerve stimulation [83] to a 15-fold increase in developed tension [84].

In addition, data from our laboratory [85] suggest that myotropic actions of angiotensins are species-specific. There is general consensus that facilitation of sympathetic neurotransmission by angiotensin II contributes greatly to its inotropic actions. The majority of studies conclude that this facilitation is based primarily on an increase in the amount of neurotransmitter released from presynaptic nerve terminals [83, 84, 86], although angiotensin II has also been shown to decrease prejunctional reuptake [87], stimulate sympathetic ganglia [88], increase catecholamine biosynthesis [89], release catecholamines from the adrenal medulla [90], and sensitize post-junctional structures [91]. We have recently reported on experiments in which the physiologic relevance of this interaction with the sympathetic nervous system was tested in the heart. Isolated perfused heart preparations with intact sympathetic cardiac nerves [92] were prepared from rabbits that has been pretreated orally with the CE inhibitor one hour before they were killed. Sympathetic nerve stimulation increased heart rate and contractility and decreased coronary flow. These effects were significantly reduced in animals pretreated with CE inhibitor. These experiments are of particular importance to the proposed cardiac renin-angiotensin system, because the observed effects must be presumed to be caused by the inhibition of locally generated angiotensin II in the absence of exogenous angiotensins.

The potential physiologic role of the cardiac renin-angiotensin system is emphasized by studies demonstrating a cardio-protective effect of CE inhibitors in subjects with regional myocardial ischemia. Ertl et al. [93] demonstrated a reduction in infarct size after coronary artery ligation in dogs treated with CE inhibitors. Their observation that the area at risk and the infarcted area were smaller than would have been expected from the concomitant augmentation of coronary flow afforded by CE indicates additional effects of these agents, possibly on myocardial metabolism. This has been confirmed by examining the effects of CE inhibitors in isolated, perfused rat hearts subjected to a 15-minute period of regional ischemia by occluding the left anterior descending artery [94]. During the subsequent reperfusion phase, lactate dehydrogenase and creatine kinase activities in the coronary effluent were significantly lower when the CE inhibitor ramiprilat was added to the perfusion medium or had been administered orally before the animal was killed. In addition, CE inhibitor administration was associated with preservation of myocardial stores of glycogen and high-energy phosphates, which were both markedly depleted in untreated hearts. These effects were accompanied by a significant reduction in the incidence and duration of ventricular arrhythmias during the reperfusion period. All effects associated with CE inhibition could be abolished by addition of angiotensin II in the perfusate. Significantly, an isolated heart preparation was used instead of the in situ-preparation used in other studies; thus, the effects of CE inhibition are presumed to be caused by their action on local, intracardiac generation of angiotensin II. This does not rule out a possibly equally important role of kinins, which would be expected to accumulate after CE inhibitor treatment, since converting enzyme is identical with the kinine- degradating enzyme kininase II.

The results of these animal studies complement the clinical observations of a decreased incidence of arrhythmias in subjects treated with angiotensin CE inhibitors [95, 96]. Given the important role of malignant ventricular arrhythmias in morbidity and mortality associated with ischemic heart disease, the suggested influence of the cardiac renin-angiotensin system assumes major clinical importance as a target for CE inhibitors.

Blood Vessels as a Target for CE Inhibitors

Renin in blood vessel walls may contribute locally to vascular tone independently of the plasma RAS [97–99]. Recently the presence of the various components of the RAS in vascular tissue has been demonstrated [101, 104]. Renin is synthesized in cultured aortic smooth muscle cells [105], and renin gene expression has been shown in cultured vascular endothelial cells [106]. The capability of the vascular RAS to generate the effector peptide ANG II independently of the hormonal RAS has been demonstrated in cultured bovine aortic endothelial cells [107] and in isolated mesenteric vessel preparations [108].

Locally generated angiotensin may act in many ways to influence vascular tone and compliance. These include a direct vasoconstriction by stimulation of angiotensin receptors on the smooth muscle cells of the vascular media [109], facilitation of adrenergic transmission leading to vasoconstriction [86, 110], and stimulation of Na^+ and Ca^{2+} transport systems acros the cell membrane [111].

The physiopathological importance of the vascular RAS has been emphasized by Okamura et al. [112], who demonstrated increased vascular CE activity and an enhanced vasoconstrictor response to ANG I in arteries isolated from hypertensive rats. Of note, both the CE inhibitor, enalapril, and an ANG II receptor antagonist lowered blood pressure in these animals, despite the fact that the plasma RAS was not stimulated. Inhibition of CE can attenuate pre- and postsynaptic sympathetic facilitation afforded by angiotensin II [28, 113, 114]. Nakamura et al. [108] demonstrated, that ANG II is released from isolated rat mesenteric arteries upon β-adrenergic stimulation and that the β-adrenoceptor mediated enhancement of vascular noradrenergic transmission is probably caused largely by a stimulation of local vascular ANG II synthesis [115, 116]. In man, local vascular ANG II generation can probably also be reduced by CE inhibitors [117].

Thus, there is accumulating evidence that inhibition of vascular CE in resistance vessels and large arteries may contribute to the therapeutic actions of CE inhibitors in cardiovascular disease. Much remains to be learned about the cellular localization, action, and regulation of the vascular RAS. Of particular interest for future studies are the possible effects on cardiac and vascular hypertrophy [118, 119], particularly in view of the actions of angiotensin as a growth factor and mitogen [56, 57].

Conclusions

Physiological, biochemical and molecular biologic studies have by now firmly established the existence of local "tissue" RAS in addition to the hormonal plasma renin-angiotensin-system. These local systems are thought to function on an autocrine or paracrine level. We submit that different roles with respect to blood pressure regulation are realized by the plasma RAS and tissue RAS, respectively. The plasma renin-angiotensin system is an important acute regulator of vascular tone and electrolyte and volume homeostasis. The tissue renin-angiotensin systems, on the other hand, probably carry out more long-term functions. Thus, modulation of tissue RASs by converting enzyme inhibitors may well be more important to their long term therapeutic effects than their interference with the hormonal plasma RAS. Hypertension is a chronic disease, and treatment of mild to moderate hypertension does not warrant acute lowering of blood pressure; thus, inhibition of the proposed long-term effects of tissue angiotensin may be more desirable and important than the acute inhibitory effects on the plasma RAS. This view is supported by preliminary data on the effects of different renin-inhibitors. It seems that those renin inhibitors which penetrate into tissue are more effective in lowering hypertension than those which do not penetrate.

The possibility that different CE inhibitors show different pharmacodynamic profiles depending on their tissue penetration and lipid solubility has been thoroughly studied so far. Studies examining effect of different CE inhibitors on the gene expression of renin and angiotensinogen in tissues are presently underway. Thus, as we learn more about the RAS and unravel an increasingly complex picture, we are presented with ever new questions and challenges to be addressed by both basic scientists and the clinical investigators.

Acknowledgement: This work was supported in part by grants from the Deutsche Forschungsgemeinschaft (DFG), SFB 317, and National Institute of Health (NIH) USA 1RO HL 35821-01. The competent secretarial help of Daniela Wirth is gratefully acknowledged.

References

1. Swales JD, Abramovici A, Beck F, Bing RF, Loudon M, Thurston H (1983) Arterial wall renin. J Hypertension 1 [Suppl I]:17–22
2. Thurston H, Swales JD (1977) Blood pressure response of nephrectomized hypertensive rats to converting enzyme inhibition: evidence for persistent vascular renin activity. Clin Sci Mol Med 55:261–270
3. Doi Y, Atarashi K, Franco-Saenz R, Mulrow P (1983) Adrenal renin: A possible regulator of aldosterone production. Clin Exp Hypertension (Theory and Practice) A5 (7 and 8):1119–1126
4. Baba K, Doi Y, Franco-Saenz R, Mulrow P (1986) Mechanisms by which nephrectomy stimulates adrenal renin. Hypertension 8:997–1002
5. Naruse M, Inagami T (1982) Markedly elevated specific renin levels in the adrenal in genetically hypertensive rats. Proc Natl Acad Sci USA 79:3295
6. Deboben A, Inagami T, Ganten D (1983) Tissue renin. In: Genest J, Kuchel O, Hamet P, Cantin M (eds) Hypertension-Physiopathology and Treatment. McGraw Hill, New York, pp 194–209
7. Jin M, Wilhelm MJ, Lang RE, Unger Th, Lindpaintner K, Ganten D (1988) Endogenous tissue renin-angiotensin systems. From molecular biology to therapy. Am J Med 84 [Suppl 3a]:28–36
8. Dzau VJ (1984) Vascular renin-angiotensin: a possible autocrine or paracrine system in control of vascular function. J Cardiovasc Pharmacol 6:377
9. Dzau VJ, Ingelfinger J, Pratt RE, Ellison KE (1986) Identification of renin and angiotensinogen messenger RNA sequences in mouse and rat brains. Hypertension 8:544
10. Ganten D, Lang RE, Lehmann E, Unger Th (1984) Brain angiotensin: on the way to becoming a well-studied neuropeptide system. Biochem Pharmacol 22:3523–3528
11. Hirose S, Yokosawa H, Inagami T, Workman KJ (1980) Renin and prorenin in hog brain: uniquitous distribution and high concentration in pituitary and pineal. Brain Res 191:489–499
12. Suzuki F, Hellmann T, Murakami K, Ludwig G (1987) Expression of the genes for renin and angiotensinogen in tissues of rats. Naunyn-Schmiedebergs Arch Pathol 335: R66
13. Campbell DJ, Bouhnik J, Menard J, Corval P (1984) Identity of angiotensinogen precursors of rat brain and liver. Nature 308: 206–208
14. Nakanishi S, Ohkubo H, Nawa H, Kitamura N, Kageyama R, Ujihara M (1983) Angiotensinogen and kininogen: cloning and sequence analysis of the cD-NAS. Clin Exp Hyper A5 (7/8):997–1003
15. Hellmann W, Suzuki F, Ohkubo H, Nakanishi S, Ludwig G, Ganten D (1988) Angiotensinogen gene expression in extrahepatic rat tissues: Application of a solution hybridization assay. Naunyn-Schmiedebergs Arch Pharmacol 338:327–331
16. Lind RW, Swanson LW, Ganten D (1985) Organization of angiotensin II immunoreactive cells and fibers in the rat central nervous system. Neuroendocrinology 40:2–24
17. Lind RW, Swanson LW, Bruhn TO, Ganten D (1985) The distribution of angiotensin II-immunoreactive cells and fibers in the paraventriculo-hypophysial system of the rat. Brain Res 338:81–89
18. Ganten D, Fuxe K, Phillips MI, Mann JFE, Ganten U (1978) The brain isorenin-angiotensin system: Biochemistry, localization and possible role in drinking and blood pressure regulation. In: Ganong WF, Martini L (eds) Frontiers in Neuroendocrinology, vol 5. Raven Press, New York, pp 61–99
19. Ganten D, Prinz M, Phillips MI, Schölkens BA (eds) The renin-angiotensin system in the brain. Exp Brain Res [Suppl 4]
20. Rettig R, Lang RE, Rascher W, Unger Th, Ganten D (1982) Brain peptides and blood pressure regulation. Clin Sci 63:269s–283s
21. Ganten D, Hermann K, Bayer C, Unger Th, Lang RE (1983) Angiotensin synthesis in the brain and increased turnover in hypertensive rats. Science 221:869–871
22. Schelling P, Meyer D, Loos HE, Speck G, Phillips MI, Johnson AK, Ganten D (1982) A micromethod for the measurement of renin in brain nuclei: its application in spontaneously hypertensive rats. Neuropharmacology R1:445–463
23. Berecek KH, Okuno T, Nagahama S, Oparil S (1983) Altered vascular reactivity and baroreflex sensitivity induced by chronic central administration of captopril in the spontaneously hypertensive rat. Hypertension 5:869–700
24. Evered MD, Robinson MM, Richardson MA (1980) Captopril given intracerebroventricularly, subcutaneously or by gavage inhibits angiotensin converting enzyme activity in the rat brain. Eur J Pharmacol 68:443–449
25. Mann JFE, Phillips MI, Dietz R, Haebara H, Ganten D (1978) Effects of central and peripheral angiotensin blockade in hypertensive rats. Am J Physiol 234:629–637
26. McDonald W, Wickre C, Aumann S, Ban D, Moffit B (1980) The sustained antihyperten-

sive effect of chronic cerebroventricular infusion of angiotensin antagonist in spontaneously hypertensive rats. Endocrinology 197:1305–1308
27. Unger Th, Kaufmann-Bühler I, Schölkens B, Ganten D (1981) Brain converting enzyme inhibition: a possible mechanism for the anthihypertensive action of captopril in spontaneously hypertensive rats. Eur J Pharmacol 70:467–478
28. Unger Th, Ganten D, Lang RE (1983) Pharmacology of converting enzyme inhibitors: new aspect. Clin Exp Hypertension A5 (7/8):1333–1354
29. Stamler JF, Brody MJ, Phillips MI (1980) The central and peripheral effects of captopril (SQ 14225) on the arterial pressure of the spontaneously hypertensive rat. Brain Res 186:499–503
30. Hutchinson JS, Mendelsohn FAO, Doyle AE (1980) Blood pressure responses of conscious normotensive and spontaneously hypertensive rats to intracerebroventricular and peripheral administration of captopril. Hypertension 2:546–550
31. Phillips MI, Kimura B (1986) Converting enzyme inhibitors and brain angiotensin. J Cardiovasc Pharmacol 8 [Suppl 10]:82–90
32. Suzuki H, Kondo K, Handa M, Saruta T (1981) Role of the brain iso-renin-angiotensin system in experimental hypertension in rats. Clin Sci 61:175–180
33. Pochiero M, Nicoletta P, Losi E, Bianchi A, Caputi AP (1983) Cardiovascular responses of conscious DOCA-salt hypertensive rats to acute intracerebroventricular and intravenous administration of captopril. Pharmacol Res Comm 15:173–182
34. Vollmer RR, Boccagno JA (1977) Central cardiovascular effects of SQ 14 225, an angiotensin converting inhibitor in chloralose anesthetized cats. Eur J Pharmacol 45: 117–125
35. Mann JFE, Rascher W, Dietz R, Schömig A, Ganten D (1979) Effects of an orally active converting enzyme inhibitor, SQ 14 255, on pressor responses to angiotensin administered into brain ventricles of spontaneously hypertensive rats. Clin Sci 56:585–589
36. Hutchinson JS, Hooper R, Jarott B, Mendelsohn FAO, Louis WJ (1982) Captopril does not cross the blood cerebrospinal fluid barrier in the spontaneously hypertensive rat after a single, intravenous injection. In: Rascher W, Clough D, Ganten D (eds) Hypertensive mechanism. Schattauer, Stuttgart, New York, pp 691–694
37. Unger Th, Ganten D, Lang RE, Schölkens BA (1984) Is tissue converting enzyme inhibition a determinant of the antihypertensive efficacy of converting enzyme inhibitors? Studies with two different compounds, Hoe-498 and MK-421, in spontaneously hypertensive rats. J Cardiovasc Pharmacol 6:872–880
38. Cohen ML, Kurz KD (1982) Angiotensin converting enzyme inhibition in tissues from spontaneously hypertensive rats after treatment with captopril or MK-421. J Pharmacol Exp Ther 220:63–69
39. Norman JA, Lehmann M, Goodman FR, Barclay BW, Zimmermann MB (1987) Central and peripheral inhibition of angiotensin converting enzyme (ACE) in the SHR: Correlation with the antihypertensive activity of the inhibitos. Clin Exp Hyper A9 (2/3):461–468
40. Nakata K, Nishimura K, Takada T, Ikuse T, Yamauchi H, Iso T (1987) Effects of an angiotensin-converting enzyme (ACE) inhibitor, SA 446, on tissue ACE activity in normotensive, spontaneously hypertensive, and renal hypertensive rats. J Cardiovasc Pharmacol 9:305–310
41. Geppetti P, Spillantini MG, Frilli S, Pietrini U, Fanciullacci M, Sicuteri F (1987) Acute oral captopril inhibits angiotensin converting enzyme activity in human cerebrospinal fluid. J Hypertension 5:151–154
42. Ganten D, Ganten U, Kubo S, Grayer P, Nowaczynski W, Bruder R, Genest J (1973) Iso-renin in rat adrenal glands: Influences of sodium, potassium and pituitary hormones. Am J Physiol 227:224–230
43. Suzuki F, Hellmann W, Paul M, Lindpaintner K, Murakami K, Ganten D (1986) Renin gene espression in rat tissue: a new quantitative assay method for rat renin mRNA using synthetic cRNA. Clin Exp Hypertension 2:345–359
44. Campell DJ, Habener JF (1986) Regional distribution of angiotensinogen messenger RNA in rat adrenal and kidney. J Hypertension 4:385–387
45. Naruse M, Takii Y, Inagami T (1981) Renin exists in high concentration in the rat adrenal gland. Biomed Res 2:583–586
46. Deschepper CF, Mellon SH, Cumin F, Baxter JD, Ganong WF (1983) Analysis by immunochemistry and in situ hybridization of renin and its mRNA in kidney, testis, adrenal and pituitary of the rat. Proc Natl Acad Sci USA 86:7552–7556
47. Peach MJ (1977) Renin-angiotensin systems: biochemistry and mechanism of action. Physiol Rev 57:313–320
48. Ganten D, Herrman K, Unger T, Lang RE (1983) The tissue renin-angiotensin system: focus on brian angiotensin, adrenal gland and aterial wall. Clin Exp Hypertension 5:1099–1118

49. Ganten D, Ganten U, Kubo S, Grayer P, Nowaczinsky W, Bruder R, Genest J (1974) Iso-renin in rat adrenal glands: Influences of sodium, potassium and pituitary hormones. Am J Physiol 227:224–230
50. Ganten D, Conn JW, Helber A, Vescei P, Hornung H, Hutchinson JS, Schelling P (1975) Evidence for a role of adrenal iso-renin for corticosteroid synthesis. Eur J Clin Invest 5:16
51. Ganten D, Hutchinson JS, Schelling P, Ganten U, Fischer H (1976) The iso-renin angiotensin system in extrarenal tissue. Clin Exp Pharmacol 3:103–106
52. Peach MJ, Bumpus FM, Kharallah PA (1971) Release of adrenal catecholamines by angiotensin I. J Pharmacol Exp Ther 176: 366–376
53. Nakamaru M, Misono KS, Naruse M, Workman RF, Inagami T (1985) A role for the adrenal renin-angiotensin system in the regulation of potassium-stimulated aldosterone production. Endocrinology 117:1772–1778
54. Mizuno K, Hoffman LH, McKenzie JC, Inagami T (1988) Presence of renin secretory granules in rat adrenal gland and stimulation of renin secretion by angiotensin II but not by adrenocorticotropin. J Clin Invest 82: 1007–1016
55. Strittmatter SM, De Souza EB, Lynch DR, Snyder SH (1986) Angiotensin-converting enzyme localized in the rat pituitary and adrenal glands by 3H captopril autoradiographz. Endocrinology 118:1690–1699
56. Schelling P, Ganten D, Speck G, Fischer H (1979) Effects of angiotensin II and angiotensin II antagonist saralasin on cell growth and renin 3T3 and SC3T3 cells. J Cellular Physiol 98:503–513
57. Gill GN, Ill CR, Simonian MH (1977) Angiotensin stimulation of bovine adrenocortical cell growth. Proc Natl Acad Sci USA 12:5563–5573
58. Jackson TR, Blair LAC, Marshall J, Goedert M, Hanley MR (1988) The mas oncogene encodes an angiotensin receptor. Nature 335:437–440
59. Gernandez LA, Twickler J, Mead A (1985) Neovascularization produced by angiotensin II. J Lab Med 105:141–145
60. Folkman J, Klagsbrun M (1987) Angiogenic factors. Science 235:442–447
61. Re R, Vizzrd DL, Brown J, Bryan SE (1984) Angiotensin II receptors in chromatin fragments generated by micrococcal nuclease. Biochem Biophys Res Commun 119: 220–227
62. Re R, Parab M (1984) Effect of angiotensin II on RNA synthesis by isolated nuclei. Life Sci 34:648–651
63. Vinson GP, Pudney JA, Whitehouse BJ (1985) The mammalian adrenal circulation and the relationship between adrenal blood flow and steroidogenesis. J Endocrinol 105: 285–294
64. Axelrod J, Reisine TD (1984) Stress hormones: their interactions and regulation. Science 224:452–459
65. Kenyon CJ, DeConti GA, Cupolo NA, Morris DJ (1981) The role of aldosterone in the development of hypertension in spontaneously hypertensive rats. Endocrinology 109/6:1841–1845
66. Aoki K, Tankawa H, Fujinami T, Miyazaki O, Hashimoto Y (1963) Pathological studies on the endocrine organs of the spontaneously hypertensive rats. Jpn Heart J 14:443
67. Iams SG, McMurtry JP, Wexler BC (1979) Aldosterone, deocycorticosterone, corticosterone and prolactin changes during the livespan of chronically and spontaneously hypertensive rats. Endocrinology 104: 1357–1363
68. Ganten D, Ludwig G, Hennhoefer C (1986) Genetic control of renin in the tissue of different strains of mice (abstr.). Naunyn Schmiedebergs Arch Pharmacol 332:R59
69. Hayduk K, Boucher R, Genest J (1970) Renin activity and content in various tissues in dogs under different pathophysiological states. Proc Soc Exp Biol Med 134:252–255
70. Ganten D, Ganten U, Granger O, Boucher R, Genest J (1972) Renin in heart muscle and arterial tissue (abstr.). Verh Dtsch Ges Kreislaufforsch 38:268
71. Re RN, Michalik RJ, Dzau VJ (1983) Cardiac myocytes contain renin (abstr.). Clin Res 31:845A
72. Dzau VJ, Ellison KE, Brody T, Ingelfinger J, Pratt RE (1987) A comparative study of the distributions of renin and angiotensinogen messenger ribonucleic acids in rat and mouse tissues. Endocrinology 120: 2334–2338
73. Auffray C, Rougeon F (1980) Purification of mouse immunoglobulin heavy chain mRNAs from total myeloma tumor RNA. Eur J Biochem 107:303–314
74. Le Muer M, Glanville N, Mandel JL, Gerlinger P, Palmiter R, Chambon P (1981) The ovealbumin gene family: hormonal control of X- and Y-gene transcription and mRNA accumulation. Cell 23:561–571
75. Lindpaintner K, Wilhelm M, Jin M, Unger Th, Lang RE, Ganten D (1987) Tissue renin-angiotensin systems: focus on the heart. J Hyper 5:S33–S38
76. Needleman P, Marshall GR, Sobel BE (1975) Hormone interactions in the isolated rabbit heart. Circ Res 37:802–808

77. Nakashima A, Angus JA, Johnston CI (1982) Chronotropic effects of angiotensin I, angiotensin II, bradykinin and norepinephrine in guinea pig atria. Eur J Pharmacol 81:479–485
78. Heeg E, Meng K (1965) Die Wirkung des Bradykinins, Angiotensins und Vasopressins auf Vorhof, Papillarmuskel, und isoliert durchströmte Herzpräparate des Meerschweinchens. Naunyn Schmiedebergs Arch Pathol 250:35–47
79. Freer RJ, Pappano AJ, Pech MJ et al. (1976). Mechanisms for the positive inotropic effect of angiotensin II on isolated cardiac muscle. Circ Res 39:178–183
80. Kobayashi M, Furukawa Y, Chiba S (1978) Positive chronotropic and inotropic effects of angiotensin II in the dog heart. Eur J Pharmacol 50:17–25
81. Dempsey PJ, McCallum ZT, Kent KM, Cooper T (1971) Direct myocardial effects of angiotensin II. Am J Physiol 220:477
82. Koch-Weser J (1964) Myocardial actions of angiotensin. Circ Res 1964, 14:337–344
83. Starke K, Werner U, Schuermann JH (1966) Wirkungen von Angiotensin auf Funktion und Noradrenalinabgabe isolierter Kaninchenherzen in Ruhe und bei Sympathikusreizung. Naunyn Schmiedebergs Arch Pharmacol 265:170–186
84. Blumberg AL, Acherly JA, Peach MJ (1976) Differentiation of neurogenic and myocardial angiotensin II receptors in isolated rabbit atria. Circ Res 36:719–726
85. Xiang J, Linz W, Becker H et al. (1984) Effects of converting enzyme inhibitors ramipril and enalapril on peptide actions and sympathetic neurotransmission in the isolated heart. Eur J Pharmacol 113:215–223
86. Malik KU, Nasjletti A (1976) Facilitation of adrenergic transmission by locally generated angiotensin II in rat mesenteric arteries. Circ Res 38:26–30
87. Khairallah PA (1972) Action of angiotensin on adrenergic nerve endings. Fed Proc 31: 1351–1357
88. Swartz SL, Williams GH, Hollenberg NK, Levine L, Denk JR, Moore TJ (1980) Captopril-induced changes in prostaglandin production. J Clin Invest 65:1257–1264
89. Roth RH (1972) Action of angiotensin on adrenergic nerve endings. Fed Proc 31: 1358–1364
90. Westfall TC (1977) Local regulation of adrenergic neurotransmission. Physiol Rev 57:659–728
91. Glough DP, Mulroy SC, Angell D, Hatton R (1983) Interference by inhibitors of the renin-angiotensin system with neurogenic vasoconstriction. Clin Exp Hypertension 5:1287–1299
92. Xiang JZ, Schoelkens BA, Ganten D, Unger Th (1984) Effects of sympathetic nerve stimulation are attenuated by the converting enzyme inhibitor Hoe-498 in isolated rabbit hearts. Clin Exp Hypertension 6:1853–1857
93. Ertl G, Kloner RA, Alexander RW, Braunwald E (1982) Limitation of experimental infarct size by an angiotensin converting enzyme inhibitor. Circulation 65:40–48
94. Linz W, Schoelkens BA, Han YF (1986) Beneficial effects of the converting enzyme inhibitor, ramipril, in ischemic rat hearts. J Cardiovasc Pharmacol 8:S91–S99
95. Cleland JGF, Dargie HJ, Hodsman GJP et al. (1984) Captopril in heart failure. A double-blind controlled trial. Br Heart J 52: 530–535
96. Webster MWI, Fitzpatrick MA, Nicholls MG, Ikram H, Wells JE (1985) Effect of enalapril on ventricular arrthythmias in congestive heart failure. Am J Cardiol 56: 566–569
97. Rosenthal J, Boucher R, Rojo Ortega JM, Genest J (1969) Renin activity in aortic tissue of rats. Can J Physil Pharmacol 47:53
98. Ganten D, Hayduk K, Brecht HM, Boucher R, Genest J (1970) Evidence of renin release of production in splanchnic territory. Nature 226:551
99. Thurston H, Swales JD (1977) Blood pressure response of nephrectomized hypertensive rats to converting enzyme inhibition: evidence for persistent vascular renin activity. Clin Sci Mol Med 52:299–304
100. Thurston H, Swales JD, Bing RF, Hurst BC, Marks ES (1979) Vascular renin-like activity and blood pressure maintenance in the rat: studies of the effect of changes in sodium balance, hypertension and nephrectomy. Hypertension 1:643–649
101. Campbell DJ, Habener JF (1986) Angiotensinogen gene is expressed and differentially regulated in multiple tissue of the rat. J Clin Invest 78:31–39
102. Dzau VJ (1987) Vascular angiotensin pathways: a new therapeutic target. J Cardiovasc Pharmacol 10:S9–S16
103. Swales JD, Heagerty AM (1987) Vascular renin-angiotensin system: The unanswered questions. J Hypertension 5:S1–S5
104. Darby I, Aldred P, Crawford RJ, Fernley RT, Niall HD, Penschow JD, Ryan GB, Coghlan JP (1985) Gene expression in vessels of the ovine cortex. J Hypertension 3:9–12
105. Re R, Fallon JT, Dzau VJ, Quay SC, Haber E (1982) Renin synthesis by canine aortic smooth muscle cells in culture. Life Sci 30:99-106
106. Lilly LS, Pratt RE, Alexander RW (1984)

Renin expression by vascular endothelial cells in culture. Circ Res 57:312–318
107. Kifor I, Dzau VJ (1987) Endothelial renin-angiotensin pathway: evidence for intracellular synthesis and secretion of angiotensins. Circ Res 60:422–428
108. Nakamura M, Jackson EK, Inagami T (1986) Beta adrenoceptor-mediated release of angiotensin II from mesenteric arteries. Am J Physiol 250:H144–H148
109. Oliver JA, Sciacca RR (1984) Local generation of angiotensin II as a mechanism of regulation of peripheral vascular tone in the rat. J Clin Invest 74:1247–1251
110. Zimmermann BG (1981) Adrenergic facilitation by angiotensin: does it serve a physiological function? Clin Sci 60:343–348
111. Kuriyama S, Nakamura A, Hopp L, Fine BP, Kino M, Cragoe E Jr, Aviv A (1988) Angiotensin II effect on $^{22}Na^+$ transport in vascular smooth muscle cells. J Cardiovasc Pharmacol 11:139–146
112. Okamura T, Myazaki M, Inagami T, Toda N (1986) Vascular renin-angiotensin system in two-kidney, one clip hypertensive rats. Hypertension 8:560–565
113. Ball SG (1989) ACE inhibitors and the nervous system. J Card Vasc Pharm (in press)
114. Schölkens BA, Xiang JZ, Tilly H (1984) Influence of the converting enzyme inhibitors Hoe 498, enalapril and captopril on vascular reactivity of isolated arterial preparations. Clin Exp Hypertension A6:1807–1813
115. Kawasaki H, Cline WH Jr, Su C (1984) Involvement of the vascular renin-angiotensin system in beta adrenergic receptor-mediated facilitation of vascular neurotransmission in spontaneously hypertensive rats. J Pharmacol Exp Ther 231:23–32
116. Göthert M, Kollecker P (1986) Subendothelial β_2-adrenoceptors in the rat vena cava: facilitation of the release via local stimulation of angiotensin II synthesis. Naunyn-Schmiedebergs Arch Pharmacol 334: 156–165
117. Webb DJ, Collier JG (1986) Vascular angiotensin conversion in humans. J Cardiovasc Pharmacol 8:S40–S44
118. Oshima T, Matsushita Y, Miyamoto M, Koike H (1983) Effect of long-term blockade of angiotensin converting enzyme with captopril on blood pressure and aortic prolyl hydroxylase activity in spontaneously hypertensive rats. Eur J Pharmacol 91:283–286
119. Henrichs KJ, Unger Th, Berecek KH, Ganten D (1980) Is arterial media hypertrophy in spontaneously hypertensive rats a consequence of or a cause for hypertension. Clin Sci 59:331s–333s

Catecholamines, Adrenergic Receptors and Exercise Capacity in Trained Subjects and in Coronary Heart Disease

M. Lehmann

Medizinische Universitätsklinik, Abt. Sport- und Leistungsmedizin, Freiburg, FRG

Summary. An activation of the sympathetic nervous system can be observed, dependent on decreasing cardiac pump capacity and decreasing exercise capacity in coronary heart disease patients. The sympathetic activation contributes to an uneconomical functioning of the damaged heart; this activation is the result and not the cause of the disease. In end-stage IV coronary heart disease, increasing exhaustion of the sympathetic system is probable with impaired neurotransmitter synthesis, storage, re-uptake and homologous desensitization of target organs. As we know from training methods, improvement in the aerobic exercise capacity – beside an increase in vagal tone – reduces sympathetic activity. This mechanism can also be observed in physical therapy of suitable heart patients, hemodynamically stage I and II. The extent is, of course, much lover, only marginal in part, or not givem, dependent on the remaining exercise capacity and the course of their disease. Thus, after one year of physical therapy, there was a mean decrease in the lactate, noradrenaline and adrenaline responses at same exercise levels with a reduction in the double product; consequently, an economization of cardiac work, which on the average favored a 25% increase in exercise capacity without direct improvement of coronary circulation or myocardial function.

Key words: Catecholamines – Adrenic receptors – Exercise capacity – Coronary heart disease

Introduction

The pathogenic importance of changes in sympathetic activity, adrenoreceptors and post-receptor mechanisms in various heart diseases has been intensively discussed in the past few years [for example 1, 4, 5, 8, 29, 34]. The purpose of this article is not to repeat this discussion, but rather to present the training results in healthy athletes which may have beneficial effects in the therapy of heart patients, especially coronary heart disease. Moreover, findings in coronary heart disease stage IV will be discussed which indicate exhaustion of the sympathetic system.

Methods

Catecholamine behavior in tissue, plasma and urine may be used to evaluate sympathetic activity, by which we mean the neural activity in sympathetic nerves. In spite of critical objections, this appears justified, since there are correlations 1. between the response of the heart to sympathetic stimulation and the noradrenaline concentration in the coronary sinus of the dog; 2. between sympathetic outflow to muscles and plasma noradrenaline concentration in venous blood in man; 3. between noradrenaline concentration simultaneously determined in the coronary sinus, aorta and peripheral veins; 4. between catecholamine concentrations determined by radioenzymatic methods or HPLC [11, 33, 37]. We measure the catecholamines radioenzymatically [10] and the beta-2-adrenoreceptors by means of tritium-labeled dihydroalprenolol or yohimbin (alpha-2-adrenoreceptors) in intact vital blood cells [20, 21].

Training and Overtraining

Braunwald was among the first to describe heart as an endocrine organ of the sympathetic system [4].

The heart is an important site of synthesis, release and re-uptake of noradrenaline,

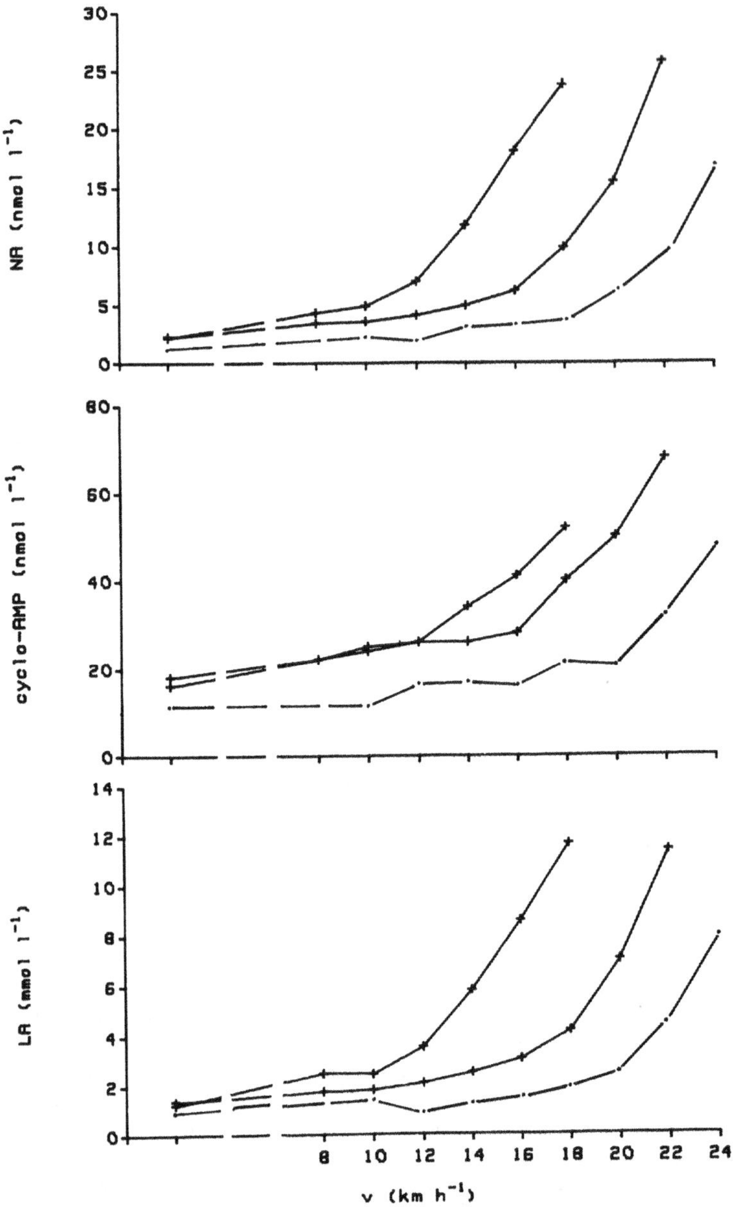

Fig. 1. Behavior of plasma noradrenaline (primary messenger), Cyclo-AMP (secondary messenger) and lactate level (substrate metabolite of anaerobic glycolysis) in incremental physical exercise (treadmill, v = velocity) in a highly-trained endurance athlete (●) and less well trained athletes (+)

Fig. 2. Decrease in plasma noradrenaline and adrenaline in physical exercise at a submaximum exercise level (above) during training of three times 30 min per week (bicycle ergometry); also decrease in catecholamine excretion after 12 weeks of training (DA = dopamine excretion in 24 h; NA = noradrenaline, A = adrenaline) ▶

Fig. 3. 24-h noradrenaline excretion in untrained control subjects (CS), endurance-trained atheletes (TS), overtrained athletes (OTS) and patients with Shy-Drager Syndrome (sympathetic insufficiency) – above- and corresponding beta-2-adrenoreceptor density on intact leukocytes (below) ▶

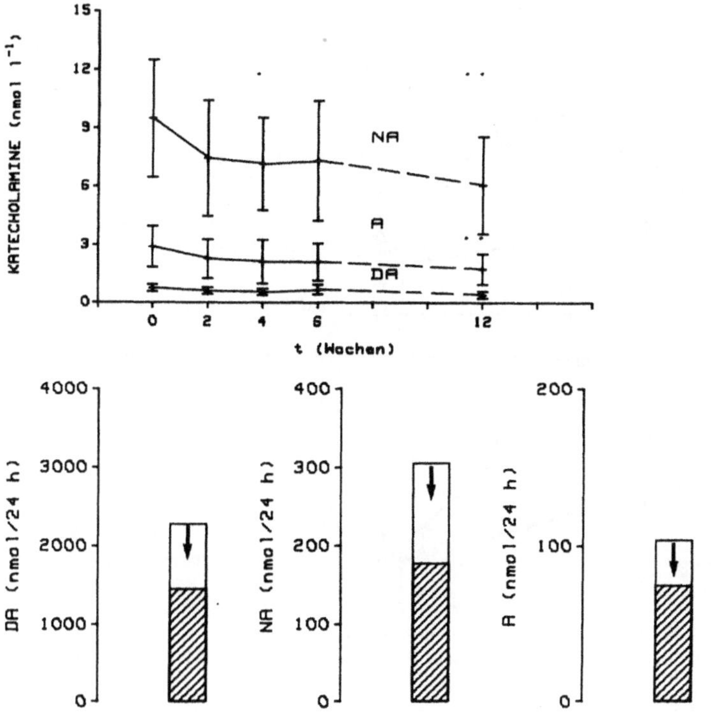
KATECHOLAMINE (nmol l⁻¹)
15
12
9
6
3
0
NA
A
DA
0
2
4
6
12
t (Wochen)
DA (nmol/24 h)
4000
3000
2000
1000
0
NA (nmol/24 h)
400
300
200
100
0
A (nmol/24 h)
200
100
0

Fig. 2

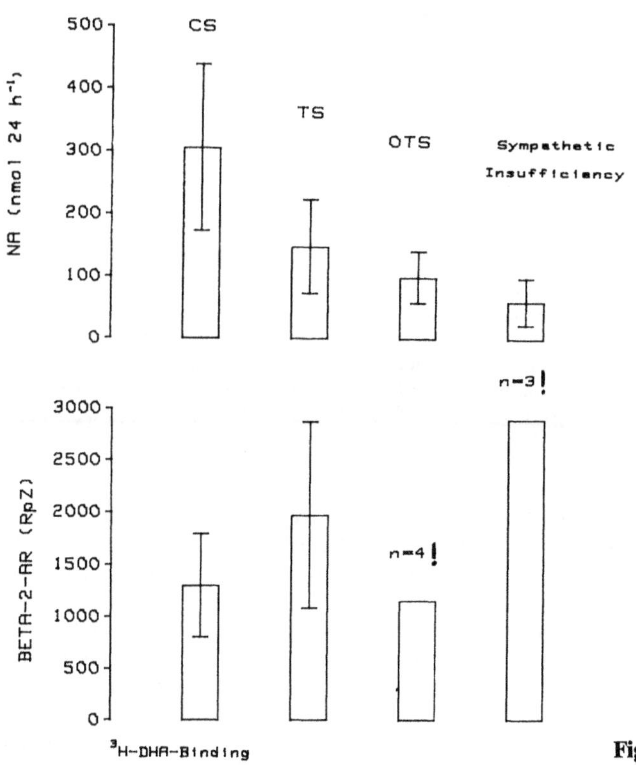
NA (nmol 24 h⁻¹)
500
400
300
200
100
0
CS
TS
OTS
Sympathetic
Insufficiency
n=3 !
BETA-2-AR (RpZ)
3000
2500
2000
1500
1000
500
0
n=4 !
³H-DHA-Binding

Fig. 3

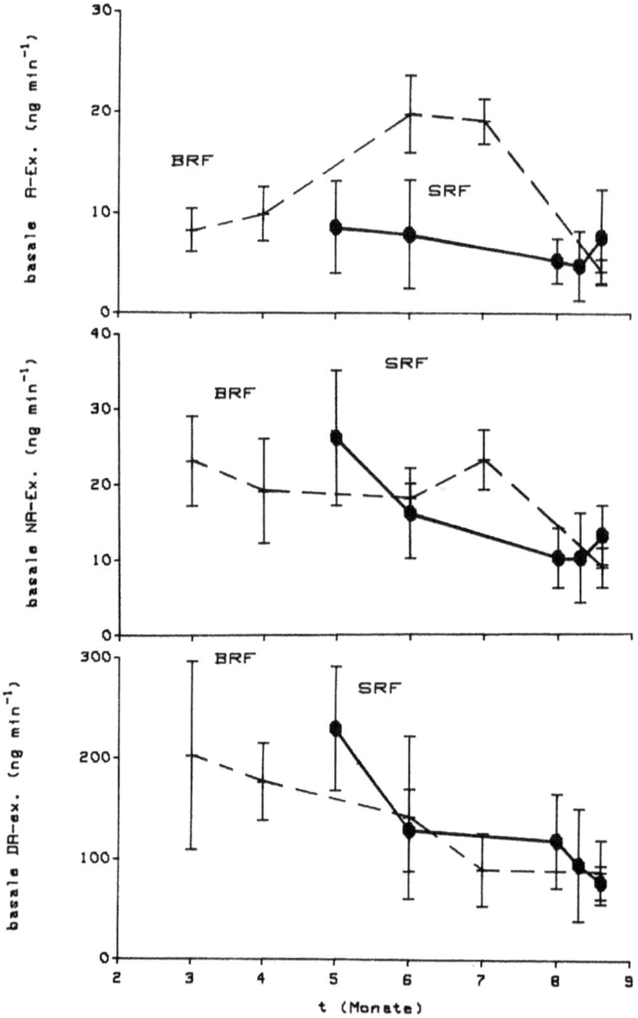

Fig. 4. Behavior of basal, nightly catecholamine excretion in track cyclists (BRF) and road cyclists (SFR) from March 1988 and May 1988, respectively to August 1988 prior to the Olympic Games. The behavior of basal adrenaline (above) indicates overexertion of the track cyclists with subsequent exhaustion (sharp decrease); these cyclists were eliminated from competition in the qualification rounds. The road cyclists (SFR) show a comparably stable adrenaline pattern and slight re-increase prior to the Games, which we interpret as a regeneration effect. This team won two medals. The basal noradrenaline (NA) and dopamine (DA) excretion do not differ as sharply between the two groups

as well as a target organ. Adequate adaptation to stress is only possible with an intact sympathetic system. This is especially clear in primary orthostatic or asympathicotonic hypotension [22, 23]. These patients show reduced sympathetic activity and increased adrenoreceptor density and sensitivity to catecholamines. The increased sensitivity cannot offset the neurotransmitter deficiency. The symptomatics represent a model for the integrative importance of the sympathicus in the regulation of the reaction to stress.

The effects of physical endurance training on sympathetic activity and catecholamine behavior have often been presented [12, 16, 17, 18, 24, 25, 35]. Catecholamine levels (primary messengers), cyclic adenosine

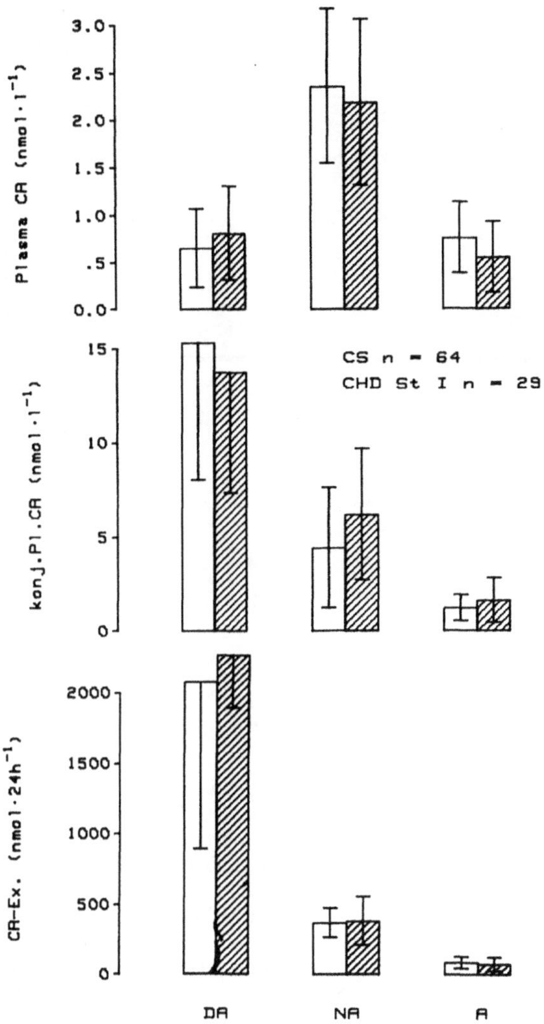

Fig. 5. Coronary heart disease patients, hemodynamic stage I or II (shaded columns) show no differences in plasma catecholamine level at rest (free catecholamine above, conjugated fractions in the middle) or in 24-h catecholamine excretion compared to healthy control subjects (unshaded columns)

monophosphate (secondary messenger) and lactate as a substrate metabolite of anaerobic glycolysis are lower in endurance trained subjects at the same, absolute exercise level than in untrained individuals (Fig. 1). This indicates economization of energy supply in trained subjects, of which the basis is the increased aerobic work capacity of the trained muscle cells.

The low catecholamine levels in trained individuals are primarily an expression of a lower excretion, not increased metabolism, since the metabolized fractions and urinary catecholamines (Fig. 2) are also reduced. The lower sympathetic activity in trained individuals, as in asympathicotonic hypotension [22, 23] is accompanied by elevated beta-2-adrenoreceptor density (Fig. 3) and sensitivity to catecholamines [25].

The change in adrenoreceptor density is the subject of controversial discussion [2, 3, 5–7, 15, 17, 25, 27, 34]. The controversy arises mostly for methodic reasons (membrane preparation vs. study of the receptor on vital, intact cells) or because the two-phase regulation of the receptors is overlooked [32]. In overtrained athletes, catecholamine excretion decreases, the

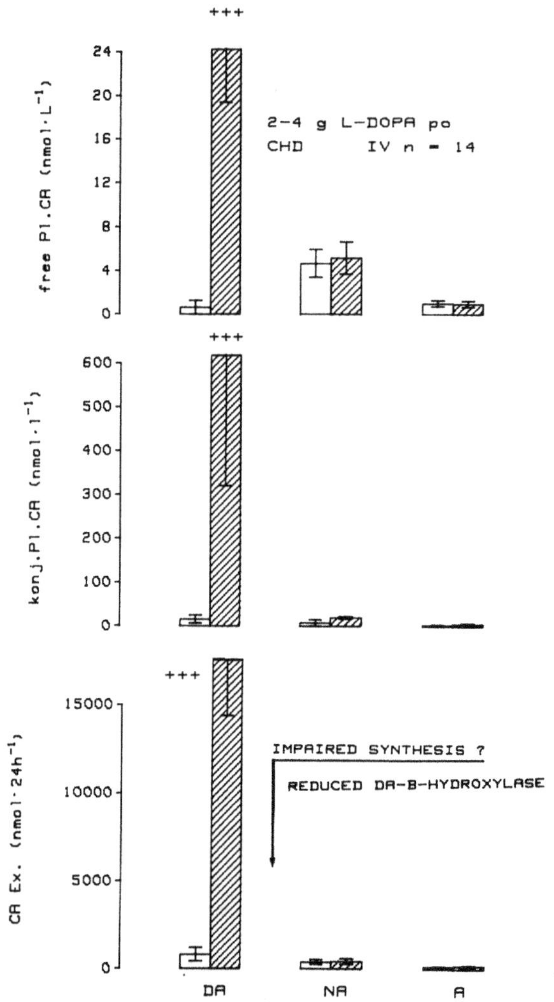

Fig. 6. After administration of 2–4 g levodopa per os to CHD patients, stage IV, there is a flooding of the organism with free dopamine (above), conjugated dopamine (middle) and marked increase in dopamine excretion (below, shaded column). No noteworthy increase in free, conjugated or urinary noradrenaline and adrenaline can be recognized

beta-2-adrenoreceptor density is normal to subnormal; the catecholamine excretion is in the same range as that of patients with A-sympathicotonic hypotension (Fig. 3). This is probably a transient exhaustion of the sympathetic system due to overload as a protective mechanism against sympathetic overstimulation of the cell.

The analysis of basal, or nightly catecholamine excretion has been proven as a parameter of chronic physical overload, for example resulting from training (Fig. 4). The marked increase in basal excretion in over-exercise [14] and the subsequent subnormal adrenaline excretion may be interpreted as an indicator of overtraining or exhaustion (Fig. 4), as we observed with Dr. G. Huber and Dr. W. Stockhausen in track cyclists in the German Olympic Team – compared to the road cyclists. The track cyclists were already eliminated from competition in the qualification rounds. Apparently, a transient insuffiency of the sympathetic system may also occur in healthy individuals as a result of physical overwork.

Heart Patients and Sympathicus

At rest, CHD patients with mild impairment of left ventricular function show no

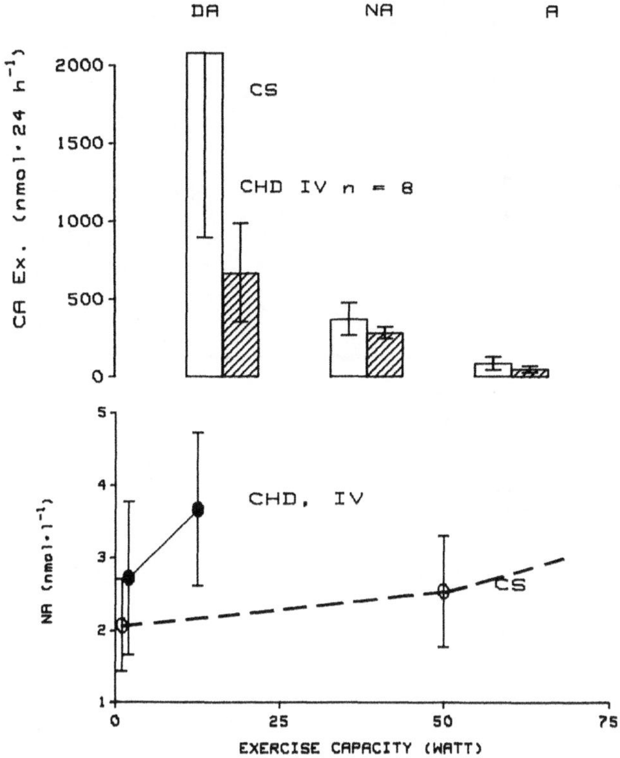

Fig. 7. CHD patients in end stage IV of the disease show a marked decrease in dopamine excretion and less marked decrease in noradrenaline and adrenaline excretion (above, shaded columns) than healthy control subjects (CS). The mean plasma noradrenaline level (below) is elevated, most likely due to impaired re-uptake

evidence of altered sympathetic activity (Fig. 5), but only in physical exercise or higher-grade impairment of the left ventricular function [28]. Noradrenaline in particular correlated to coronary score [11], angina pectoris index [28], key hemodynamic parameters [19, 29], exercise capacity [26] and prognosis [9]. As we see it today, elevated sympathetic activity is the result of left ventricular dysfunction, and not its cause. Initially, increased catecholamine release is probably decisive for the elevated plasma catecholamine concentration and urinary catecholamine elimination [17–19, 29]; in advanced stages, impaired re-uptake also plays a role [29]. In the end stage, there ist evidence of impaired synthesis, that is reduced activity of the rate-limiting enzyme [30] (Fig. 6), cardiac catecholamine deficiency [4, 5, 8], reduced catecholamine excretion (particularly dopamine) in 24 h (Fig. 7), and homologous desensitization (beta-2-adrenoreceptors) [2, 5, 16, 17]. The myocardium and sympathetic system appear equally "burned out".

Physical Therapy

Dosed and controlled physical therapy may result in relief of heart strain and improvement in the exercise capacity of about 50% of the CHD patients, hemodynamic stage I and II of the disease [16] through endurance training of the skeletal muscles, improvement in flexibility and coordination (Fig. 8), in other words, in an economization of cardiac work [13, 31] (Fig. 9). Favorable influence on the prognosis remains debatable.

References

1. Andersson KE (1986) Adrenergic mechanisms in congestive heart failure. Acta Med Scand [Suppl] 707:37–44
2. Baumann G, Rieß G (1982) Verhalten kardialer β-Rezeptoren bei akutem Myokardin-

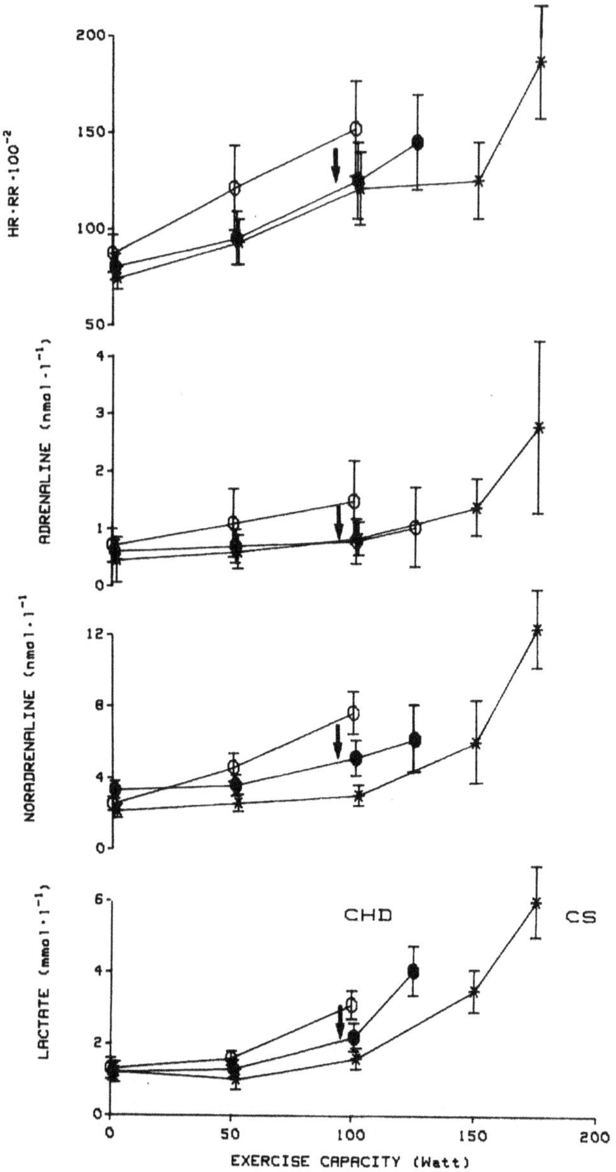

Fig. 8. Behavior of the lactate level, noradrenaline and adrenaline plasma concentrations and double product during incremental bicycle ergometry, supine, in 20 post-infarction patients (exercise capacity >1 watt per kg body weight) prior to (○) and 1 year after outpatient physical therapy (●). Also shown are the data of healthy control subjects (CS *)

farkt und chronischem Herzversagen. Mögliche Rolle von H2-Rezeptor-Agonisten im Katecholamin-refraktären Myokard. Herz Kreisl 14:169–178
3. Bieger W, Zittel R (1982) Effect of physical activity on beta-receptor activity. In: Knuttgen HG, Vogel JA, Poortmans J (eds) Biochemistry of exercise. Human Kinetics Publishers, Champain-Ill. USA: 205–211
4. Braunwald E (1964) The heart as an endocrine organ. Am J Med 36:1–3
5. Bristow MR, Ginsburg R, Minobe W (1982) Decreased catecholamine sensitivity and β-adrenergic receptor density in failing human hearts. New Engl J Med 307:205–211
6. Brodde OE, Daul A, O'Hara N (1984) β-Adrenoceptor changes in human lymphocytes induced by dynamic exercise. Naunyn-Schmiedebergs Arch Pharmacol 325: 190–192
7. Butler J, O'Brian M, O'Malley K, Kelle JG (1982) Relationship of β-adrenoceptor de-

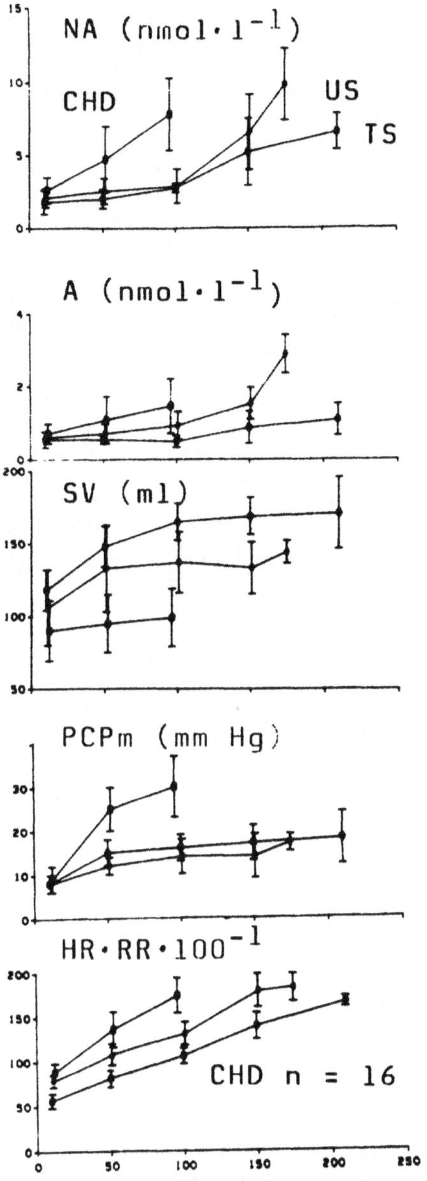

Fig. 9. Behavior of noradrenaline (NA), adrenaline (A), stroke volume (SV), wedge pressure (PCPm) and double product during incremental bicycle ergometry, supine, in post-infarction patients (exercise capacity >1 watt per kg body weight), untrained control subjects (CS) and healthy endurance athletes of comparable age (TS)

nsity to fitness in athletes. Nature 298:60–61
8. Chidsey CA, Braunwald E, Morrow AG (1965) Catecholamine excretion and cardiac stores of norepinephrine in congestive heart failure. Am J Med 39:442–451
9. Cohn JN, Levine TB, Olivari MT, Graberg V, Lura D, Francis GS, Simon AB, Rector T (1984) Plasma norepinephrine as a guide to prognosis in patients with chronic congestive heart failure. New Engl J Med 311:819–823
10. DaPrada M, Zürcher G (1976) Simultaneous radioenzymatic determination of plasma and tissue adrenaline, noradrenaline and dopamine within the fentomole range. Life Sci 19:1161–1174
11. Dominiak P, Schulz W, Delius W, Kober G, Grobecker H (1981) Catecholamines in patients with coronary heart disease. In: Delius W, Gerlach E, Grobecker H, Kübler W (eds) Catecholamines and the heart. Springer, Berlin Heidelberg New York, pp 223–233
12. Hartley LH, Mason JW, Hogan RP, Jones LG, Kotchen TA, Mougey EH, Wherry FE, Penington LL, Ricketts PT (1972) Multiple hormonal response to graded exercise in relation to physical training. J Appl Physiol 33:602–606
13. Heiss HW, Barmeyer J, Wink K, Huber G, Breiter J, Keul J, Reindell H (1975) Durchblutung und Substratumsatz des gesunden menschlichen Herzens in Abhängigkeit vom Trainingszustand. Verh Dtsch Ges Kreislaufforsch 41:247
14. Jakob E, Lehmann M, Huber G, Rokitzki L, Stockhausen W, Keul J (1988) The role of basal catecholamine excretion as a parameter in training management. Int J Sports Med 9:392
15. Krawietz W, Klein EM, Unterberg C, Ackenheil (1985) Physical activity decreases the number of β-adrenergic receptors on human lymphocytes. Klin Wochenschr 63: 73–78
16. Lehmann M, Keul J (1988) Sympatho-vagal changes induced by physical training in cardiac patients. Eur Heart J 9 [Suppl F]:55–62
17. Lehmann M, Rühle K, Schmid P, Klein H, Matthys K, Keul J (1983) Hämodynamik, Plasmakatecholaminverhalten und β-Adrenorezeptorendichte bei Trainierten, Untrainierten und Herzinsuffizienten. Z Kardiol 72:529–536
18. Lehmann M, Dickhuth HH, Franke T, Huber G, Keul J (1983) Simultane Bestimmung von zentraler Hämodynamik und Plasmakatecholaminen bei Trainierten, Untrainierten und Patienten mit Kontraktionsstörungen des Herzens in Ruhe und während Körperarbeit. Z Kardiol 72: 561–568

19. Lehmann M, Keul J (1982) Die Beziehung der Plasmakatecholamine zur Herzgröße, Förderleistung und zum Füllungsdruck des insuffizienten Herzens. Herz Kreisl 14: 142–148
20. Lehmann M, Schmid P, Porzig H, Keul J (1983) Bestimmung von Beta-Rezeptoren an polymorphkernigen intakten Leukozyten im autologen Plasma. J Clin Chem Clin Biochem 21:805–811
21. Lehmann M, Hasler K, Bergdolt E, Keul J (1986) Alpha-2-Adrenoreceptor density on intact platelets and adrenaline-induced aggregation in endurance- and nonendurance-trained subjects. Int J Sports Med 7:172–176
22. Lehmann M, Gastmann U, Tauber R, Weiler C, Pilot R, Hirsch FH, Auch-Schwelk W, Keul J (1986) Katecholaminverhalten, Adrenorezeptordichte an intakten Zellen und Katecholamin-Empfindlichkeit bei einer Patientin mit orthostatischer Hypotonie. Klin Wochenschr 64:1249–1254
23. Lehmann M, Hirsch FW, Auch-Schwelk W, Alnor J, Ochs A, Gastmann U, Keul J (1986) Primäre orthostatische Hypotonie. Ein Fallbericht. Z Kardiol 75:117–121
24. Lehmann M, Keul J (1986) Free plasma catecholamines, heart rates, lactate levels, and oxygen uptake in competition weight lifters, cyclists and untrained control subjects. Int J Sports Med 7:18–21
25. Lehmann M, Dickhuth HH, Schmid P, Porzig H, Keul J (1984) Plasma catecholamines, β-adrenergic receptors, and isoproterenol sensitivity in endurance trained and non-endurance trained volunteers. Eur J Appl Physiol 52:362–369
26. Lehmann M, Keul J (1985) Basale sympathische Aktivität und Belastbarkeit von 47 Gesunden und 59 Herzkranken. Dtsch Z Sportmed 36:305–309
27. Lehmann M, Keul J (1986) Trainings-induzierte Variabilität von Adrenorezeptoren. In: Schölmerich P, Holtmeier HJ (Hrsg) Kardiovaskuläre Rezeptoren. Thieme, Stuttgart, S 139–147
28. Lehmann M, Gastmann U, Keul J (1987) Sympathische Aktivität bei Koronarinsuffizienz. Anwendung von Beta-Rezeptorenblockern. In: Brisse B, Bender F (Hrsg) Autonome Innervation des Herzens. Steinkopff, Darmstadt, S 119–135
29. Mäurer W, Tschada R, Manthey J, Ablasser A, Kübler W (1981) Catecholamines in patients with heart failure. In: Delius W, Gerlach W, Grobecker H, Kübler W (eds) Catecholamines and the heart. Springer, Berlin Heidelberg New York, pp 236–245
30. Penttilä O, Merikallio E, Pispa J, Klinge E, Siltanen P, Kyösola K (1978) Auricular tyrosine hydroxylase and dopamine-β-hydroxylase activities and noradrenaline content in ischaemic heart disease. Acta Med Scand 203:161–166
31. Sarnoff SJ, Braunwald E, Welch jr GH, Case RB, Stainsby WN, Marcruz R (1958) Hemodynamic determinants of oxygen consumption of the heart with special reference to the tension-time-index. Am J Physiol 12:148–158
32. Tohmeh JF, Cryer PE (1980) Biphasic adrenergic modulation of β-adrenergic receptors in man. J Clin Invest 65:836–840
33. Wallin BG (1981) Relationship between sympathetic outflow to muscles, heart rate and plasma noradrenaline in man. In: Delius W, Gerlach E, Grohbecker H, Kübler W (eds) Catecholamines and the heart. Springer, Berlin Heidelberg New York, pp 11–17
34. Willerson JT (1982) What is wrong with the failing heart? New Engl J Med 307:243–245
35. Winder WW, Hickson RC, Hagberg JM, Ehsani AA, McLane JA (1979) Training induced changes in hormonal and metabolic responses to submaximal exercise. J Appl Physiol 46:766–771
36. Yakovlev NN, Viru AA (1985) Adrenergic regulation of adaptation to muscular activity. Int J Sports Med 6:255–265
37. Yamaguchi N, deChamplain J, Nadeau R (1975) Correlation between the response of the heart to sympathetic stimulation and the release of endogenous catecholamines into the coronary sinus of the dog. Circ Res 36:662–668

Discussion

Hollmann: I thank you very much for these interesting findings. Are there comments, questions, remarks?
Kokot: May I ask you, do you have some data on the influence of anabolic steroids on sympathetic activity in these patients?
Lehmann: No, we do not have any results in this field. But there are results of Scandinavian authors, who discussed decrease of catecholamine excretion in weight lifters in relation to anabolic steroids. This may be a general inhibiting effect on the adrenal glands by anabolic steroids. However, this is only a hypothesis.
Addicks (Köln): I would like to give a comment to Dr. Lehmann and Dr. Koppert. We did train mice for 6 weeks and observed the catecholamine with the microscopy and the

sympathetic neurons in the myocardium with the electrone microscope. And my comment is the following point. This topic is not only the density in receptors, but also in the damage in the adrenergic neurons. If you train mice for one week, you have an increase in the amounts of fluescing fibers, that means sympathetic fibers spread out through the tissue. But if you are training for 3 weeks, you have a decrease in the amount of fluescing fibers, and after 6 weeks you have an increase again. Either structurally you see after 1 week axinal profiles with neuronal damaged cell sites. And after 6 weeks you have both, growing in volume in the axels as well as sites of damages. And to the question of Dr. Kokot. If you apply e.g. dianabol, or some forms of anabole steroids you can see quite the same, if you train mice; but if you give both the trained model and the additionally the anabole steroids you have the damages also in one week. This means you can see the same if you train mice or if you apply anabole steroids. If you combine both you have a decrease in the fibers.

Lehmann: Thank you for your comment, but we do not train mice, that is, we have no experience of our own in this field. Apart from that, you should consider, that training of mice for some weeks may be quite different from training of humans for some years. Nevertheless, I have some reservations about speaking of "damage in the adrenergic neurons" in connection with physiological training measures, except of course in overtraining or use of anabolic agents. I also have methodical reservations about quantitative statements based on the "amount of fluescing fibers".

Short Communications

ANP: Experimental Studies

Is the Hypothalamus Involved in the Regulation of the Kidney Excretory Function and ANP Secretion in Chronically Sodium-Loaded Rats?

N. Natcheff[1], N. Belova[1], O. Ikonomov[1], A. Stojnev[1], T. Avramova[1], I. Damova[1], H.-G. Klein[2], K. Thurau[2], and M. Davidov[3]

[1] Department of Physiology, Medical Academy, Sofia 1431
[2] Institute of Physiology, University of Munich
[3] Central Laboratory of Regeneration, Bulgarian Academy of Sciences, Sofia, Bulgaria

Key words: Hypothalamus – Kidney excretory function – ANP secretion – Sodium

The discovery of the atrial natriuretic peptide (ANP) has put new light on control of water and salt excretion by the kidney. At the same time our knowledge of the mechanisms which ensure the integration of the water-salt homeostasis becomes more complicated. In the last two decades, publications have appeared which have doubtlessly shown the key role of the hypothalamus in the control of water-salt homeostasis and the production of renal hormons [1, 2, 3].

The concept of the current work is to attain more clarity about the role of the hypothalamus and the participation of ANP in the regulation of the excretory function of the kidney under chronic salt loading.

Material and Methods

The experiment were performed on male Long-Evans rats weighing 220–250 g. The animals were housed singly 10 days in plastic cages at room temperature between 22–24°C, relative humidity 60% and a dark/light periodicity of 12/12 hr. Prior to the experiments standard food and tap water were allowed ad libitum. After that one half of the animals was subjected to electrocoagulation on both sides in the area of the posterior hypothalamus (Nuclei supramammillares and Nuclei mammillares laterales). One week later the rats were divided into four groups:

A. Control rats, kept on tap water
B. Rats with lesions in the hypothalamus, kept on tap water
C. Intact rats, kept on 1% saline solution
D. Rats with lesions, kept on 1% saline solution.

The hypothalamic lesions were carried out with stereotaxic apparatus with coordinates of the Szentagothai atlas [4] being set at: 0.9 mm laterally from the Sutura sagitalis; 4.5 mm dorsally from the Sutura coronaria and at a depth of 8.8 mm from the surface of the skull. The glass insulated cantal electrodes had an external diameter of 0.35 mm, the length of the free tip was 0.1 mm and the thickness 0.25 mm. The lesions were effected with anode direct current 1.5 mA for 15 sec.

Experimental Protocol

The rats were kept in metabolic cages from 8 to 14.00, without food. They drank tap water or 1% solution, according to the above named groups. The urine collected was examined for volume, electrolytes and endogeneous creatinine. 10 days later the rats were decapitated (without anesthesia) and the blood collected and analysed for electrolytes, creatinine and ANP.

Results

All parameters are calculated based on 100 g. B. W. per minute. The data are represented in Table 1 as average values ± SEM[1].

Table 1

V µl	UNaV nmol	UKV nmol	UClV nmol	GFR µl	E/FNa %	Hct %	ANP pg/ml
A.2,94 ±0,40	264 ±40	570 ±60	339 ±31	314 ±38	1,2 ±0,4	47 ±1,4	705 ±47
B.3,18 ±0,40	146⁺ ±14	572 ±96	359 ±49	314 ±78	0,4⁺ ±0,1	46 ±0,8	635 ±81
C.2,97 ±0,40	542 ±95	411 ±72	504 ±72	248 ±48	1,3 ±0,2	44 ±0,8	575 ±48
D.2,90 ±0,10	663 ±73	460 ±61	798⁺ ±78	341 ±33	1,7⁺ ±0,3	44 ±0,3	460 ±57

The histological verification of 6 randomly chosen animals from groups B. and D. showed that all lesions were localised in the area of the Supramammillary and Lateromammillary nuclei and had a size of 1 mm³ approximately.

Discussion

The data obtained show that the intake of 1% saline solution over 10 days caused a moderate, but significant, enlargement of the ECV. At the same time, a tendency in the reduction of the plasma ANP level can be observed, although this cannot ve verified statistically. It is ineresting to observed that lesions of the posterior hypothalamus of rats drinking tap water caused a distinct inhibition of sodium excretion. This result correspond to our earlier experiments on rats in acute experiments [5]. However, the observed discrepency in the change of Na- and Cl-excretion still remains unclear.

In the salt loaded rats the damage in these hypothalamic areas potentiated the excretion of Na and Cl in that GFR does not change and the ANP plasma level decreases. This loss is compensated for by an increased uptake of saline, as the body weight does not show any tendency to decrease. These data lend further support to the assumption that the posterior hypothalamic region is critical for the maintenance of salt-water balance. As the measurement of ANP had been performed 10 days after the animals were put on saline as drinking water, we did not expect any significant increase in this peptide [6, 7]. The fact that the ANP levels remained comparable between rats with and without hypothalamic lesions indicates that this area of the hypothalamus plays no major role in the regulation of ANP plasma level under these experimental conditions.

[1] The results are statistically evaluated by Stüdent's t-test. A. versus B. and C. versus. D. groups are compared and the significant differences are marked with +.

References

1. Logophetov AP, Natcheff ND (1974) Erythropoietic activity of plasma in rats with erythropoietin application to the posterior hypothalamus. Compt Rend Acad Bulg Sci 27: 133–136
2. Natcheff ND, Logophetov A, Tzaneva N (1977) Hypothalamic control of plasma renin activity. Pflügers Arch 371:279–283
3. Hansel P, Göransson A, Leppäluoto J, Arjamma O, Ulfendahl HR (1987) CNS-induced natriuresis is not mediated by the atrial natriuretic factor. Acta Physiol Scand 129: 221–227
4. Szentagothai J, Flerko B, Mess B, Halast B (1962) Hypothalamic control of the anterior pituitary. Kiado, Budapest
5. Natcheff ND, Piryova B, Girchev R, Kirkova L (1975) Influence of the hypothalamic mammillary area on the kidney function in rats. Agressology 16/6:367–372
6. Luft FC, Sterzel RB, Lang RE, Trabold EM, Veelken R, Ruskoaho H, Gao Yi, Ganten D, Unger T (1986) Atrial natriuretic factor determinations and chronic sodium homeostasis. Kidney Int 29:1004–1010
7. Sakata M, Greenwald JE, Needleman P (1988) Paradoxal relationship between atriopeptin-plasma levels and diuresis-natriuresis induced by acute volume expansion. Proc Natl Acad Sci USA 85/9:3155–3160

Regulation of Rat Vascular ANP Receptors during Chronic Salt-Loading

H. Michel, H. Meyer-Lehnert, A. Bäcker, H. Stelkens, and H. J. Kramer

Medizinische Universitäts-Poliklinik, Bonn, FRG

Key words: ANP – Aortic receptors – Chronic salt-loading

Introduction

In numerous studies, atrial natriuretic peptides (ANP) have been shown to be involved in the regulation of electrolyte balance, extracellular fluid volume (ECFV) and blood pressure [1, 2, for review see Ref. 3]. Receptors, mediating the effects of ANP have been identified in renal, vascular and other tissues. Concerning the vascular site of action, ANP receptors were shown to be regulated differently in volume-dependent and non-volume-dependent models of hypertension [3, 4, 5, 6]. The role of ANP in the long-term regulation of blood pressure, electrolyte balance and ECFV, however, requires further elucidation. Thus, our study was performed to examine the effects of chronic salt-loading on regulation of vascular ANP receptors and on potentially associated changes in systemic hemodynamics and in renal function in male Sprague-Dawley rats.

Materials and Methods

^{125}I-labeled rANP was obtained from NEN-DU PONT (Boston, MA; USA). Unlabeled rANP was purchased from Peninsula Lab., England.

Animal Experiments

Studies were performed after 2 (n = 8), 10 (n = 6) and 35 (n = 10) days in salt-loaded and control rats (= NaCl and C-rats) which were fed the same diet (0.2% Na) except that NaCl-rats received 0.9% saline as drinking fluid and C-rats received deionized water. All rats were kept in metabolic cages and blood pressure was measured by tail-cuff plethysmography daily for the first 7 days and every 3rd day thereafter. Sodium intake was 9.7–12.3 mmol/24 h in NaCl-rats and 1.4–1.7 mmol/24 h in C-rats. At the end of the experiments average weight of rats was 370 g within all experimental groups. Blood and last 24 h urine were collected for measurements of plasma ANP and cGMP, sodium balance, and GFR (creatinine clearance).

Tissue Preparation and Receptor assay

Thoracic aortas were excised from decapitated animals and were dissected free from fat and connective tissue. After rinsing in ice-cold phosphate buffered saline (PBS) aortas were cut in several sections and each section in several rings (up to 50/aorta). To rule out inhomogenous receptor distribution within one aorta, each assay sample contained tissue from all sections.

The assay was performed in Hank's balanced salt solution (HBSS) containing bovine serum albumin (200 mg/dl), Hepes (10 mM), glucose (5.5 mM) and phenylmethylsulfonylfluoride (PMSF, 1 mM). Competitive binding inhibition was performed with 15–20 fmol ^{125}I-rANP and varying concentrations of unlabeled ANP (0.1 ml of 10^{-10}–10^{-8} M). Unspecific binding was calculated as cpm obtained in the presence of 10^{-6} M unlabeled ANP. Bound and free radioactivity were separated by rapid filtration in a Millipore® filtration unit on nylon filters (mesh size = 20 µm). Filters were rinsed four times with 3 ml of ice-cold PBS. Receptor characteristics were calculated by Scatchard analysis of competitive binding inhibition data. Maximal binding (B_{max}) is expressed in fmol/g dry weight (d.w.) and dissociation constant (K_d) in nM. All data are presented as means ± SEM. Statistical comparison was performed using two-tailed Student's t-test for unpaired data.

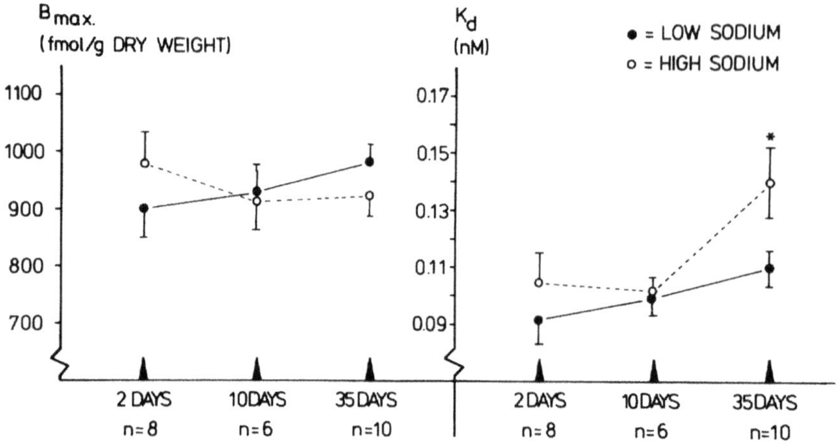

Fig. 1. Rate aortic receptors during chronic low and high sodium intake. Presented are data for maximal binding (B_{max}) after 2, 10 and 35 days on the left side and corresponding values of dissociation constant (K_d) on the right side. B_{max} and K_d were evaluated by Scatchard-analysis of competitive binding inhibition of ^{125}I-labeled rANP and unlabeled rANP. * $0.05 < p < 0.1$

Results

At days 2 and 10, salt-loading did not affect receptor characteristics (Fig. 1). After 35 days of salt-loading, the dissociation constant in NaCl-rats was slightly increased (140 ± 10 vs 110 ± 5 pM, $0.05 < p < 0.1$). B_{max} after 35 days, however, remained unaltered (935 ± 35 fmol/g d.w. in NaCl-rats versus 975 ± 40 in C-rats). Plasma ANP after 2 and 10 days of salt-loading was not different from controls. After 35 days, plasma ANP was slightly elevated in NaCl-rats (530 ± 52 vs 390 ± 40 pmol/l). During the entire period, sodium balance was maintained. Plasma concentration of cGMP and GFR did not differ between experimental groups. Mean systolic blood pressure was mildly elevated beginning from the 3rd week of high sodium intake, without reaching significance (134 ± 9 vs 121 ± 4 mmHg in NaCl-rats and C-rats, respectively, after 35 days).

Discussion

The present study demonstrates that under the condition of chronic salt-loading no alteration in density of aortic ANP receptors occurs. Elevated dissociation constant after 35 days of salt-loading, however, indicates a decrease in affinity of vascular ANP receptors. This may represent a response to increased plasma ANP levels. Other studies performed in vascular tissue homogenates demonstrated a decrease of receptor density in models of volume-expanded hypertension [3, 4, 7]. This decrease in receptor number in the presence of an elevated affinity was associated with increased plasma ANP levels. Studies in a non volume-expanded, renin dependent model of hypertension showed no alteration in receptor density and ANP plasma levels, respectively [3, 5]. Thus, it seems that changes in vascular responsiveness to ANP are not always accompanied by changes in receptor density. Despite slightly elevated plasma ANP concentrations we did not observe a down-regulation of receptor binding sites. Although the use of aortic rings in our study should mimic the in vivo situation, we cannot differentiate between endothelial and vascular smooth muscle receptors which may be regulated differently. Further studies are in progress investigating the regulation of ANP receptors in suspensions of smooth muscle cells and smooth muscle homogenates, respectively.

It is of interest to note, however, that besides the receptor density altered receptor affinity (expressed as K_d) may play a crucial role in mediating effects of ANP. Thus, in glomerular ANP receptor studies we could demonstrate that the rise in affinity during chronic salt-loading may contribute to the maintenance of body sodium and ECFV balance despite marked down-regulation of B_{max}. This inverse regulation has already been shown by Ballermann et al. [8].

This inverse receptor regulation was not observed in our aortic receptor study. In contrast, vascular receptor affinity decreased during chronic salt-loading. Thus, we suggest that ANP may only play a minor role in the long-term regulation of blood pressure, at least under condition of salt-loading. ANP may be more important in the renal regulation of body sodium and fluid volume.

References

1. Currie MG, Geller DM, Cole BR, et al. (1983) Bioactive cardiac substances: potent vasorelaxant activity in mammalian atria. Science 221:71–73
2. Garcia R, Thibault G, Cantin M, Genest J (1984) Effects of a purified atrial natriuretic factor on rat and rabbit vascular stripes and vascular beds. Am J Physiol 247:R34–R39
3. Kramer HJ (1988) Atrial natriuretic hormones. Gen Pharmac 19:747–753
4. Schiffrin EL, St. Louis J, Garcia R, Thibault G, Cantin M, Genest J (1986) Vascular and adrenal binding sites for atrial natriuretic factor: Effects of chronic sodium and hypertension. Hypertension 8 [Suppl I]:I141–I145
5. Garcia R, Gutkowska J, Genest J, Cantin M, Thibault G (1985) Reduction of blood pressure and increased diuresis and natriuresis during chronic infusion of atrial natriuretic factor (ANF/Arg 101-Tyr 126) in conscious one kidney one clip hypertensive rats. Proc Soc Exp Biol Med 179:539–545
6. Schiffrin EL, Tremblay J, Hamet P, St. Louis J (1986) Vascular binding sites for atrial natriuretic peptide in rats: down-regulation in volume expanded states is mediated by ANP (Abstract). Clin Res 32:486A
7. Schiffrin EL, Chartier L, Thibault G, St. Louis J, Cantin M, Genest J (1985) Vascular and adrenal receptors for atrial natriuretic factor in the rat. Circ Res 56:801–807
8. Ballermann BJ, Hoover RL, Karnovsky MJ, Brenner BM (1985) Physiologic regulation of atrial natriuretic peptide receptors in rat renal glomeruli. J Clin Invest 76:2049–2056

Renal Function after Renal Ischemia in Dogs Infused with Atrial Natriuretic Peptide (ANP)

D. Dimitrov[1], H. G. Klein[2], I. Atanasova[1], K. Thurau[2], and N. Natcheff[1]

[1] Department of Physiology, Medical Academy Sofia, Bulgaria
[2] Department of Physiology, University of Munich, FRG

Key words: Renal function – Renal ischemia – ANP

Introduction

Application of atrial natriuretic peptides (ANP) has been shown to ameliorate acute renal failure in the rat. The beneficial effect is explained by renal vasodilation, enhancement of glomerular filtration rate and lowering energy-dependent ion transport across the tubular membrane [4, 5]. This study was performed to evaluate the effects of a low and a medium dose of ANP-infusion on the initial postischemic renal functional parameters under the condition of a mild ischemic kidney damage.

Methods

15 mongrel dogs, weighing 15.2 + 5.8 kg were randomly divided into 3 groups and anesthetized with Nembutal (30 mg/kg bw i.v.). Surgical preparation included cannulation of both ureters for urine collections, both femoral arteries for blood pressure monitoring and arterial blood sampling and both femoral veins for infusions of saline (group I = control) or ANP for 45 min (group II = 20 ng/min/kg bw, group III =

100 ng/min/kg bw). The left renal artery was exposed by flank incision. Renal blood flow (RBF) was measured by an electromagnetic flowmeter. Ischemic renal failure was induced by clamping the artery for 45 min. Following parameters were determined: blood pressure (BP), heart rate (HR), left kidney renal blood flow (RBF), kidney excretory function (V, $U_{Na}V$, U_KV, FE_{Na}, creatinine), creatinine clearance (C_{Cr}), hematocrit (Hct), plasma levels of Na, K, ANP, renal vascular resistance (RVR) was calculated from BP and RBF.

Experimental Protocol

After a 45 min control period, left renal artery was clamped for 45 min. Immediately after the beginning of reperfusion, saline or ANP-infusion was started for 45 min. Recovery period lasted 90 min. Urine collections were taken every 15 min, arterial blood was obtained in the midpoint of every period.

Statistical analysis was performed by MANOVA. Results are presented as means ± SEM.

Results

Right kidney (non-ischemic): Filtration and excretory functions tended to compensate left kidney failure during ischemia. ANP-infusion caused a significant increase in V and $U_{Na}V$ only in the 100 ng group (22 ± 10 to 94 ± 35 µl/min/kg, 4.0 ± 1.2 to 14.9 ± 4.5 µmol/min/kg respectively). Left kidney (ischemic): Parameters are shown in the table.

Table 1. Effects of ANP on left renal function after a 45 min ischemia

	time (min)	0.9% NaCl	20 ng ANP	100 ng ANP
RBF (ml/min/kg)	− 15	6.7 ± 0.7	5.8 ± 0.6	5.6 ± 0.8
	ischemia			
	+ 30	8.3 ± 1.2	5.2 ± 0.6	5.3 ± 0.7
	+ 75	7.6 ± 0.9	5.5 ± 0.7	3.9 ± 1.0[b]
	+120	7.2 ± 0.8	5.7 ± 0.6	4.2 ± 1.0[a]
RVR (mmHg/ml/min)	− 15	1.3 ± 0.1	1.6 ± 0.2	1.6 ± 0.2
	ischemia			
	+ 30	1.2 ± 0.3	1.9 ± 0.3	1.8 ± 0.3
	+ 75	1.2 ± 0.3	1.8 ± 0.3	2.9 ± 0.7[b]
	+120	1.2 ± 0.2	1.7 ± 0.2	2.2 ± 0.8
C_{Cr} (ml/min/kg)	− 15	1.5 ± 0.2	1.1 ± 0.1	1.4 ± 0.3
	ischemia			
	+ 30	0.6 ± 0.2	0.5 ± 0.2	1.1 ± 0.3[a]
	+ 75	0.6 ± 0.2	0.7 ± 0.2	0.4 ± 0.1
	+120	0.7 ± 0.2	0.8 ± 0.2	0.6 ± 0.1
V (µl/min/kg)	− 15	15 ± 4	11 ± 3	16 ± 3
	ischemia			
	+ 30	8 ± 4	23 ± 12	114 ± 55[b]
	+ 75	12 ± 4	18 ± 7	31 ± 5[a]
	+120	11 ± 4	9 ± 3	29 ± 6
$U_{Na}V$ (µmol/min/kg)	− 15	1.5 ± 0.3	1.7 ± 0.4	2.8 ± 0.3
	ischemia			
	+ 30	1.7 ± 0.3	3.1 ± 2.0	15.1 ± 7.0[b]
	+ 75	1.1 ± 0.4	2.4 ± 1.2	3.9 ± 0.4
	+120	1.3 ± 0.5	1.2 ± 0.2	3.1 ± 0.5
IR-ANP (pg/ml)	+ 15	15 ± 1	14 ± 1	46 ± 22
	ischemia			
	+ 30	13 ± 4	184 ± 109	761 ± 455
	+ 75	18 ± 1	24 ± 4	233 ± 152
	+120	19 ± 2	19 ± 2	81 ± 7

[a] $p < 0.08$; [b] < 0.05

Discussion

Clamping of the renal artery for 45 min caused a mild reversible renal failure manifested by an impaired glomerular function as previously described [6]. The suppression of reactive hyperaemia in the ischemic kidney during ANP-infusion [2] and the sustained C_{Cr} in the initial postischemic period resulted in a normal postischemic filtration fraction. This observation is consistent with the assumption that ANP has led to a normalization of pre- and postglomerular resistances as compared to the untreated postischemic kidney. These events might be due to a shift in the tone of intrarenal resistance vessels [1, 2, 7], namely a vasodilation in the afferent and vasoconstriction in the efferent arteriole [3]. The excretory responsiveness of the postischemic kidney to ANP was demonstrated by the same extent of diuresis and natriuresis compared to those of the non-ischemic kidney. It appears therefore, that the receptor mediated cellular response to ANP is not affected by this type of ischemia.

Acknowledgements. This work was supported by grants of the Deutsche Forschungsgemeinschaft and of the Friedrich-Baur-Stiftung.

References

1. Huang CL, Lewicki J, Johnson LK, Cogan MG (1985) Renal mechanism of action of rat atrial natriuretic factor. J Clin Invest 75:769–773
2. Maack T, Atlas SA, Camargo MJF, Cogan MG (1986) Renal hemodynamic and natriuretic effects of atrial natriuretic factor. Fed Proc 45:2128–2132
3. Marin-Grez M, Fleming JT, Steinhausen M (1986) Atrial natriuretic peptide causes preglomerular vasodilation and post-glomerular vasoconstriction in rat kidney. Nature 324:473–476
4. Nakamoto M, Shapiro JI, Shanley PF, Chan L, Schrier RW (1987) In vitro and in vivo protective effect of atriopeptin III on ischemic acute renal failure. J Clin Invest 80:698–705
5. Shaw SG, Weidmann P, Hodler J, Zimmermann A, Paternostro A (1987) Atrial natriuretic peptide protects against acute ischemic renal failure in the rat. J Clin Invest 80:1232–1237
6. Thurau K, Mason J, Gstraunthaler G (1985) Experimental acute renal failure. In: Seldin DW, Giebisch G (eds) The Kidney, pp 1885–1899
7. Veldkamp PJ, Carmines PK, Inscho EW, Navar LG (1988) Direct evaluation of the microvascular actions of ANP in juxtamedullary nephrons. Am J Physiol 254:F440–F444

Atrial Natriuretic Peptide (ANP) Protects Cells against Injury by Hypoxia and Hypochlorous Acid

A. A. von Ruecker, R. Pella, and F. Bidlingmaier

Institut für Klinische Biochemie der Universität Bonn, FRG

Key words: Atrial natriuretic peptide – Cell protection – Hypoxia – Reactive oxygen

Recent reports show that ANP protects against post-ischemic renal failure in vivo and in the isolated perfused kidney [4, 8]. Since ANP has been shown to be a potent renal vasodilatator, this protective effect may be mediated exclusively by improving hemodynamics. To determine if ANP also has a protective effect at the cellular level, studies were performed in hepatocyte cell cultures. Hepatocytes showed a considerable increase in cellular cGMP content after ANP stimulation, suggesting the presence of ANP receptors. Cell cultures were exposed to hypoxia and reactive oxygen (hypochlorous acid, HClO), which cause cell damage similar to postischemic injury in vivo [3]. The following report demonstrates that ANP can protect cell cultures.

Methods

Male Sprague-Dawley rats, weighing 150–200 g, were used. Hepatocyte cultures were prepared as described previously [7].

In *hypoxia experiments*, 20 h-old cell cultures were divided into a 20%-O_2 (control) group and a 0.5%-O_2 (hypoxic) group. After addition of drugs, both groups were placed in incubators equilibrated with the desired oxygen concentration. An oxygen electrode was used to monitor the O_2 concentration in the medium. After 4 h of hypoxia, reoxygenation occured for 20 h at 20% O_2. Cell damage was assayed by trypan blue exclusion and release of glutamate transaminase (SGOT) (for details cf. [1]). In *experiments with HClO,* 20 h-old hepatocyte cultures were washed with a modified Krebs-Henseleit buffer containing 2% dialyzed bovine serum albumin, 15 mM glucose, 20 mM Hepes, pH 7.4 and incubated in the same buffer at 37°C under an atmosphere of 95% O_2, 5% CO_2 for 2 h without further additions. HClO (100 μM) and other agents were then added to intact cultures as indicated without further change of medium. Cell demage was assessed by determining a) trypan blue exclusion, b) the percent increase in membrane blebs [6], c) the release of SGOT into the supernatant [1], and d) the rate of intracellular proteolysis [7]. All assays were done in triplicate.

Cellular cGMP content was measured with the help of commercially available radioimmunoassay kits (New England Nuclear, Dreieich).

Materials: ANP, hypochlorous acid, and sodium nitroprusside were from Sigma Chemicals, Munich. Cell culture medium was from Seromed, Munich. Other solvents and chemicals were from Merck, Darmstadt. Ly 83583 (6-anilino-5,8-quinolinedione) was a generous gift from Lilly Research Laboratories, Indianapolis, Ind.

Results

Fig. 1a shows the increase in cellular cGMP content in cultured hepatocytes in response to different ANP concentrations. At concentrations 100 nM ANP increased cellular cGMP content 12–15-fold. Ly 83583 (10 μM), which interferes with activation of the particulate guanylate cyclase [5], completely blocked the ANP-induced increase in cGMP (data not shown).

To determine if ANP can protect cultured hepatocytes after hypoxic injury, a procedure was applied described in detail by Costa et al. [1]. Hepatocyte cultures were first exposed to 0.5% oxygen for 4 h in the presence and absence of ANP and Ly 83583. Fig. 1b shows that with no reoxygenation period after hypoxia, the cells remained intact as judged by trypan blue exclusion. Pretreatment of cells with ANP (1 μM) and/or Ly 83583 (10 μM) did not change the survival rate. These results were quite different, if the cells were exposed to a prolonged 20h-reoxygenation period. In this case (Fig. 1b), the survival rate of cells without ANP (1 μM) pretreatment was less than 15%, whereas approx. 70% of the ANP-treated cells survived. This beneficial effect of ANP was largely blocked by Ly 83583 (Fig. 1b), which suppressed the ANP-mediated formation of cGMP. Ly 83583 did not influence controls without ANP (data not shown).

Similar results were obtained if the release of SGOT into the supernatant was used to monitor hypoxic cell damage. No major increase in SGOT leakage was observed in control and drug-treated cells immediately after hypoxia. After a 20 h-reoxygenation period, more than 75% of total cellular SGOT was found in the supernatant of cells without ANP pretreatment. In the ANP (1 μM) treated cells, only 30–35% of total SGOT had leaked into the supernatant. Ly 83583 (10 μM) inhibited this benefical effect of ANP by 85–95%.

These results show that detectable damage to the cells occured after the normal oxygen concentration had been restored, rather than during the hypoxic period itself. This reoxygenation effect after hypoxia is well known and has been attributed to increased formation of reactive oxygen that induces lipid peroxidation after reoxygenation (for review see ref. [3]). We found that ANP can also protect cultured hepatocytes after treatment with hypochlorous acid, which also forms reactive oxygen ($HClO \longrightarrow O + HCl$) (Fig. 1c). Hepatocyte cell cultures were exposed to HClO (100 μM) for 30 min in the absence and presence of ANP (1 μM). Bleb formation, trypan blue uptake, release of SGOT and proteolysis of cellular proteins were considered indices of cell damage. ANP prevented cell damage as

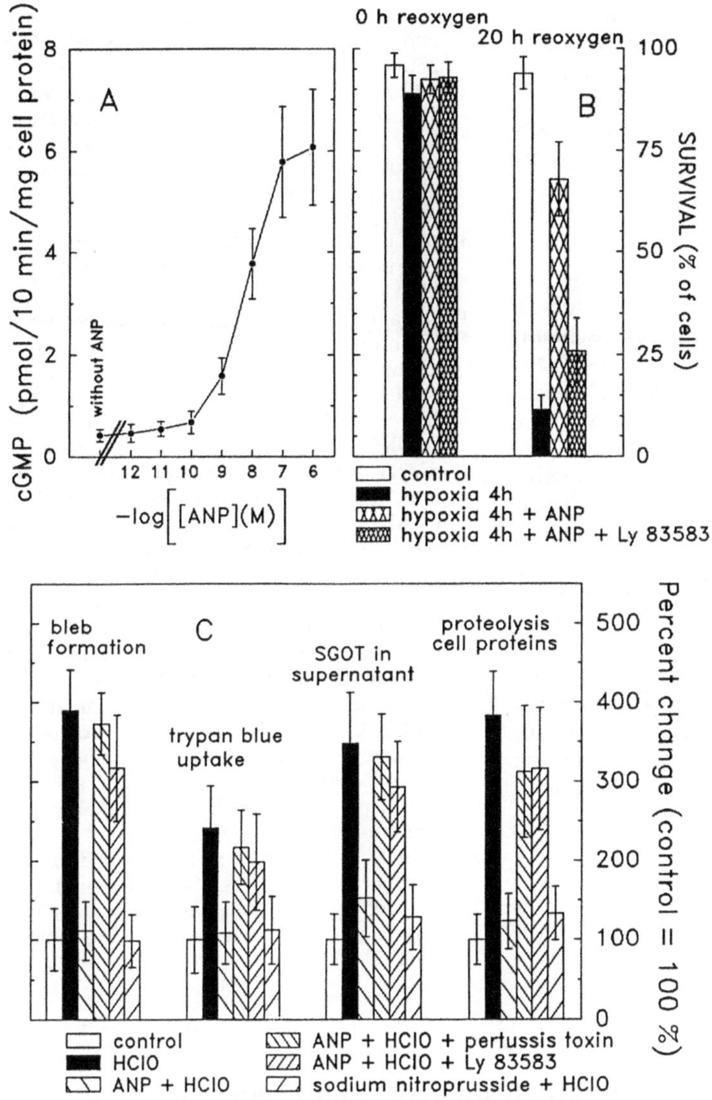

Fig. 1 A–C. Effect of ANP and various agents on hepatocytes before and after damage by hypoxia and hypochlorous acid. **A** Increase of cellular cGMP at different ANP concentrations. Isolated hepatocytes were incubated at 37°C for 10 min with and without ANP as described by Leitman et al. [2]. cGMP was measured by radioimmunoassay (Methods). Values represent the mean ± SE of 4 separate experiments performed in triplicate. **B** Cell protection by ANP after hypoxia and reoxygenation. Hepatocytes were exposed to hypoxia (0.5% O_2) and reoxygenation (20% O_2) for 0 and 20 h as indicated. ANP (1 μM) was added to the cells immediately before hypoxia was introduced. Ly 83583 (10 μM) was added to the medium 5 min before ANP. Cell survival was assessed by trypan blue exclusion. Values are the mean ± SE of 3 separate experiments performed in triplicate. **C** Cell protection by ANP after treatment of cells with HClO. Hepatocyte cultures were exposed to HClO (100 μM) for 30 min at 37°C in the absence and presence of ANP (1 μM), pertussis toxin (200 ng/ml), Ly 83583 (10 μM) and sodium nitroprusside (10 μM) as indicated. These agents were added to the medium 5, 30, 10 and 5 min prior to HClO, respectively. Cell damage was assessed by the percent increase of the parameters indicated. Controls in the presence of the mentioned agents but in the absence of HClO were not significantly different from controls without these agents. Values are the mean ± SE of 3 separate experiments performed in triplicate

judged by these indices. This beneficial effect was prevented by pertussis toxin (200 ng/ml) and Ly 83583 (10 μM), and was mimicked by nitroprusside (10 μM), which, like ANP, increased cellular cGMP content >40-fold in hepatocyte cultures (data not shown).

Discussion

Our results demonstrate that the beneficial effects of ANP observed in acute ischemic renal failure [8] and in the isolated perfused kidney [4] may not only be due to ANP-induced vasodilatation and improved hemodynamics, but also to ANP-mediated protection at the cellular level. The protective effect of ANP was inhibited by pertussis toxin in hepatocytes. This suggests that a guanine nucleotide binding protein (G protein) may be involved in the action of ANP. Since the protective actions of ANP were largely inhibited by Ly 83583 (which blocks particulate guanylate cyclase) and could be mimicked by nitroprusside (which increases cellular cGMP), a cGMP-dependent mechanism seems important for cytoprotection by ANP. The exact mechanism remains to be elucidated.

References

1. Costa AK, Heffel DF, Schieble TM, Trudell JR (1987) Toxicity of t-butylhydroperoxide in hepatocyte monolayers exposed to hypoxia and reoxygenation. In Vitro Cell Develop Biol 23:501–506
2. Leitman DC, Agnost VL, Tuan JJ, Andresen JW, Murad F (1987) Atrial natriuretic factor and sodium nitroprusside increase cyclic GMP in cultured rat lung fibroblasts by activating different forms of guanylate cyclase. Biochem J 244:69–74
3. McCord JM (1985) Oxygen-derived free radicals in postischemic tissue injury. N Engl J Med 312:159–163
4. Nakamoto M, Shapiro JI, Shanley PF, Chan L, Shrier RW (1987) In vitro and in vivo protective effect of atriopeptin III on ischemic acute renal failure, J Clin Invest 80:698–705
5. O'Donnell ME, Owen NE (1986) Role of cyclic GMP in atrial natriuretic factor stimulation of Na^+, K^+, Cl^- cotransport in vascular smooth muscle cells. J Biol Chem 261: 15461–15466
6. Rao GS, Lemoch H, Kessler H, Damm I, Eiermann V, Koll S, Zarbock J, Usadel KH (1986) Prevention of phalloidin-induced lesions in isolated rat hepatocytes by novel synthetic analogues of somatostatin. Klin Wochenschr 64 [Suppl VII]:79–86
7. von Ruecker AA, Rao G, Bidlingmaier F (1988) Cyclosporin A inhibits proteolytic cleavage and degradation of membrane bound protein kinase C in hepatocytes after stimulation by phorbol ester. Biochem Biophys Res Commun 151:997–1003
8. Shaw SG, Weidmann P, Hodler J, Zimmermann A, Paternostro A (1987) Atrial natriuretic peptide protects against acute ischemic renal failure in the rat. J Clin Invest 80:1232–1237

Atrial Natriuretic Factor Protects against Angiotensin II – Induced Deterioration in Isolated Working Rat Hearts

R. H. A. Becker, U. Albus, W. Linz, and J. Knolle

Hoechst AG, Frankfurt/M, FRG

Key words: h-ANF (103–126) – Angiotensin II – Arrhythmia – Cardioprotection – Ischemic heart Rat

Introduction

In congestive heart failure, infusion of human atrial natriuretic factor (h-ANF) has shown to be of benefit, and converting enzyme inhibition which decreases angiotensin II (ANG II) formation improved symptoms and reduced mortality. Therefore we investigated the interaction between h-ANF and ANG II in the isolated ischemic rat heart.

Table 1. Duration and Incidence of Ventricular Fibrillation during 30 min Reperfusion after 15 min Coronary Ligation in Isolated Working Rat Hearts

	Duration (min)	p	Incidence
control	16.9 ± 2.5	–	10/10
h-ANF	2.7 ± 0.9	*	3/10
ANG II	$>30.0 \pm 0.0$	*	10/10
h-ANF + Ang II	7.7 ± 2.9	*	7/9

h-ANF: 1×10^{-7} mol/l human atrial natriuretic factor (103–126); ANG II: 1×10^{-9} mol/l angiotensin II; *: $p < 0.05$ compared to controls

Materials and Methods

Isolated working heart preparations from Wistar rats were perfused, as previously described [1], for an initial 20 min pre-ischemic period followed by a 15 min ischemic period by left coronary artery occlusion, and a 30 min reperfusion period. Left ventricular pressure (LVP), LV dp/dt max, heart rate (HR), coronary flow (CF) and an epicardial ECG were continously determined. Lactate, lactate dehydrogenase (LDH) and creatine kinase (CK) were measured in the perfusate and levels of lactate, glycogen, adenosine triphosphate (ATP) and creatine phosphate (CP) in the myocardial tissue. h-ANF (103–126) was perfused at a concentration of 1×10^{-7} mol/l and ANG II at a concentration of 1×10^{-5} mol/l.

Results are given as means ± SEM.

Results

Effects of h-ANF and/or ANG II on duration and incidence of ventricular fibrillation are given in Table 1.

After release of coronary occlusion in h-ANF perfused hearts the restoration of CF was more pronounced than in control hearts but LVP and dp/dt_{max} were decreased, whereas HR did not differ between both groups. Release of lactate, CK and LDH was less than in control hearts, and myocardial tissue levels of glycogen, ATP and CP were increased and lactate levels decreased.

Perfusion with ANG II produced opposite effects. CF was reduced and release of lactate and enzymes increased. Myocardial tissue levels of glycogen, ATP and CP were lower than in control hearts. These ANG II-induced effects were antagonized by simultaneous perfusion with h-ANF.

Conclusion

h-ANF functionally antagonizes the effects of ANG II in the ischemic reperfused rat heart. These effects of h-ANF could be mediated by inhibiting changes in Ca^{2+}-flux, cyclic nucleotide levels or other post-receptor events believed to mediate the actions of ANG II.

Reference

1. Linz W, Schölkens BA, Han YF (1986) Beneficial effects of the converting enzyme inhibitor ramipril in ischemic rat hearts. J Cardiovasc Phyrmacol 8 [Suppl 10]:91–99

Does Atrial Natriuretic Factor (ANF) Affect Changes of Myocardial Extracellular K^+ and H^+ Concentrations ($[K^+]_e$; $[H^+]_e$) and Noradrenaline (NA) Release During Global Ischaemia (GI)?

A. Hilger, H. Hirche, H. Knopf, C. H. Moon, and R. Theising

Department of Applied Physiology, University of Cologne, FRG

Key words: ANF – Myocardial K^+ and H^+ concentrations – Noradrenaline – Ischaemia

Introduction

An increased release of ANF (atrial natriuretic factor) during myocardial infarction due to atrial distension or hypoxia has been observed (Dietz 1984; Ledsome et al. 1985). Furthermore, an ANF induced decrease of coronary vascular resistance (Otero et al. 1987) and a raised plasma level of ANF has been described in patients with coronary heart disease (Porter B. et al. 1987).

It was the purpose of this study to investigate, whether ANF influences transmembrane net-ion-fluxes of ischaemic myocardium and ischaemia induced myocardial noradrenaline release.

Methods

Isolated rat hearts were perfused at constant flow (6–8 ml/g heart) according to the Langendorff technique. The perfusate [modified Krebs-Henseleit solution (KHS): NaCl 120, $NaHCO_3$ 23.8, $NaH_2PO_4 \times H_2O$ 0.44, Na-pyruvate 1.82, Na_2-EDTA $\times$ $2H_2O$ 0.027, KCl 4, $CaCl_2 \times 2\,H_2O$ 1.85, $MgCl_2O \times 6\,H_2O$ 1.05, glucose 11,1 mM/l] was heated (37 °C) and gassed with carbogen (95% O_2; 5% CO_2). The hearts were set up to allow the recording of left ventricular pressure (LVP), the first derivative (dp/dt), coronary perfusion pressure (CPP) and the heart rate (HR) according to a "systemic circulation" (Bardenheuer and Schrader 1983).

Tetramethylammoniumchloride (TMA; 100 μM/l) was used as marker to measure the decrease of the extracellular space (ECS) during global ischaemia (gI).

The extracellular concentrations of K^+, Na^+, Ca^{2+}, H^+ and TMA were measured using double barreled ion selective PVC-mini-electrodes (outer tip diameter 350 μm, Hill et al. 1978) in the left mid-ventricular myocardium. The hearts with the electrodes in place were immersed in warm oil (37 °C) to prevent cooling and desiccation during ischaemia.

Two randomised groups of hearts were chosen: Control hearts (n = 6–24) were perfused with KHS until reaching stable hemodynamics. Perfusion was switched in treated hearts (n = 10–19) to KHS containing ANF 20 ng/ml (= 6.99 nM/l; Peninsula Lab., Inc., USA; 8–33, 101 Arg-126 Thy; MW: 2862.65; rat) and maintained for 15 minutes. Subsequently both groups of hearts were submitted to 60 minutes of gI induced by clamping the aortic canula. Following gI the hearts were reperfused with the pre-ischaemic perfusate. During the first 10 minutes of reperfusion the effluent was collected in 1 minute periods to determine the NA overflow. NA concentration was measured using HPLC.

Results

The administration of ANF (20 μg/l) 15 min. before the onset of global ischaemia decreased the efflux of K^+ (from 7.18 to 4.8 mM/l ECS/h), the influx of Na^+ and Ca^{++} (from −89.6 to −47.6 and from −1.02 to −0.51 mM/l ECS/h, respectively), the shrinkage of ECS (50% versus 66% in control hearts) and noradrenaline overflow during gI (155 versus 295 ng/g in control hearts). During preocclusion period ANF increased coronary perfusion pressure (45 ± 1.7 to 46 ± 2 mmHg), left ventricular pressure (46 ± 1.7 to 50 ± 1.7 mmHg) and dp/dt (1633 ± 100 to 1822 ± 104 mmHg/s).

Conclusion

The lowered intracellular Na^+ concentration may be the cause of diminished noradrenaline release (Schömig et al. 1988), shrinkage of the ECS and of increased Na^+/Ca^{2+} exchange mechanism which would explain decreased Ca^{2+} net influx.

Thus ANF might have a protective effect on ischaemic myocardium.

References

Bardenheuer H, Schrader J (1983) Relationship between myocardial oxygen consumption, coronary flow, and adenosine release in an improved isolated working heart preparation of guinea pigs. Circ Res 51:263–271

Dietz JR (1984) Release of natriuretic factor from rat heart-lung preparation by atrial distension. Am J Physiol 16:R1093–1096

Ledsome JR, Wilson N, Courneya CA, Rankin AJ (1985) Release of natriuretic peptide by atrial distension. Can J Physiol Pharmacol 63:739–742

Hill JL, Gettes LS, Lynch MR, Herberg NC (1978) Flexible valinomycin electrodes for on line determination of intravascular and myocardial K^+. Am Physiol 235:H455–H459

Otero HO, Wangler RD, Sparks HV, Chimoskey JE (1987) Alpha human atrial natriuretic peptide is a coronary vasodilator in the Langendorff-perfused guinea pig heart. Life Sciences 42:695–700

Porter B, Gumprecht E, Geer PG, Goetz KL (1987) Plasma atrial peptide concentration during acute changes in cardiac filling pressure induced by a contrast agent. Clin Cardiol 10:289–292

Schömig A, Kurz TH, Richardt G, Schömig E (1988) Neuronal sodium homoeostasis and axoplasmic amine concentration determine calcium-independent noradrenaline release in normoxic and ischemic rat heart. Circ Res 63:1–13

The Roles of Atrial Natriuretic Peptide (ANP) and of Dopamine Receptors in Mediating the Natriuresis during Head-Out Water Immersion of Healthy Subjects

H.-G. Predel, M. Erkeling, H. Meyer-Lehnert, and H. J. Kramer

Medizinische Poliklinik, University of Bonn, FRG

Key words: ANP – Dopamine receptors – Natriuresis – Head- out water immersion

Introduction

Previous experimental findings in rats suggested that the renal dopaminergic system may function as a mediator of atrial natriuretic peptide (ANP)-induced diuresis and natriuresis. After pharmacological blockade of dopamine (DA)-1 receptors in rats the diuretic and natriuretic responses to an infusion of ANP was blunted significantly [8].

The purpose of the present study was, first, to stimulate the endogenous ANP secretion by thermoneutral head-out water immersion (HWI) and to evaluate the effects on renal excretory function, and second, to investigate the effects of an unselective blockade of DA-1 and DA-2 receptors on HWI-induced diuresis and natriuresis in six healthy male volunteers.

Methods

Thermoneutral HWI in sitting position with a duration of 240 minutes with a control period (pre-HWI) and a recovery period (post-HWI) of each 60 minutes was performed in six male healthy volunteers aged 26.3 ± 1.6 years.

The identical protocol was repeated 48 hours later after an intravenous (i.v.) administration of 15 µg/kg of haloperidol, an unselective DA-1 and DA-2 receptor antagonist. The protocol was outlined to all subjects and they gave their informed consent according to the declaration of Helsinki. Urine flow and urinary sodium excretion were measured every 30 minutes by spontaneous voiding.

Plasma concentrations of α-hANP and cGMP were measured during the control period, after 60 and 240 minutes of HWI and during the recovery period. Plasma α-hANP was extracted according to Kohno et al. [6]. Radioimmunoassay (RIA) was performed using an antibody against ANP from the Peninsula Laboratories (St. Helens, UK) as described previously [10]. Plasma concentrations of cGMP were determined with a commercially available RIA-Kit (DRG, Marburg, FRG).

For statistical analysis a rank-signed Wilcoxon test was used. Values are given as means ± SEM.

Results

In the absence of pretreatment with haloperidol plasma α-hANP and cGMP concentrations during the pre-HWI period averaged 8.4 ± 1.6 pmol/l and 16.6 ± 1.1 pmol/ml, respectively. Similar control plasma concentrations of 9.7 ± 2.2 pmol/l and 17.1 ± 1.9 pmol/ml, respectively, were found after pretreatment with haloperidol (Fig. 1).

Urinary volume and sodium excretion during the pre-HWI period were 105.8 ± 26.9 ml/h and 14.4 ± 3.1 mmol/h in the absence and were 89.2 ± 15.2 ml/h and 15.1 ± 3.1 mmol/h, respectively, in the presence of haloperidol (Fig. 1).

During HWI plasma α-hANP and cGMP concentrations rose significantly ($p < 0.05$) to 32.9 ± 3.0 pmol/l and 32.5 ± 1.9 pmol/ml in the absence and to 30.5 ± 7.2 pmol/l and 29.6 ± 3.1 pmol/ml, respectively, in the presence of haloperidol. Highest ANP and cGMP plasma levels were reached within 60 minutes of HWI. They persisted during HWI and rapidly declined to basal values within 30 minutes after cessation of HWI (Fig. 1).

During HWI urinary volume and sodium excretion increased significantly ($p < 0.05$) to 222.5 ± 56.6 mol/h and 19.5 ± 2.0 mmol/h in the absence and to 250.5 ± 58.7 mol/h and 22.1 ± 3.3 mmol/h, respectively, in the presence of haloperidol. They rapidly returned to basal values during the post-HWI period (Fig. 1).

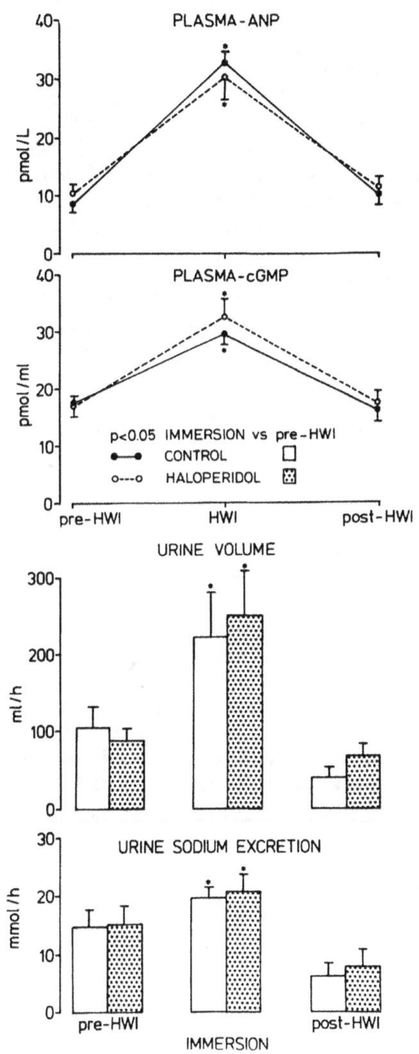

Fig. 1. Mean ANP and cGMP plasma concentrations, mean urine volume and urine sodium excretion 60 minutes before, during, and after head-out water immerson (HWI)

Discussion

In agreement with previous studies HWI proved to be an adequate stimulus of ANP secretion [2]. The increase in ANP plasma levels was accompanied by a comparable rise in cGMP plasma concentrations, the proposed second messenger of ANP. The increases in α-hANP and cGMP plasma concentrations during HWI were similar in the absence and presence of pretreatment with haloperidol.

In parallel there was a significant increase in urine volume and sodium excretion during HWI which was similar without or with concomitant administration of haloperidol. dol.

Previous investigations on the effects of DA-receptor blockade have revealed controversial results. Marin-Grez et al. performed bolus injections of ANP in anesthetized rats with or without pretreatment with metoclopramide, sulpiride, chlorpromazine or haloperidol. The authors demonstrated that haloperidol and chlorpromazine blunted the ANP-induced diuresis and natriuresis [8]. Similar results were obtained by Petterson et al. [9] and Webb et al. [11] using various DA-receptor antagonists in different animal models. However, the blunted natriuresis and diuresis were consistently accompanied by a significant fall in blood pressure, which may have led to decreased renal perfusion pressure and may have activated sodium retaining neuro-hormonal systems. Therefore, it may be difficult to differentiate between the effects of these physiological counter-regulatory mechanisms and the effects of the DA-receptor blockade itself.

In contrast, our findings are in agreement with more recent studies performed in man [1] and in monkeys [6]. These studies did not reveal an inhibitory influence of various DA-receptor antagonists on ANP-mediated diuresis and natriuresis.

The conflicting results may be explained first, by the different mode of raising ANP plasma concentrations, i.e. administration of exogenous ANP, on the one hand, and stimulation of endogenous ANP secretion, on the other hand. In our present experiments endogenous ANP secretion was stimulated by HWI over a period of 240 minutes without changes in blood pressure. This prolonged physiological rise in ANP plasma concentrations may itself have suppressed the activity of sodium retaining neuro-hormonal systems in our subjects, whereas they may be stimulated when acute hemodynamic changes occur with intravenous administration of exogenous ANP. Second, there may be species differences responsible for the differing effects of DA-receptor blockade.

In summary, we conclude that HWI is a physiological stimulus of ANP secretion. The renal dopaminergic system does not seem to be involved in the diuresis and natriuresis induced by HWI in healthy man. The accompanying rise in ANP secretion may contribute at least in part to the renal response to head-out water immersion.

Acknowledgments: This study was supported in part by a grant from the Ministerium für Wissenschaft und Forschung des Landes Nordrhein-Westfalen, FRG (FA-8871 and IV A6-402-046-87) and was presented in part at the 3rd World Congress On Biologically Active Atrial Peptides, New York, June 1988 and at the 12th Meeting of the Gesellschaft für Nephrologie, Göttingen, September 1988.

The authors gratefully acknowledge the excellent technical assistance of Mrs. A. Bäcker and Mrs. H. Stelkens.

References

1. Allen MJ, Bennett D (1987) The renal effects of atrial natriuretic peptide are not inhibited by the dopamine antagonist domperidone (Abstract). Circulation 76:268
2. Anderson JV, Miliar ND, O'Hare JP, Mackenzie JC, Corrall RJM, Bloom SR (1986) Atrial natriuretic peptide: physiological release associated with natriuresis during water immersion in man. Clin Science 71:319–322
3. Frederickson ED, Bradley T, Goldberg LI (1985) Blockade of renal effects of dopamine in the dog by the DA-1 antagonist, SCH-23390. Am J Physiol 249:F236–F240
4. Goldberg LI (1972) Cardiovascular and renal effects of dopamine: potential clinical applications. Pharmacol Rev 24:1–29
5. Goldberg LI, Kohli JD (1981) Agonists and antagonists of peripheral postsynaptic dopamine receptors: clinical implications. In: Gessa G, Corsini GU (eds) Apomorphine and other dopaminomimetics: Basic pharmacology. Raven Press, New York, pp 273–284
6. Kastner PR, Ertel MA, Bohnke RA, Emmert LW, Burkhard TA (1986) Dopamine (DA-1) receptor blockade does not inhibit the diuretic/natriuretic (D/N) effects of (Ile 12) 5–28 atrial natriuretic peptide in rhesus monkeys. (Abstract) Fed Proc 46:1296
7. Kohno M, Takaori K, Matsuura T, Murakawa K, Kanayama Y, Takeda T (1986) Atrial natriuretic polypeptide in atria and plasma in experimental hyperthyroidism and hypothyroidism. Biochem Biophys Res Commun 134:178–183
8. Marin-Grez M, Briggs JP, Schubert G, Schnermann J (1985) Dopamine receptor antagonists inhibit the natriuretic response to atrial natriuretic factor (ANF). Life Sci 36:2171–2176
9. Petterson A, Hedner J, Hedner T (1986) The diuretic effects of atrial natriuretic peptide (ANP) is dependent on dopaminergic activation. Acta Physiol Scand 126:619–621
10. Predel HG, Kipnowski J, Bäcker A, Stelkens H, Jürgens U, Düsing R, Kramer HJ (1988) Elevated plasma concentrations and molecular weight heterogeneity of human atrial natriuretic peptide in patients with progressive chronic renal failure. Z Kardiol 77 [Suppl 2]:65–71
11. Webb RL, Della Puca R, Manniello J, Robson RD, Zimmerman MB, Ghai RD (1986) Dopaminergic mediation of the diuretic and natriuretic effects of ANP in the rat. Life Sci 38:2319–2327

Increased Sympathetic Stimulation Does Not Increase Plasma Levels of Human Atrial Natriuretic Factor

K. Kienast, A. Daul, K. Cissewski, G. Benker and D. Reinwein

Abteilung für Endokrinologie, Medizinische Klinik und Poliklinik, Universitätsklinikum (GHS) Essen, FRG

Key words: Atrial Natriuretic Factor (ANF) – Central Sympathetic Stimulation (CSS) – Hypoglycemia

Introduction

In vivo evidence suggests that atrial distention is the major regulator of ANF release [1]. Sympathetic denervation, leading to a reduce in heart rate and blood pressure, abolishes the ANF secretion induced by volume expansion [4]. Alpha-adrenergic stimulation is found to increase plasma ANF in humans [4], and neuronal influences are also important in the volume-induced ANF release in denervated heart preparations [3]. Thus, it has to be discussed that besides atrial distention, CSS or CSS-dependent alterations may be indirectly involved in ANF secretion.

Methods

Insulin (0.1 I.U./kg body weight) or isotonic saline were administered intravenously to 7 healthy volunteers (aged 24–32 years). To monitor sympathetic activation, plasma levels of adrenaline and noradrenaline, lymphocyte, β_2-adrenoceptor density and isoprenalin-induced lymphocyte cAMP were measured. ANF was assessed by radioimmunoassay with 125-Jodotyrosil-28 ah ANF and rabbit anti-ah-ANF (Amersham). Lymphocytes were isolated from 30 ml EDTA blood. Lymphocyte β_2-adrenoceptor density was determined by (−) – $I^{125}I$-iodocyanopindolol (ICYP) binding at 6 concentrations ranging from 10-150 pM. Lymphocyte cyclic AMP content was determined by protein binding assay, as described by Brodde et al. [2].

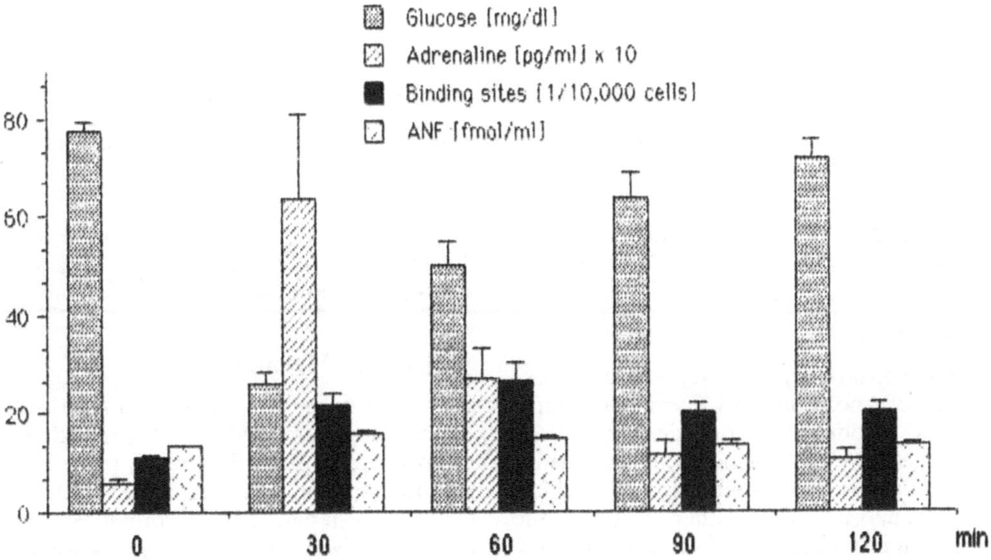

Fig. 1. Blood glucose, plasma adrenaline, ANF and β2-adrenoceptor density during hypoglycemia-induced sympathetic stimulation

Statistical evaluations: All values are given as ± SEM.

Results

Within 30 minutes after injection of insuline blood glucose levels decreased from 77 ± 3 to 26 ± 6 mg/dl. Concomitantly heart rate increased from 62 ± 5 to 76 ± 4/min, systolic pressure from 117 ± 7 to 131 ± 8 mmHg, while diastolic blood pressure fell from 73 ± 6 to 63 ± 7 mmHg. Plasma adrenaline rose from 56 ± 1.4 to 622 ± 249 pg/ml, plasma noradrenaline from 323 ± 44 to 541 ± 61 pg/ml. Lymphocyte β_2-adrenoceptor density increased by about 250–300%, this increase was accompanied by a similar rise in the 10 μM isoprenaline induced lymphocyte cAMP accumulation, indicating a real increase in functional β-adrenoceptors. Basal ANF was 13.5 ± 0.5 fmol/ml there was a discret elevation up to 16 ± 1 fmol/ml after 60 minutes.

Central sympathetic stimulation by hypoglycemia, documented by elevated plasma catecholamines, increased lymphocyte β_2-adrenoceptor density and increased lymphocytic cAMP production could not induce a significant release of ANF. The observed action in ANF plasma concentrations appears to be mediated by hemodynamic changes.

References

1. Arendt RM et al. (1986) Atrialer natriuretischer Faktor. DWM 111: 1849–1854
2. Brodde OE et al. (1985) Terbatuline-induced Desensitisation of Human Lymphocyte β_2-Adrenoceptors. J Clin Invest 76: 1096–1101
3. Eskay R et al. (1986) Circulating Atrial Natriuretic Peptides in Conscious Rats: Regulation of Release by Multiple Factors. Science 232:636–639
4. Sanfield JA et al. (1986) Alpha-Adrenergic Stimulation of Immunoreactive Atrial Natriuretic Hormone Levels in Humans. Clin Res 34 (2):433 A

Hemodynamic and Diuretic Effects of Two Consecutive Bolus Applications of Atrial Natriuretic Peptide (α-hANP) in Healthy Volunteers

M. Kentsch, G. Müller-Esch, D. Ludwig, J. Potratz, P. Ball, R. Gerzer, and P. C. Scriba

Medizinische Universität Lübeck und Medizinische Klinik Innenstadt der Universität München, FRG

Key words: Atrial Natriuretic Peptide – Hemodynamics – Diuresis – Natriuresis

Introduction

Human atrial natriuretic peptide (α-hANP) is a cardiac hormone with diuretic, natriuretic and vasodilating properties [1, 6, 7]. It has been given intravenously as a bolus injection or as a constant infusion. Vasodilating actions [3] as well as other hemodynamic [3, 6] and diuretic effects of α-hANP may depend on the application scheme and the given dose [8]. With regard to a possible therapeutic role in congestive heart failure, we investigated the hemodynamic and diuretic effects of two consecutive high dose bolus injections of α-hANP in normal man.

Subjects and Methods

Six healthy male volunteers on non-salt-restricted diet were studied in the unsedated postabsorptive state. Urine was passed before the study and then after 30 minute intervals. Systemic arterial pressures and heart rate were measured noninvasively (Automatic cuff, Dynamap), pulmonary artery pressures were recorded via a Swan-Ganz catheter and cardiac output was determined by thermodilution method (Recomed, Hellige). Cyclic GMP was measured by radioimmuno assay.

Two bolus injections of 200 μg α-hANP were given at a 30-minute interval (time of injection: t0.0 and t0.30). Data were recorded 20, 10 and 0 minutes before the study, and 2, 5, 10, 20 and 30 minutes after the first and second α-hANP bolus as well as 45 and 60 minutes after the second bolus.

Results are expressed as mean and standard deviation. Areas under the response curve (t0.0, t0.30; t0.30, t0.60) were computed according to the trapezoidal rule. Statistical analysis was performed by analysis of variance for repeated measures, paired t-test (individuals basal versus maximum values) and Dunnett t-test for comparison with the control group.

Results

After the first and second α-hANP bolus cardiac output (l/min; B1:8.3 ± 1.0 to 11 ± 1.1, $p < 0.001$; B2: 8.5 ± 0.66 to 11 ± 1.7, $p < 0.01$) and heart rate (bpm; B1: 69.7 ± 10.1 to 84.7 ± 12.1, $p < 0.01$; B2: 70.2 ± 5.3 to 79.0 ± 9.6, $p < 0.05$) were significantly higher than baseline values. Systolic arterial pressure (mmHG, B1: 129.0 ± 10.2 to 114.8 ±1 2.6, $p < 0.01$; B2: 125.7 ± 14.8 to 110.3 ± 13.4, $p < 0.01$), systolic pulmonary arterial pressure (mmHg; B1: 18.2 ± 2.5 to 16.8 ± 2.6, $p < 0.05$; B2: 18.0 ± 2.1 to 14.8 ± 2.5, $p < 0.05$) and systemic arterial resistance (dyn-sec-cm-5; B1: 845 ± 195 to 555 ± 79, $p < 0.01$; B2: 820 ± 174 to 571 ± 59, $p < 0.01$) were significantly lower than baseline values after both hANP bolus injections. As determined by the area under the response curve, increase of cardiac output was less pronounced after the second hANP bolus (Area. 2: 276 ± 28) than after the first bolus (Area. 1: 295 ± 19, $p < 0.05$).

Hematocrit constantly increased during the first 60 minutes of the study ($r = 0.8988$, $p < 0.001$) from 40.5 ± 2,6% before the first bolus to 42.3 ± 2.4% 30 minutes after the second bolus ($p < 0.01$). Cyclic GMP levels were elevated after both bolus injections (pMol/ml; B1: 4.9 ± 1.3 to 26 ± 6.9, $p < 0.001$; B2: 17 ± 5.6 to 29 ± 7.5, $p < 0.01$). As 30 minutes after the first injection the cyclic GMP levels were still higher than before the study ($p < 0.01$), the area under the response curve for cGMP was greater after the second (701.8 ± 183.1) than after the first bolus (600.5 ± 165.4, $p < 0.05$).

Compared to the 30 minute control period before the first injection, urine volume (ml/min; 1.2 ± 0.8) was significantly higher 30 minutes after the first injection (22.4 ± 10.7), 30 minutes after the second hANP bolus (20.5 ± 7.1) and 60 minutes after the second bolus (11.8 ± 6.4; Dunnett t-tests, $p < 0.01$). Also urine sodium excretion (mmol/h; 6.3 ± 6.5) was significantly higher at t0.30 (70.6 ± 24.5), t0.60 (69.5 ± 27.9) and t0.90 (50.0 ± 31.9) than during the control period ($p < 0.01$).

Discussion

Like others [4, 6], in the present study we observed diuretic, natriuretic and cardiovascular effects after α-hANP bolus injection.

Cyclic GMP is referred to as a marker [4] and may be a mediator of α-hANP activity [5]. Experimental data gave evidence that the excretion of cGMP is attenuated by prior exposure to α-hANP [5]. In contrast, in the present study with repeated α-hANP bolus injection the second α-hANP bolus produced an even higher peak plasma cGMP concentration, while cGMP levels were still elevated from the first bolus. Diuresis increased 18-fold and natriuresis 11-fold after the first α-hANP bolus and increases of both parameters persisted after the second α-hANP bolus.

The hemodynamic profile of repeated high dose bolus injection of α-hANP can be characterized by a significant reduction of cardiac afterload as measured by systemic vascular resistance. Concomittant increase of cardiac output is most likely due to reduced afterload but reflex mediated catecholamine activation may also play a role [9]. Together with assumed reduction in preload due to sustained diuresis and additional plasma volume shift to extravascular compartments [2, 10], the changes might be of therapeutical benefit in the treatment of patients with congestive heart failure.

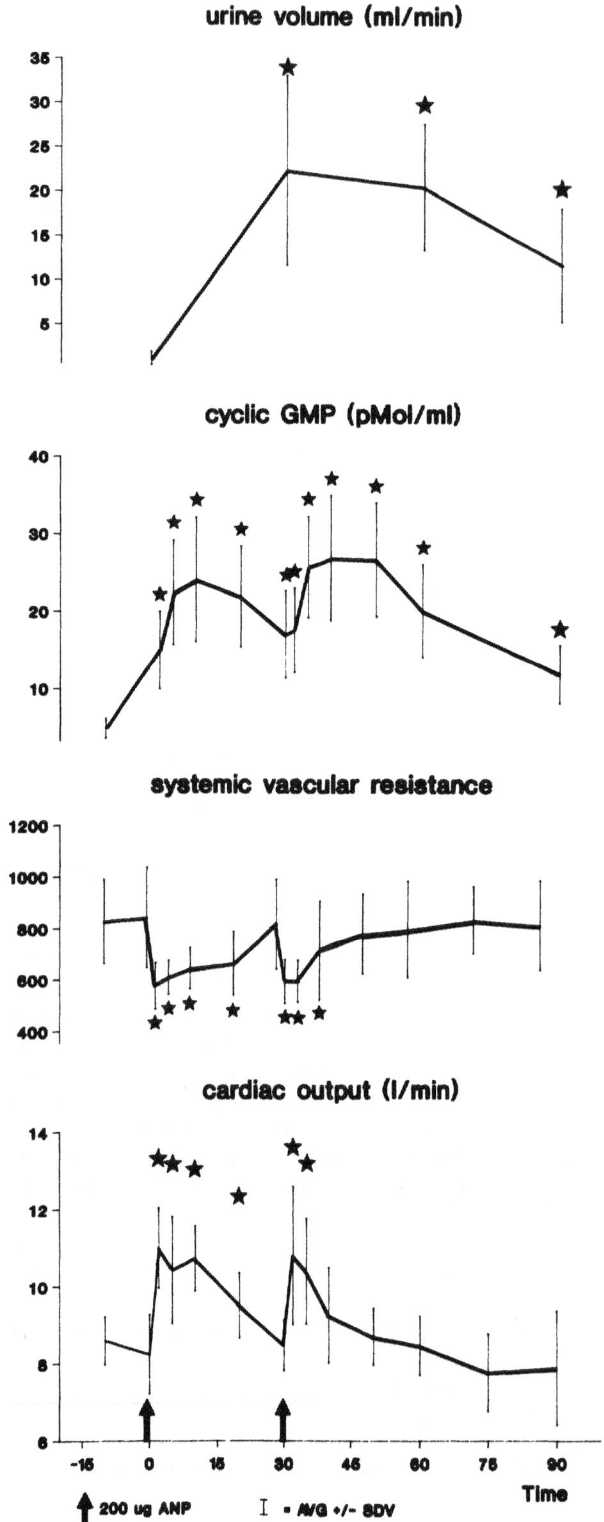

Fig. 1. Effect of two consecutive α-hANP bolus injections on urine volume, cyclic GMP, systemic vascular resistance and cardiac output (* $p < 0.01$, Dunnett t-test)

References

1. Bolli P, Müller FB, Lindner L, Raine AEG, Resink TJ, Erne P, Kiowski W, Ritz R, Bühler FR (1987) The vasodilator potency of atrial natriuretic peptide in man. Circulation 75:221–228
2. Cody RC, Atlas SA, Laragh JH, Kubo SH, Covit AB, Ryman KS, Shaknovich A, Pondolfino K, Clark M, Camargo MJF, Scarborough RM, Lewicke JA (1986) Atrial natriuretic factor in normal subjects and heart failure patients. J Clin Invest 78:1362–1374
3. Cuneo RC, Espiner RA, Nicholls MG, Yandle TG, Joyce SL, Gilchrist NL (1986) Renal, hemodynamic, and hormonal response to atrial natriuretic peptide infusions in normal man, and effect of sodium intake. J Clin Endocrinol Metab 63:946–953
4. Gerzer R, Witzgall H, Tremblay J, Gutkowska J, Hamet P (1985) Rapid increase in plasma and urinary GMP after bolus injection of atrial natriuretic factor in man. J Clin Endocrinol Metab 61:1217–1219
5. Hamet P, Tremblay J, Pang SC, Shuherska R, Schiffrin EL, Garcia R, Cantin M, Genest J, Palmour R, Ervin FR, Martin S, Goldwater R (1986) Cyclic GMP as mediator and biological marker of atrial natriuretic factor. J Hypertension 4 [Suppl II]:49–56
6. Richards AM, Nicholls MG, Ikram H, Webster MWI, Yandle TG, Espiner EA (1985) Renal, haemodynamic and hormonal effects of human alpha atrial natriuretic peptide in healthy volunteers. Lancet 1:545–549
7. Tikkanen I, Fyhrquist F, Metsarinne K, Leidenius R (1985) Plasma atrial natriuretic peptide in cardiac disease and during infusion in healthy volunteers. Lancet 1:66–69
8. Waldhäusl W, Vierhapper H, Nowotny P (1986) Prolonged administration of human atrial natriuretic peptide in helathy men: evanescent effects on diuresis and natriuresis. J Clin Endocrinol Metab 62:956–959
9. Weidman P, Gnädinger MP, Ziswiler HR, Shaw S, Bachmann C, Rascher W, Uehlinger DE, Hasler L, Reubi FC (1986) Cardiovascular, endocrine and renal effects of atrial natriuretic peptide in essential hypertension. J Hypertension 4 [Suppl II]:71–83
10. Weidmann P, Hasler L, Gnädinger MP, Lang RE, Uehlinger DE, Shaw S, Rascher W, Reubi FC (1986) Blood levels and renal effects of atrial natriuretic peptide in normal man. J Clin Invest 77:734–742

Circadian Rhythm of Atrial Natriuretic Peptide in Normal Subjects

K. Ehlenz, H. Schneider, P. Tremmel, P. Schmidt, and H. Kaffarnik

Abteilung für Endokrinologie und Stoffwechsel, Zentrum für Innere Medizin der Universität Marburg, FRG

Key words: ANP – Circadian rhythm

Introduction

ANP plays an important role in the regulation of volume and sodium homeostasis and can influence blood pressure. Changes of ANP levels under physiological and pathological states could be demonstrated. Studies about circadian secretion patterns can be helpful to clarify the physiological role of a hormone and can also elucidate mechanisms important in hormone secretion. As there exists little information about diurnal changes of ANP plasma levels, we studied the circadian variation of ANP in normal subjects.

Protocol and Methods

4 healthy medical students with a mean age of 26 participated in this study. Blood samples were taken every 30 minutes between 8 a.m. and 11 p.m. while the subjects were in a sitting position. Breakfast was at 8 a.m., dinner at 12:30 a.m. and supper at 6 p.m. Fluid intake was ad libitum. From 9:30 p.m., probands were in a supine position. At eleven o'clock, lights were turned off. Thereafter, blood samples were taken every 20 minutes without disturbing sleep. ANP was determined with a commercially available radioimmunoassay (IBL; Hamburg) after extraction of 1 ml plasma with Sep pak (Waters Associates) according to a procedure from Hartter et al. (1986). Intraassay

variability was 8% and lower detection limit 2.5 pg/ml plasma. The obtained values were transformed by the so-called Z score transformation according to the following equation:

$$Z = [x(t) - \bar{X}]/SD$$

where x(t) is the ANP level at time point t and $\bar{X}$ and SD are the arithmetic mean respectively standard deviation of all values from one subject.

Results

All probands show a significant diurnal variation in plasma ANP levels between 8 and 50 pg/ml. In the morning, ANP levels increase to a maximum at 11 a.m. Thereafter, we saw a decline, which was interrupted by a slight increase shortly after lunch. Between 2 and 4 p.m., we found a through. Thereafter, ANP showed an increase lasting until 8 p.m. A slight decrease in the early evening was followed by an increase about 10 p.m. related to the time of change in body position. This elevation lasted about 3 hours and was followed by a trough between 1 and 4 p.m. In the early morning, plasma ANP again showed a slight increase between 4 and 6 a.m. (see Fig. 1).

Discussion

In a short communication, Donckier et al. (1986) reported an increase of ANP in the evening and higher levels at night. After wake up, ANP levels decreased. But during daytime, he found no changes in subjects performing their normal daily activity. Although he measured ANP during sleep only three times, his results are well corresponding to ours. We also found higher levels after sleep onset and in the early morning. But we found clear changes in plasma ANP levels during daytime too. The different protocol could be an explaination as our probands were in a sitting position most of the time and the subjects in Donckiers paper performed a normal daily work.

The decrease of ANP in the early afternoon is possibly related to postprandial changes in hemodynamics. Increase of bloodflow in the intestinal circulation may lead to a decrease in central blood volume, which in turn leads to a decrease of atrial distension and consequently of ANP secretion. The increase of ANP in the late evening is clearly related to the change in position; it was seen in all subjects before sleep onset. So, the increased venous return may

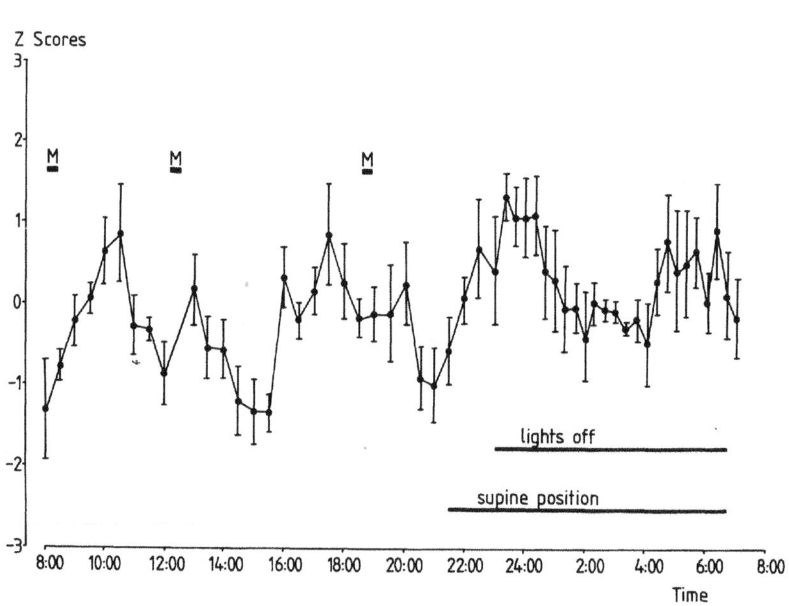

Fig. 1. Circadian changes in ANP plasma levels in four healthy men. The data were transformed to Z scores (mean ± SEM). M = time of meal

be the cause for this effect. In contrast to the short half life of ANP, this peak lasted about 3 hours. We should have expected that a new steady state of blood distribution between peripheral and central volume was reached faster. But reabsorption of extracellular fluid can possibly explain the phenomenon. The decrease of ANP levels in the early night indicates a new state of volume distribution.

In another study, Richards et al. (1987) saw only small changes in plasma levels with a significant trough at 7 p.m. But in his investigation volunteers were in a supine position throughout the whole day.

Follenius et al. (1988) found no significant changes of ANP during sleep and also no dependency from sleep stages. But in their experiments, probands were in a supine position for about 2 hours before the beginning of blood sampling. Comparing our results with the results of the other cited groups, the differences can only be explained by changes in body position and hemodynamics.

References

Donckier J, Anderson JV, Yeo T, Bloom SR (1986) Diurnal rhythm in the plasma concentration of atrial natriuretic peptide. N Engl J Med 315:710–711

Follenius M, Brandenberger G, Simon C (1988) Nocturnal fluctuations of plasma atrial natriuretic peptide in normotensive and hypertensive men. Life Sci 42:1635–1639

Hartter E, Woloszczuk W, Stummvoll HK (1986) Radioimmunoassay of atrial natriuretic peptides in human plasma. Clin Chem 32:441–445

Rankin AJ (1987) Mechanisms for the release of atrial natriuretic peptide. Can J Physiol Pharmacol 65:1673–1679

Richards AM, Tonolo G, Fraser R, Morton JJ, Leckie BJ, Ball SG, Robertson JIS (1987) Diurnal change in plasma atrial natriuretic peptide concentrations. Clin Sci 73:489–495

Effect of Low-Dose ANF Infusion on Renin and Aldosterone Secretion in Man*

W. Oelkers, S. Kleiner, H. Tuchelt, G. Eschenhagen, and V. Bähr

Division of Endocrinology, Department of Medicine, Klinikum Steglitz, Freie Universität Berlin

Key words: ANF – Low dose infusion – Renin – Aldosterone

Introduction

Early studies on the effects of infused atrial natriuretic factor (ANF) in man were performed using large doses that raised ANF plasma levels far above the physiological range (Weidmann et al. 1986; Cuneo et al. 1986). We attempted to find out at what ANF plasma concentration – attained by infusion of the peptide – blood pressure, plasma renin activity (PRA), and plasma aldosterone (P-Al) would be affected. A second part of the study was to answer the question as to whether "sensitization" of the zona glomerulosa of the adrenal cortex to angiotensin II (AII) in the sodium deplete state (Oelkers et al. 1974) was due to changes in ANF plasma concentration.

Methods

Study 1: 6 normal young males received ANF or placebo infusions in the sodium deplete state (for details see Oelkers et al. 1988). Between 4.00 and 6.00 p.m., 0.1 µg/min or 0.3 µg/min or 1.0 µg/min of human α ANF (99–126) or placebo were infused intravenously after 2 hours of recumbency. From 5.20 to 6.00 p.m., an AII-infusion (6 ng/kg/min) was superimposed. Plasma ANF, AII, P-Al, PRA, blood pressure, and heart rate were measured at appropriate intervals.

* Supported by a grant from the Deutsche Forschungsgemeinschaft (Oe 47/9)

Study 2: 6 other normal young males received stepwise increasing doses of AII (1, 3, and 6 ng/kg/min) between 3.00 and 6.00 p.m. under 3 different conditions: a) after sodium loading (5 days, 200 mM Na^+/day), b) after sodium depletion, and c) after sodium depletion plus an infusion of 0.12 µg/min of ANF from 10.00 a.m. until 6.00 p.m. on the AII infusion day. Plasma levels of the same hormones as in study 1 were measured.

Results

Study 1: Fig. 1a shows the plasma levels of ANF attained by infusion of the peptide itself. Normal levels (sodium deplete, placebo) were around 26 pg/ml. The lowest dose of ANF raised plasma ANF within the physiological range (ca. 68 pg/ml). The two higher doses were supraphysiological (ca. 220 and 650 pg/ml ANF respectively). Systolic blood pressure (BP) tended to fall and diastolic BP to rise with increasing ANF doses. PRA and P-Al dropped significantly (compared with placebo) with the two higher ANF doses infused. The trend with the lowest dose pointed into the same direction (Fig. 1b and 1c). P-Al was markedly increased during the final AII infusion when placebo was infused instead of ANF. The highest dose of ANF blunted the effect of AII on P-Al significantly (Fig. 1c) with a similar trend upon infusion of lower ANF doses.

Study 2: After sodium loading and sodium depletion, plasma ANF levels were around 55 pg/ml and 20 pg/ml respectively. During infusion of AII in sodium deplete state, the dose-response curve (dose of AII vs. the increment of P-Al) was significantly steeper in the sodium deplete than in the loaded state, as expected (Oelkers et al. 1974 and 1983). Additional ANF infusion in the sodium deplete state raised plasma ANF levels into the range of sodium-loaded subjects. ANF infusion induced a fall in the high aldosterone levels, but the steepness of the AII-P-Al dose response curve was only slightly diminished.

Discussion

Our study, together with other recent publications (Cuneo et al. 1987; Anderson et al. 1987), shows that ANF infusions start to inhibit renin and aldosterone secretion when plasma ANF levels were increased by infusion into the high-physiological range. Higher doses are more inhibitory. Thus, ANF may be of physiological importance in the regulation of renin and aldosterone secretion, at least acutely. As shown in studies 1 and 2, the effect of ANF on *basal* PRA and P-Al levels seems to occur at lower ANF plasma concentrations than the effect of ANF on AII-stimulated aldosterone secretion. This suggests that lowering of renin secretion (with a secondary fall of P-Al) is the more physiological effect of ANP and that the inhibition of the effect of AII on the zona glomerulosa occurs at slightly higher ANF plasma concentrations only. Furthermore, "sensitization" of the adrenal cortex to AII by sodium depletion is probably not caused

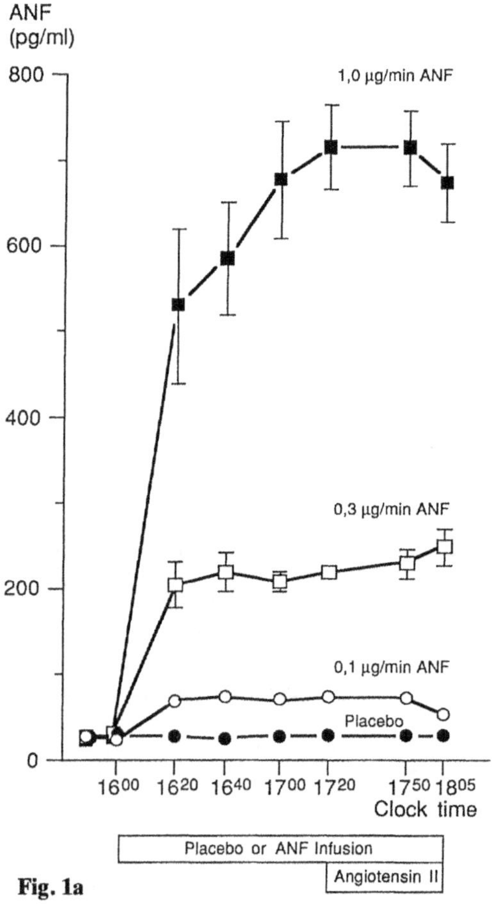

Fig. 1a

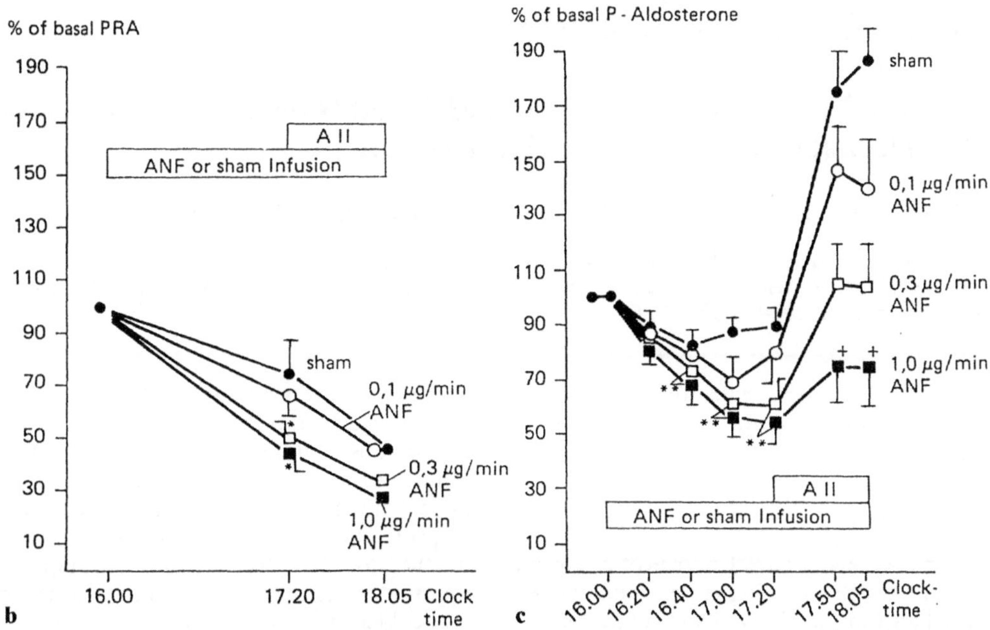

Fig. 1. Plasma levels of ANF obtained during ANF or placebo infusion **(a)** and relative changes of PRA **(b)** and plasma aldosterone **(c)** during the same infusion. Angiotensin II infusions were superimposed during the last 45 min of ANF infusion. Asterisks indicate that the percentage falls in PRA and aldosterone are significantly greater than on placebo day (*$p < 0.05$; ** $p < 0.001$). Dagger ($^{+}$) indicates significantly smaller rise in p-Al between 5.20 p.m. and later measurements than on placebo day

by removal of a tonic inhibitory effect of ANF on the zona glomerulosa (ANF levels are higher in the sodium-loaded state). Possible other causes of "sensitization" were discussed extensively in a previous publication (Oelkers et al. 1983).

References

Anderson JV, Donckier J, Payne NN, Beacham J, Slater JDM, Bloom SR (1987) Atrial natriuretic peptide: evidence of action as a natriuretic hormone at physiological plasma concentrations in man. Clin Sci 72:305–312

Cuneo RC, Espiner EA, Nicholls MG, Yandle TG, Joyce St, Gilchrist SL (1986) Renal, hemodynamic, and hormonal responses to atrial natriuretic peptide infusion in normal man, and effect of sodium intake. J Clin Endocrinol Metab 63:946–953

Cuneo RC, Espiner EA, Nicholls MG, Yandle TG, Liversey JH (1987) Effect of physiological levels of atrial natriuretic peptide on hormone secretion: inhibition of angiotensin-induced aldosterone secretion and renin release in normal man. J Clin Endocrinol Metab 65:765–772

Oelkers W, Brown JJ, Fraser R, Lever AF, Morton JF, Robertson JIS (1974) Sensitization of the adrenal cortex to angiotensin II in sodium deplete man. Circ Res 34:69–77

Oelkers W, Schöneshöfer M (1983) Acute and chronic regulation of aldosterone secretion in man. In: Kaufmann W et al. (eds) Mineralocorticoids and Hypertension. Springer, Berlin Heidelberg New York, pp 51–61

Oelkers W, Kleiner S, Bähr V (1988) Effects of incremental infusions of artrial natriuretic factor on aldosterone, renin and blood pressure in humans. Hypertension 12:462–467

Weidmann P, Hellmüller B, Uehlinger D (1986) Plasma levels and cardiovascular, endocrine, and excretory effects of atrial natriuretic peptide during different sodium intakes in man. J Clin Endocrinol Metab 62:1027–1036

ANP and Cardiac Diseases

Basal and Exercise Plasma Levels of Atrial Natriuretic Peptide and Noradrenaline in Congestive Heart Failure

I. Tikkanen[1,3], H. Leinonen[2], H. Näveri[2], A. Sovijärvi[4], and F. Fyhrquist[1,3]

[1] The Minerva Foundation Institute for Medical Research, Helsinki, and the [2] First and [3] Fourth Departments of Medicine and [4] Department of Pulmonary Medicine, Helsinki University Central Hospital, Helsinki, Finland

Key words: Atrial natriuretic peptide – ANP – Noradrenaline – Heart failure – Exercise

Introduction

Plasma levels of atrial natriuretic peptide (ANP) are elevated in patients with congestive heart failure (CHF) and related to the severity of the disease, judged by functional capacity of the patients [9] and by direct measurements of cardiac preload [8]. Thus, plasma ANP measurements have been suggested to be useful in the evaluation of the degree of cardiac impairment [4, 6, 8]. Plasma noradrenaline (NA) levels have also been shown to increase in proportion to the severity of CHF, and high NA levels are associated with increased mortality [1]. In the present study, plasma ANP and NA levels were measured at rest and during maximal exercise in patients with chronic CHF to see if there is a correlation between ANP, NA, and the severity of heart failure, assessed by maximal oxygen consumption ($\dot{V}O_2$max).

Patients and Methods

We studied 10 men patients, aged 37 to 57 years (mean 47 years) with chronic class II to IV (New York Heart Association classification) CHF and 6 healthy controls (4 males and 2 females, aged 28–45 years). Eight patients had idiopathic dilated cardiomyopathy (three with mild mitral valve regurgitation and two with severe mitral and tricuspid valve regurgitation), one had ischemic cardiomyopathy, and one hade mitral valve regurgitation. All patients were treated with digoxin, diuretics and vasodilators at constant doses. Both the patients and the controls underwent maximal upright bicycle ergometer exercise test with continuous analysis of expired gas to determine $\dot{V}O_2$max. The achievement of anaerobic threshold was determined by a disproportionate rise in carbon dioxide production relative to oxygen consumption (ventilatory exchange ratio) and by a rise in blood lactate level. The level of anaerobic threshold was reached in all cases before termination of exercise. Arterial blood samples for determination of ANP (radioimmunoassay method [9]) and NA (radioenzymatic method) were taken in the supine position, in the upright position on the bicycle, during the last minute of maximal exercise, and 10 minutes after exercise in the supine position. Data were analyzed by Student's *t*-test for paired or non-paired observations and are presented as mean ± SEM.

Results

The mean $\dot{V}O_2$max of the patients was 14.9 ml/min/kg (range 6.5 to 21.3 ml/min/kg). The basal plasma ANP levels of the patients were markedly elevated (311 ± 58 pg/ml) as compared with controls (49.0 ± 6.2 pg/ml, $p<0.001$). In the patient group, there was a significant negative correlation between $\dot{V}O_2$max and basal ANP ($r = -0.78$, $p < 0.01$, Fig 1) and NA ($r = -0.79$, $p < 0.01$) concentrations. Moreover, there was a correlation between basal ANP and NA levels ($r = 0.73$, $p < 0.02$, Fig. 1).

Plasma ANP increased during exercise both in the patients (to 568 ± 128 pg/ml) and in the controls (to 69.7 ± 10.9 pg/ml, $p < 0.02$), but there was a great interindividual variability in the magnitude of this response. During maximal exercise, plasma

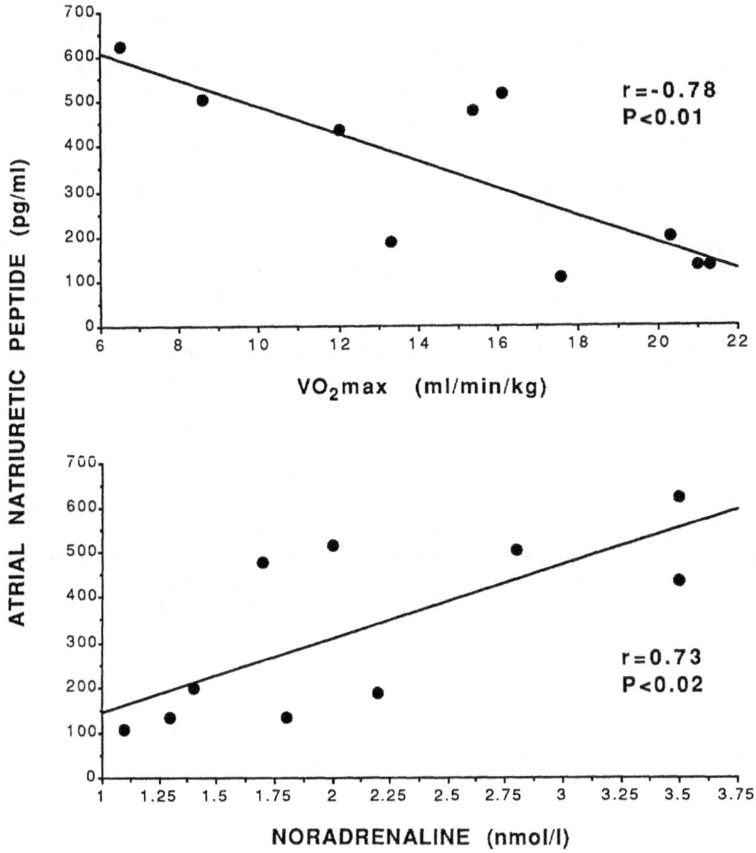

Fig. 1. Correlation between basal plasma atrial natriuretic peptide levels and maximal oxygen consumption (upper panel) and basal plasma noradrenaline levels (lower panel) in patients with congestive heart failure

levels of ANP had no correlation with heart rate or plasma NA levels. Furthermore, there was no relationship between exercise-induced increments in plasma ANP, NA, and heart rate.

Discussion

This study shows that basal plasma ANP levels increase with decreasing $\dot{V}O_2$max, which is considered to be the most objective measure of the severity of heart failure [3]. Thus, our study confirms and extends the previous findings indicating that in CHF, the plasma ANP levels increase in parallel to the severity of the disease [4, 5, 8, 9]. This is also supported by the present finding that the basal plasma ANP levels increase in close relationship with plasma NA levels.

During exercise, plasma ANP levels increased both in healthy controls and in patients with heart failure confirming previous results [4, 5, 6, 7]. However, the magnitude of exercise-induced ANP elevation varied markedly among patients with CHF. Contrary to findings in healthy individuals [4], and in patients with myocardial infarction [6], the increase in plasma ANP levels did not correlate with the increase in heart rate during exercise. Furthermore, there was no relationship between plasma ANP and NA levels during exercise. Clearly further studies are needed to elucidate the significance of plasma ANP changes due to exercise in patients with CHF.

Earlier studies have demonstrated that both quantitative exercise tolerance test [2] and determination of plasma NA concentration [1] may be used as means of predicting prognosis in CHF. The data presented here show that both ANP and NA are elevated in CHF in close relation to the severity of heart failure. Therefore, plasma ANP determination may prove to be a useful adjunct in the evaluation of patients with CHF, and high ANP levels may predict poor prognosis in these patients.

Acknowledgements: This study was supported by grants from the Finska Läkaresällskapet, the Paavo Nurmi Foundation, the Sigrid Jusélius Foundation, Helsinki, and the Nordisk Insulinfond, Copenhagen.

References

1. Cohn JN, Levine TB, Olivari MT, Garberg V, Lura D, Francis GS, Simon AB, Rector T (1984) Plasma norepinephrine as a guide to prognosis in patients with chronic congestive heart failure. N Engl J Med 311:819–823
2. Cohn JN, Ziesche S, Archibald DG (1986) Quantitative exercise tolerance test as a predictor of mortality in congestive heart failure: the V-HeFT study (Anstract). Circulation 74 [Suppl II]:447
3. Franciosa JA (1984) Exercise testing in chronic congestive heart failure. Am J Cardiol 53:1447–1450
4. Fyhrquist F, Tikkanen I, Tötterman KJ, Hynynen M, Tikkanen T, Andersson S (1987) Plasma atrial natriuretic peptide in health and disease. Eur Heart J 8 [Suppl B]:117–122
5. Leinonen H, Näveri H, Tikkanen I, Sovijärvi A, Fyhrquist F (1988) Basal and exercise plasma levels of atrial natriuretic factor in congestive heart failure. Am Heart J 116:209–211
6. Nishikimi T, Kohno M, Itagane H, Hirota K, Akioka K, Teragaki M, Yasuda M, Oku H, Takeuchi K, Takeda T (1988) Influence of exercise on plasma atrial natriuretic factor levels in patients with myocardial infarction. Am Heart J 115:753–760
7. Petzl DH, Hartter E, Osterode W, Böhm H, Woloszczuk W (1987) Atrial natriuretic peptide release due to physical exercise in healthy persons and in cardiac patients. Klin Wochenschr 65: 194–196
8. Richards AM, Cleland JGF, Tonolo G, McIntyre GD, Leckie BJ, Dargie HJ, Ball SG, Robertson JIS (1986) Plasma α natriuretic peptide in cardiac impairment. Br Med J 293:409–412
9. Tikkanen I, Fyhrquist F, Metsärinne K, Leidenius R (1985) Plasma atrial natriuretic peptide in cardiac disease and during infusion in healthy volunteers. Lancet II:66–69

Plasma Norepinephrine and Atrial Natriuretic Peptide Levels During Exercise Stress Test of Patients with Ischemic Heart Disease

W. Osterode, D. H. Petzl, E. Hartter, and H. Böhm

I. Medizinische Universitätsklinik, Division of Clinical Endocrinology and Diabetes mellitus, Vienna, Austria and Clinic of Occupational Medicine, Vienna, Austria, and Rehabilitationszentrum für Herz- und Kreislauferkrankungen Bad Tatzmannsdorf, Austria

Key words: Plasma norepinephrine – ANP – Exercise – Dipyridamole – Cardiac patients

Introduction

In patients with coronary heart disease venous human atrial natriuretic polypeptide (hANP) and plasma norepinephrine (NE) are increased depending on the severity of the disease. It was postulated that the hANP and NE have a noninvasive diagnostic value since elevated NE levels are thought to be a sympathetic compensatory mechanism in impaired left ventricular function while increased hANP is thought to be caused by atrial stretch (Ledsome et al. 1985). The validity of the assumption of a noninvasive diagnostic value of these hormones was studied investigating hANP and NE levels in 95 patients who had either a reversible (REV) or an irreversible (IR) perfusion defect in the thallium-201 myocard stress (upright bicycle ergometry) scintigraphy. 46 of the patients were in addition to physical stress also subjected to a pharmacological stress with

Dipyridamole, a strong coronary vasodilatator Aldor et al. [1]. The results of these groups were compared with those NE and hANP levels of 16 healthy volunteers.

Patients and Methods

55 patients (38 male 58 ± 8a and 17 female 54 ± 10a) 10 ± 2 weeks after acute myocardial infarction and 40 patients (26 male 54 ± 11a and 14 female 53 ± 7) with exercise induced angina pectoris were tested by a symptom limited upright bicycle ergometry using a specially developed protocol which allows interindividual comparisons at the attained stress level (Osterode et al. 1987). About half of these patients were investigated with additional application of dipyridamole (DIP) 0.5 mg/kg body weight within the first 4 min of exercise. On the day of investigation no medication were taken. ECG and blood pressure were measured at the end of each stress level (2 min duration). Blood samples were collected from peripheral veins to determine hANP (Hartter et al. 1986) and NE (HPLC with electrochemical detector). Gamma camera pictures (three projections: AP, LAO, LAT) were taken immediately after the exercise test in a supine position and 3–4 h later after rest. Additionally, as a control group 8 males 34 ± 10a and 8 females 35 ± 9a healthy volunteers were exercised up to their expected maximal work load (eMWL) according to their age, sex and bodysurface (Böhm et al. 1978).

Results

a) Normals: The determined hANP and NE values rose exponentially with work load. While NE was elevated significantly already at the half of the eMWL the hANP was not significantly altered. No difference was seen between the males and females. This is due to the specially developed protocol (Osterode et al. 1987). In the postexercise period NE decreased immediately exponentially while hANP showed a s-shaped decay. For both hormones the base line was reached about 30 min after exercise.

b) Patients: The patients attained about 82% of the eMWL. The mean values of NE and hANP at rest and after work load were significantly higher in comparison to those of normals. The significance level between healthy persons and patients was better at maximal work load ($p < 0.01$) than at rest ($p < 0.05$).

DIP did not influence the NE levels. On average in all patient groups the same NE concentrations at symptom limited work load were reached. In patients after myocardial infarction no differences with and without DIP were seen. Patients with a reversible perfusion defect in the myocard scan showed significantly lower levels ($p < 0.01$) of hANP with DIP at MWL. No significant difference could be calculated between the other three groups.

Discussion

In the present study short physical exercise produced an exponential increase of NE and hANP in healthy as well as in cardiac patients depending on the work load level. That NE is increased with impaired left ventricular function is well known and is thought to be a sympathetic compensatory mechanism (Lehmann et al. 1984). The mechanism of hANP release seems to be

Table 1

	Rest		mWL/2		mWL	
	hANP	NE	hANP	NE	hANP	NE
G_0	16 ± 6	0.36 ± 0.09	19 ± 8	0.46 ± 0.09	33 ± 13	1.34 ± 0.38
G_1	31 ± 19	0.49 ± 0.12	33 ± 22	0.71 ± 0.20	73 ± 48	2.16 ± 0.82
G_2	37 ± 23	0.49 ± 0.21	44 ± 29	0.82 ± 0.29	71 ± 43	2.10 ± 0.91
G_3	36 ± 28	0.51 ± 0.24	47 ± 36	0.76 ± 0.27	109 ± 78	1.93 ± 0.92
G_4	30 ± 21	0.45 ± 0.15	30 ± 21	0.83 ± 0.25	56 ± 42	2.03 ± 0.76

G_0: n = 16 healthy voluntiers, G_1: n = 33 patients after myocardial infarction. G_2: n = 22 patients after myocardial infarction with Dipyridamol (DIP). G_3: n = 16 patients with reversible perfusion defects (REV). G_4: n = 24 patients with REV and DIP. hANP in ng/l, NE in ng/ml, mWL: maximal work load; values: mean ± SD caused mainly by atrial stretch (Ledsome et al. 1985) which occurs for example in the event of increased central blood volume at physical effort.

No significant difference was seen on average in patients after myocardial infarction and in patients with reversible perfusion defects at rest as regards NE and hANP assuming that during conditions with long-lasting increase of preload compensatory higher hANP and NE levels are reached for balance. In our investigated group (NYHA I–II) the hANP increase at maximal workload was about two-fold in comparison with the control group whereas Pettersson et al. 1986 found a three-fold increase in patients with more severe congestive heart failure (NYHA III–IV).

Remarkable was that in the patients who only had reversible perfusion defects in the myocard scan during physical stress the hANP was significantly elevated in comparison to the group after myocardial infarction. We may speculate that an acute reduction in left ventriculare function at maximal work load due to a dynamic stenosis results in a pronounced increase of hANP. Dipyridamole, a strong coronary vasodilatator, seems to counteract this mechanism.

In conclusion we may say that hANP an ne are additional valuable but not very strong parameters in the preliminary investigation of coronary heart disease especially if stress tests are used.

References

Aldor E, Blazek G, Gaul G, Heger H, Kahn P (1979) Die 201-Thalliumszintigraphy des Myokards unter Ruhe- und Belastungsbedingungen. Fortschr Röntgenstr 128:41–48

Böhm H, Bürklen R, Dienstl F, Ehrenböck G, Gaul W, Herbinger E, Kiss E, Kubicek F, Kühn P, Kummer F, Niederberger M, Schlick W (1978) Empfehlungen für eine standardisierte Ergometrie. Öst Ärztez 33:333–344

Hartter E, Woluszczuk W, Stummvoll HK (1986) Radioimmunoassay of atrial natriuretic peptides in human plasma. Clin Chem 32:441–445

Ledsome JR, Wilson N, Courneay CA, Rankin AJ (1985) Release of atrial natriuretic peptide by atrial distension. Can J Pharmacol 63: 739–742

Lehmann M, Schmid P, Keul J (1984) Sympathische Aktivität bei Patienten mit Koronarinsuffizienz. Z Kardiol 73:428–433

Osterode W, Böhm H, Schober H (1987) Plasmaadrenalin- und Noradrenalinkonzentrationen gesunder, untrainierter Personen bei fahrradergometrischen Bedingungen unter individueller Anpassung der Belastungsstufen an Körperoberfläche, Alter und Geschlecht. Herz/Kreislauf Austria 2:122–128

Pettersson A, Hedner J, Hedner T, Held P, Swedberg K, Towle AC (1986) Increased plasma levels of atrial natriuretic peptide in patients with congestive heart failure. Eur Heart J 7:693–696

Plasma Levels of Atrial Natriuretic Peptide (ANP) and Hemodynamics During Rest and Exercise*

H. M. Steffen, G. Wambach, H. J. Schäfer, R. Griebenow, V. Hossmann, and W. Kaufmann

Medizinische Klinik II der Universität Köln

Key words: Human atrial natriuretic peptide – Hemodynamics – Exercise – Chronic heart failure – Resetting phenomenon

Plasma levels of ANP correlate with central hemodynamics and the degree of cardiac dysfunction [1, 2, 4–7, 9]. There is some evidence, that in advanced cardiac failure ANP secretion may be reduced due to a depletion of atrial stores [3, 8]. To determine the diagnostic value of ANP measurements in a clinical routine setting we studied a

* Supported by a grant from Ministerium für Wissenschaft und Forschung, Düsseldorf

group of unselected patients referred for right heart catheterization during rest and standardized exercise conditions. In addition, we were interested whether stimulation of ANP secretion by exercise is reduced in patients with chronic heart failure.

Methods

In 49 patients (39 males, 10 females; age 30–75 years) plasma levels of ANP were measured in venous samplings from the pulmonary artery under resting conditions. Bicycle exercise testing in supine position at 50 W for 5 minutes was done in 32/49 patients, when plasma levels of ANP were measured again. PAMP was determined during quiet respiration, cardiac output by thermodilution technique. All patients were on a regular diet without sodium or water restriction. ANP was measured radioimmunologically after extraction of the plasma by SEP-PAK-C_{18} cartridges (for details see [10]). According to hemodynamic data patients were grouped as follows: group I = normal hemodynamics ($CI_{rest} > 2.8$ l/min/m^2 and $PAMP_{rest/exercise} \leq 18/28$ mmHg; n = 14), group II = heart failure with exercise ($CI_{rest} > 2.8$ l/min/m^2 and $PAMP_{rest/exercise} \leq 18/>28$ mmHg; n = 10), group III = heart failure ($CI_{rest} \leq 2.8$ l/min/m^2 or $PAMP_{rest} > 18$ mmHg; n = 20). In 5 patients with normal hemodynamics at rest exercise testing was not possible, they were excluded from the final evaluation. Statistical analysis was done using the Wilcoxon, Mann and Whitney test for unpaired data for between-group comparisons.

Results

Under resting conditions mean ANP plasma levels in patients with heart failure already at rest (245 ± 224 pg/ml) were significantly higher compared to those with normal hemodynamics (56 ± 29 pg/ml; $p < 0.01$) or heart failure with exercise (104 ± 103 pg/ml; $p < 0.05$). With exercise mean ANP plasma levels increased to 117 ± 119 pg/ml in group I, 226 ± 201 pg/ml in group

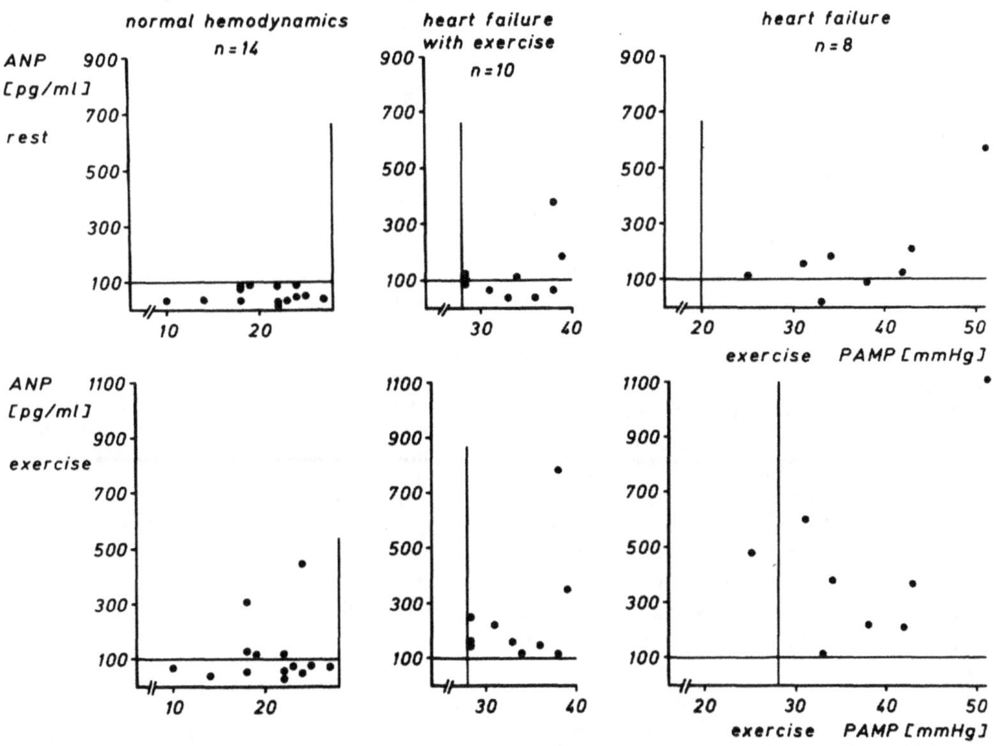

Fig 1. Plasma concentrations of atrial natriuretic peptide during rest and exercise in patients with normal hemodynamics, heart failure with exercise and heart failure already at rest

II, and 432 ± 316 pg/ml in group III. The mean absolute value of stimulated ANP plasma levels as well as the relative increase with exercise was significantly higher for patients with heart failure already at rest compared to those with normal hemodynamics ($p < 0.05$). Even with markedly increased basal ANP plasma levels there was a 2–4 fold increase during exercise. In patients with normal hemodynamics basal plasma levels of ANP were always below 100 pg/ml. During exercise the absolute value as well as the increase in ANP plasma concentrations showed a great variability. Though all patients with impaired cardiac function had ANP plasma levels increased above 100 pg/ml, this was also true for 5/14 patients with normal hemodynamics (see Fig. 1).

Discussion

In patients with chronic heart failure the hormone secretion of the atria can be stimulated by exercise. The highest mean plasma levels of basal and stimulated ANP as well as the highest mean relative increase during exercise were observed in this group. This is in agreement with findings observed by others [2] that there is no resetting of atrial ANP secretion in patients with chronic cardiac dysfunction. However, considering individual ANP plasma levels in patients with chronic heart failure reaching from 12 to 560 pg/ml under basal conditions and from 102 to 1106 pg/ml during exercise, a decreased hormone secretion in cases of chronic elevated atrial pressure may occur. Followup studies with repeated measurements of ANP plasma concentrations are necessary to answer the question definetely whether or not there is a resetting phenomenon. The diagnostic value of measurements of ANP plasma concentrations is limited as it is not possible to predict the degree of cardiac dysfunction for the individual patient due to the great variation in basal and stimulated ANP plasma levels as well as in the relative increase with exercise. This variability may be explained by differences in the underlying cardiac disease, relative contribution of both left and right atrial hormone secretion, damage of atrial myocardium due to fibrosis and differences in plasma volume. However, basal plasma levels of ANP above 100 pg/ml indicate impaired cardiac function. For patients with stimulated ANP plasma concentrations below 100 pg/ml cardiac dysfunction can be ruled out and right heart catheterization seems to be renouncable.

References

1. Dietz R, Lang RE, Purgaj J, Merkel A, Schömig A, Kübler W (1986) Relationship between hemodynamic parameters and concentrations of atrial natriuretic peptide (ANP) in human plasma. J Hypertens 4 [Suppl 6]:S512–S515
2. Dietz R, Purgaj J, Lang RE, Schömig A (1986) Pressure dependent release of atrial natriuretic peptide (ANP) in patients with chronic cardiac diseases: does it reset? Klin Wochenschr 64 [Suppl VI]:42–46
3. Drexler H, Finckh M, Lang RE, Just H (1987) Untersuchungen zum atrialen natriuretischen Peptid (ANP) bei experimenteller Herzinsuffizienz. In: Kreye VAW, Bussmann WD (Hrsg) ANP – Atriales natriuretisches Peptid und das kardiovaskuläre System. Steinkopff, Darmstadt, S 109
4. Hara H, Ogihara T, Shima J, Saito H, Rakugi H, Iinuma K, Kumahara Y, Minamino T (1987) Plasma atrial natriuretic peptide level as an index for the severity of congestive heart failure. Clin Cardiol 10:437–442
5. Nakaoka H, Imataka K, Amano M, Fujii J, Ishibashi M, Yamaji T (1985) Plasma levels of atrial natriuretic factor in patients with congestive heart failure. N Engl J Med 313:892–893
6. Raine AEG, Erne P, Bürgisser E, Müller FB, Bolli P, Burkart F, Bühler FR (1986) Atrial natriuretic peptide and atrial pressure in patients with congestive heart failure. N Engl J Med 315:533–537
7. Riegger AJG, Kromer EP, Kochsiek K (1985) Der natriuretische Vorhoffaktor bei schwerer kongestiver Herzinsuffizienz. Plasmaspiegel, hämodynamische, hormonale und renale Effekte. Dtsch Med Wochenschr 110:1607–1610
8. Rippegather G, Lang RE, Saggau W, Späth J, Forssmann WG (1986) Pathomorphologie des endokrinen Herzens. Z Kardiol 75 [Suppl 1]:27
9. Tikkanen I, Metsärinne K, Fyhrquist F, Leidenius R (1985) Plasma atrial natriuretic peptide in cardiac disease and during infusion in healthy volunteers. Lancet II:66–69
10. Wambach G, Kaufmann W (1988) Standardisierung der Plasmabestimmung des atrialen natriuretischen Peptids (ANP). Z Kardiol [Suppl 2]:31–35

Diagnostic Value of Plasma Levels of Atrial Natriuretic Peptide (ANP) in Different Cardiac Diseases

H. M. Steffen, G. Wambach, R. Griebenow, G. Bönner, L. Krämer, and W. Kaufmann

Medizinische Klinik II der Universität Köln

Key words: Human atrial natriuretic peptide – Cardiac dysfunction – Coronary heart disease – Congestive cardiomyopathy

Several authors found a correlation of plasma levels of ANP with the impairment of cardiac function [1–3, 5–8]. In order to assess its diagnostic value in a clinical routine setting we measured plasma levels of ANP in a group of unselected patients referred for cardiac workup.

Methods

In 100 consecutive patients (75 males, 25 females; mean age 55 ± 9.4 years) plasma levels of ANP were measured in peripheral venous samplings at 8.00 the day of a diagnostic left heart catheterization. 8 patients had to be excluded from evaluation because of unsatisfying LV-pressure tracings or severe renal insufficiency. The ventricle was divided into 3 anterior and inferior segments in RAO-projection, and 1 septal and posterolateral segment in LAO-projection. In patients with regional wall motion abnormalities the number of akinetic segments was derived from the ventriculogram. LVEDP, systolic, and diastolic pressures were taken from the left ventricle and aortic pressure tracings. All patients were on a regular diet without sodium or water restriction. ANP was measured radioimmunologically after extraction of the plasma by SEP-PAK-C_{18} cartridges (for details see [9]). The following diagnoses were angiographically confirmed: normal (n = 12), coronary heart disease (CHD) without wall motion abnormalities (n = 23), CHD with 2 or less akinetic segments (n = 20), CHD with 3 or more akinetic segments (n = 17), CHD and aneurysm (n = 6), congestive cardiomyopathy (n = 4), aortic valve disease (n = 2), mitral valve disease (n = 2), aortic and mitral valva disease (n = 3), carditis (n = 2). Due to the small size of the latter groups we finally evaluated only patients with CHD or congestive cardiomyopathy. Statistical analysis was done using linear regression analysis and the Wilcoxon, Mann and Whitney test for unpaired data for between-group comparisons.

* Supported by a grant from Ministerium für Wissenschaft und Forschung Düsseldorf

Results

Mean LVEDP and mean plasma levels of ANP were similiar in patients with normal angiographic findings, CHD without wall motion abnormalities and CHD with 2 or less akinetic segments. However, mean LVEDP and mean plasma levels of ANP were elevated in patients with CHD and 3 or more akinetic segments, aneurysm, and congestive cardiomyopathy (see Fig. 1). Plasma levels of ANP were always below 100 pg/ml in patients without cardiac disease, while they were increased above this value in all patients with aneurysm or congestive cardiomyopathy. In patients with CHD with or without wall motion abnormalities a great variability in ANP plasma levels was found. 20/23 patients with CHD, 17/20 patients with CHD and 2 or less akinetic segments and 5/17 patients with CHD and 3 or more akinetic segments showed ANP plasma levels within the normal range. There was a correlation between plasma levels of ANP and LVEDP for the whole study population ($r = 0.54$; $p < 0.001$), whereas no correlations were found for plasma levels of ANP and age, systolic or diastolic pressure.

Discussion

Even so we found a positive correlation between plasma levels of ANP and LVEDP

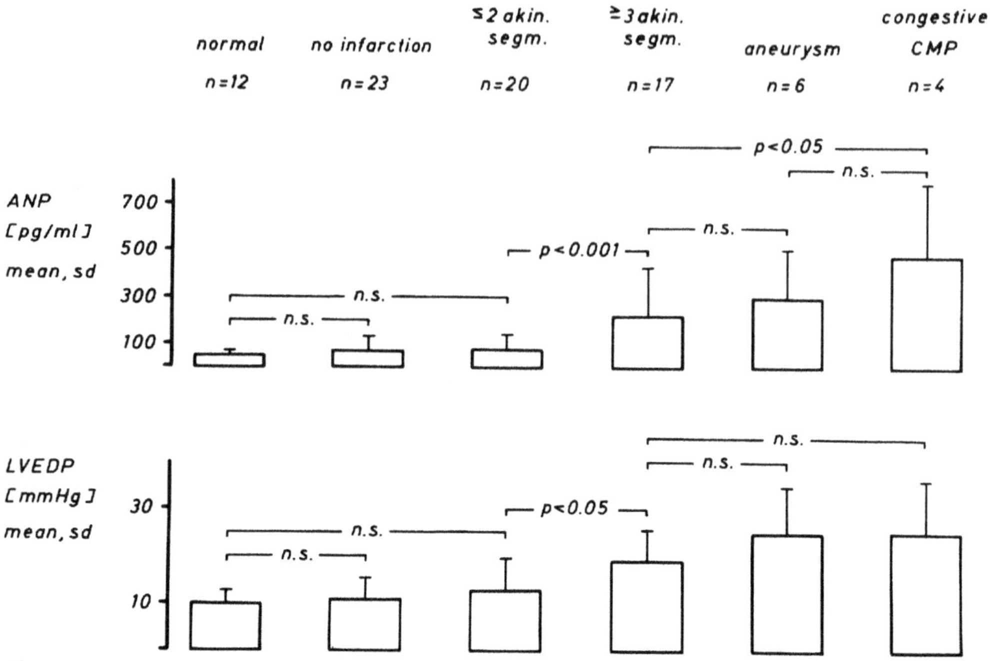

Fig 1. Plasma concentrations of atrial natriuretic peptide and LVEDP in patients with different cardiac diseases

for the whole study population there was a great variation in plasma concentrations of ANP for a given filling pressure. This may be explained by differences in both right and left atrial pressures as LVEDP is only a rough estimate of left atrial stretch during enddiastole. Because we wanted to assess the diagnostic value of measurements of ANP plasma levels in a clinical routine setting, patients were on an unrestricted diet. By that, differences in ANP plasma levels for a given LVEDP may be due to differences in plasma volume at the time of blood sampling which in addition took place some time before the left heart catheterization. The duration of the underlying cardiac disease might also be of importance in this regard. In patients with CHD the degree of cardiac dysfunction is related to the myocardial damage due to infarction. Accordingly, we found elevated mean ANP plasma levels only for patients with aneurysm or extended infarctions. Nevertheless, nearly one third of the patients with 3 or more akinetic segments showed values of the ANP plasma level within the normal range. In accordance with others we found the highest mean plasma concentrations of ANP in patients with congestive cardiomyopathy [2]. The great variability in plasma levels of ANP with normal values even for patients with marked myocardial damage and cardiac dysfunction limits the diagnostic value of a single measurement of the plasma concentration of ANP under resting conditions. For the individual patient it is impossible to predict the degree of cardiac dysfunction from the height of the basal plasma level of ANP. Plasma concentrations of ANP above 100 pg/ml in patients, where other reasons for a plasma volume overload can be excluded, can serve as a marker for cardiovascular diseases with poor sensitivity but good specifity. There are some reports showing a decrease in ANP plasma levels with improved central hemodynamics during treatment of congestive heart failure [2, 4]. However, it remains to be clarified whether measurements of ANP plasma levels may be of value in the followup of patients with cardiovascular diseases.

References

1. Dietz R, Lang RE, Purgaj J, Merkel A, Schömig A, Kübler W (1986) Relationship between hemodynamic parameters and concentrations of atrial natriuretic peptide (ANP) in human plasma. J Hypertens 4 [Suppl 6]: S512–S515
2. Haas M, Dietz R, Kübler W (1988) Hat die Plasma-ANP-Bestimmung eine diagnostische oder prognostische Bedeutung bei Patienten mit Herzvitien? Z Kardiol 77 [Suppl 2]:55–60
3. Hara H, Ogihara T, Shima J, Saito H, Rakugi H, Iinuma K, Kumahara Y, Minamino T (1987) Plasma atrial natriuretic peptide level as an index for the severity of congestive heart failure. Clin Cardiol 10:437–442
4. Katoh Y, Kurosawa T, Takeda S, Kurokawa S, Sakamoto H, Marumo F, Kikawada R (1986) Atrial natriuretic peptide in treated congestive heart failure (Letter). Lancet I:851
5. Nakaoka H, Imataka K, Amano M, Fujii J, Ishibashi M, Yamaji T (1985) Plasma levels of atrial natriuretic factor in patients with congestive heart failure. N Engl J Med 313: 892–893
6. Riegger AJG, Kromer EP, Kochsiek K (1985) Der natriuretische Vorhoffaktor bei schwerer kongestiver Herzinsuffizienz. Plasmaspiegel, hämodynamische, hormonale und renale Effekte. Dtsch Med Wochenschr 110: 1607–1610
7. Raine AEG, Erne P, Bürgisser E, Müller FB, Bolli P, Burkart F, Bühler FR (1986) Atrial natriuretic peptide and atrial pressure in patients with congestive heart failure. N Engl J Med 315:533–537
8. Tikkanen I, Metsärinne K, Fyhrquist F, Leidenius R (1985) Plasma atrial natriuretic peptide in cardiac disease and during infusion in healthy volunteers. Lancet II:66–69
9. Wambach G, Kaufmann W (1988) Standardisierung der Plasmabestimmung des atrialen natriuretischen Peptids (ANP). Z Kardiol 77 [Suppl 2]:31–35

Cyclic Guanosine Monophosphate Concentrations in Type 1 Diabetic Patients in Different Stages of Diabetic Nephropathy

L. Heinemann, P. T. Sawicki, G. Stroka, C. Angenvoort, A. Hohmann, and M. Berger

Department of Nutrition and Metabolic Diseases, University of Düsseldorf, FRG

Key words: Cyclic Guanosine Monophosphate – Atrial natriuretic factor – Diabetic nephropathy – Insulin-dependent diabetes mellitus

Introduction

Type 1 (insulin-dependent) diabetic patients exhibit elevated plasma ANF concentrations in the stage of incipient or overt diabetic nephropathy, or even when they show glomerular hyperfiltration only (Sawicki et al. 1988).

Cyclic guanosine monophosphate (cGMP) is proposed to mediate the cellular actions of atrial natriuretic factor (ANF) as its second messenger (Gerzer et al. 1987). Shortly after the discovery of ANF, it was demonstrated that increases in ANF concentrations resulted in similar increases of cGMP in plasma and urine (Gerzer et al. 1985; Heim et al. 1988). In fact, plasma cGMP concentrations correlate with plasma concentrations of ANF (Fujio et al. 1987; Gerbes et al. 1988) and ANF was shown to selectively activate guanylate cyclase in a concentration- and time-dependent fashion and hence to increase the concentration of intracellular cGMP (Waldman et al. 1984). cGMP exhibits a remarkable stability in plasma and urine samples and is therefore probably useful as a marker of ANF action in clinical routine (Heim et al. 1988).

The aim of this study was to determine plasma cGMP concentrations in Type 1 diabetic patients with glomerular hyperfiltration and in different stages of diabetic nephropathy.

Patients and Methods

Venous fasting blood samples were drawn from 71 Type 1 diabetic patients who par-

Table 1. Parameter and results of diabetic patients in different stages of diabetic nephropathy; mean (SD)

Parameter	Unit	No nephropathy	Hyperfiltration	Incipient nephropathy	Overt nephropathy
n (female/male)		33 (13/20)	15 (6/9)	14 (6/8)	9 (3/6)
Age	years	30 (10)	27 (9)	32 (8)	31 (11)
Body mass index	kg/m^2	22.5 (2.5)	22.7 (3.0)	22.6 (2.9)	24.2 (3.2)
Duration of diab.	years	8 (6)	10 (8)	9 (6)	16 (8)
Systolic RR	mmHg	110 (11)	110 (10)	121 (10)	133 (17)
Diastolic RR	mmHg	70 (9)	73 (9)	73 (11)	83 (15)
Serum-creat.	µmol/ml	82.2 (11.6)	83.6 (11.0)	82.7 (13.2)	104.0 (30.0)
Creat.-clear.	ml/min	104 (20)	158 (12)	142 (33)	87 (32)
Proteinuria	mg/24 h	38 (14)	42 (14)	133 (82)	1890 (2460)
HbA1C	%Hb	7.5 (1.6)	6.8 (1.0)	7.8 (1.9)	8.9 (0.7)
Blood glucose	mmol/l	9.9 (4.2)	10.0 (4.5)	8.6 (3.4)	9.9 (4.4)
cGMP	pmol/l	2.9 (0.9)	3.8 (1.4)	3.6 (1.9)	3.9 (1.1)

ticipated in our diabetes treatment and teaching program (Mühlhauser et al. 1983). These patients were allocated to four groups according to their renal parameters: 33 patients showed no sign of diabetic nephropathy. Glomerular hyperfiltration (creatinine clearence >140 ml/min/1.73 m^2) as the only sign of diabetic nephropathy was found in 15 patients. 14 patients with a proteinuria >60 and <500 mg/24h were classified as having incipient diabetic nephropathy, 9 patients with proteinuria >500 mg/24h as having an overt diabetic nephropathy (Table 1). The four groups were comparable with respect to age and body mass index. Patients with overt nephropathy had longer duration of diabetes, higher pressure readings, serum creatinine and HbA1c values than the other three groups of diabetic patients.

Blood for determination of plasma cGMP concentrations was collected in chilled tubes with 0.3 ml Aprotinin (= 6,000 KIE) and 0.3 ml 2.4% Na-EDTA. Samples were stored in ice-cold water and were separated by centrifugation at 4°C within one hour and plasma was stored at − 20°C until assayed.

For cGMP estimations plasma was extracted with ethanol before being measured by radio-immunoassay (IBL, Hamburg, West Germany).

HbA1c levels were determined by HPLC chromatography with a normal range of 4.2 to 5.6% Hb. All other measurements were performed with routine clinical chemistry methods. Blood pressure values are means of three to six measurements.

Because of the skewed distribution of cGMP values we used non-parametric tests (Kruskal-Wallis test and Spearman's rank correlation test) for statistical analysis. A P-Value <0.05 was deemed as significantly different.

Results

cGMP concentrations of the patients in the four groups were significantly different ($P < 0.05$). The patients in the groups without diabetic nephropathy had lower cGMP concentrations then those with hyperfiltration ($P < 0.05$) and overt diabetic nephropathy ($P < 0.01$, Table 1).

In patients with incipient, or overt diabetic nephropathy cGMP concentrations were significantly correlated with systolic blood pressure readings ($n = 23$, $r = 0.63$, $p < 0.002$).

Discussion

cGMP plasma concentrations were decreased in diabetic patients without nephropathy, a finding which is in accordance with recent results from this department indicating elevated ANF plasma concentrations in patients with hyperfiltration, incipient and overt diabetic nephropathy (Sawicki et al. 1988).

In conclusion, cGMP could be a useful alternative for assessment of ANF action in diabetic patients.

References

Fujio N, Ohashi M, Nawata H, Kato KI, Ibayashi H, Matsuo H (1987) Relationship between atrial natriuretic polypeptide and cycliy 3'5'-guanosine monophosphate in human plasma. J Lab Clin Med 109:706–710

Gerbes AL, Arendt RM, Gerzer R, Schnizer W, Jüngst D, Paumgartner G, Wernze H (1988) Role of atrial natriuretic factor, cyclic GMP and the renin-aldosterone system in acute volume regulation of healthy subjects. Eur J Clin Invest 18:425–429

Gerzer R, Witzgall H, Tremblay J, Gutkowska J, Hamet P (1985) Rapid increase in plasma and urinary cyclic GMP after bolus injection of atrial natriuretic factor in man. J Clin Endocrinol Metab 61:1217–1219

Heim JM, Gottmann K, Weil J, Haufe MC, Gerzer R (1988) Is cyclic GMP a clinically useful marker for ANF action? Z Kardiol 77 [Suppl 2]:41–46

Mühlhauser I, Jörgens V, Berger M, Graninger W, Gürtler W, Hornke L, Kunz A, Schernthaner G, Scholz V, Voss HE (1983) Bicentric evaluation of a teaching and treatment programme for type 1 (insulin dependent) diabetic patients: Improvement of metabolic control and other measures of diabetic care for up to 22 month. Diabetologia 25:470–476

Sawicki P, Heinemann L, Rave K, Berger M (1988) Atrialer natriuretischer Faktor bei Patienten mit Typ-1-Diabetes mellitus in verschiedenen Stadien der diabetischen Nephropathie. Z Kardiol 77 [Suppl 2]:111–113

Waldman SA, Rapoport RM, Murad F (1984) Atrial natriuretic factor selectively activates particulate guanylate cyclase and elevates cyclic GMP in rat tissues. J Biol Chem 259:14 332–14 334

Atrial Natriuretic Peptide as a Humoral Marker in 157 Children with Congenital Heart Diseases

J. Talartschik[1], G. Eigster[2], and T. Eisenhauer[1]

[1] Departments of Nephrology and [2] Pediatric Cardiology, University Clinic, Göttingen, FRG

Key words: Congenital heart disease – Congestive heart failure – Atrial natriuretic peptide – Children

Distension of the atria seems to be the principal stimulus for ANP secretion from myoendocrine cells [1, 7, 9, 10]. In congestive heart failure (CHF) and volume overload atrial distension is caused by an increased preload [4–6, 11, 12, 14]. Elevated ANP plasma concentration have also been reported in children with congenital heart disease (CHD) and broncho-pulmonary dysplasia [7, 9, 17, 18, 19].

Abbreviations: VSD = ventricular septal defect; PDA = patent ductus arteriosus; ASD = atrial septal defect; TA = tricuspid atresia; TAPVR = total anomalous pulmonary venous return; EFE = endocardfibroelastosis; DCM = dilatative cardiomyopathy; BWG = Bland-White-Garland syndrome; Pst = pulmonary stenosis; LV = left ventricle; TGA = transposition of the great arteries

To elucidate the diagnostic value of ANP in children with CHD ANP plasma concentrations were correlated with the type of cardiac disease and the degree of cardiac decompensation.

Patients and Methods

Diagnostic cardiac catheterization according to standard techniques was performed in 157 pediatric patients (95 boys, 62 girls) with CHD, aged 1 day to 25 years. Depending on the age and disease of the patient up to 9 samples for the determination of ANP were drawn from the peripheral vein, superior or inferior caval veins, right atrium, pulmonary artery, left atrium, right or left ventricles and aorta (n = 499).

ANP was analysed by radioimmuno-assay after extraction on a reversed-phase octadecylsilan column (Sep-Pak C 18, Waters, Mass.) and lyophilisation as described [5]. According to our normal range of healthy controls (n = 50) and to data in children

Table 1. Heart diseases with hemodynamically significant left to right shunt volume ($Q_P : Q_S >$ 1,5) and ANP plasma concentrations; VSD n = 23, PDA n = 4, AV-Canal n = 4, ASD n = 6

total	$Q_P : Q_S < 1{,}5$		$Q_P : Q_S > 1{,}5$	
n = 47	n = 15	100%	n = 32	100%
ANP < 30 f mol/min	n = 11 73,3%		n = 4 12,5%	
ANP > 30 fmol/ml	n = 4 26,7%		n = 28 87,5%	

Q_P: flow rate pulmonic circulation (l/min)
Q_S: flow rate systemic circulation (l/min)

[7–9, 13, 16, 18, 19] ANP values below 30 fmol/ml were considered normal.

Results

As depicted in Table 1 heart diseases with hemodynamically significant left to right shunt volume (Q Pulmonary: Q Systemic >1.5; n = 32) such as ASD, VSD, AV-Canal and patent ductus arteriosus (PDA) were associated with elevated ANP levels in 87.5%, whereas 73.3% of these patients with an insignificant shunt volume ($Q_P : Q_S < 1.5$; n = 15) had normal ANP plasma concentrations. There was no correlation between plasma ANP and the pressure gradient across the valve in aortic or pulmonary stenoses. 91% of the children with clinical signs and symptoms of CHF showed elevated ANP plasma levels, as did 81% who proved to be candidates for cardiac surgery. All patients with extremely elevated ANP concentrations (>300 fmol/ml) had CHF and a high mortality rate, since 5 out of this group (n = 11) died post OP (Table 2).

During catheterization lowest ANP levels were detected in the superior or inferior caval veins, whereas highest ANP concentrations could be found in the right/left atria and ventricles. All 8 patients with tricuspid atresia (TA) showed increased ANP levels, but apart from TA there were no *specific* cardiac lesions with elevated ANP plasma concentrations.

Discussion

Two mechanisms for an increased secretion of ANP from the atria in children with CHD [7, 13, 15, 17–19] have to be discussed: a, The development of CHF leads to an increased preload and filling pressure [1, 6, 9, 11, 14]. In this study patients with aortic or pulmonary stenoses did not correlate with the degree of stenosis but with the severity of CHF in view of their ANP levels. b, The specific hemodynamic situation in TA, transposition of the great arteries (TGA) [3] or a cardiac disease with a significant shunt volume (PDA, VSD, ASD, AV-Canal) [7, 13] may be the cause for left and/or right atrial distension.

Table 2. Outcome of patients (n = 11) with congenital heart diseases and high ANP plasma concentrations (>300 fmol/ml). All patients had evidence for CHF (+)

Age	Diagnosis	ANP (fmol/ml)	CHF	Outcome
3 days	Cor triatriatum TAPVR	413	+	† post OP
1 week	EFE LV, PDA	>666	+	† post OP
2 weeks	Shone Compl. + coarctatio + PDA	>666	+	OP, good result
3 weeks	AV-Canal + Pst	>666	+	OP planned
4 weeks	AV-Canal + Pst	>666	+	OP, good result
4 weeks	AVD + Pst	430	+	OP, good result
4 weeks	EFDE + DCM + PDA	>666	+	† post OP
6 weeks	BWG + DCM	>666	+	† post OP
4 months	AV-Canal + Pst	521	+	OP, good result
20 years	corr. TGA + VSD + Pst	317	+	† post OP
25 years	TGA + VSD + Pst (Rastelli)	423	+	OP planned

Both mechanisms induce atrial distension stimulating the release of ANP into the circulation [3, 15]. It has already been demonstrated that the atrioseptostomy in TGA patients is followed by a fall in ANP levels [3], as well as the ligation of a PDA leads to a decrease in ANP plasma concentrations [2, 13], whereas the Fontan procedure induces an increase in right atrial pressure and a rise in ANP [15].

Despite of this inhomogeneous group of CHD patients the intracardial distribution pattern of ANP with low concentrations in the caval veins and elevated ANP levels in the atria and ventricles is similar to that seen in adult patients [12, 17, 19]. Cardiac catheterization remains necessary for the precise hemodynamic evaluation in children with CHD. Since 91% of the patients with CHF showed increased ANP plasma concentrations periodic controls of ANP may be an additional non-invasive diagnostic tool in monitoring cardiac decompensation [1, 7, 17, 18]. The findings that elevated ANP plasma levels correlate with the indication for cardiac surgery and that extremely high ANP concentrations indicate a severe outcome of the patients underline the prognostic value of this new hormone to evaluate hemodynamic disturbances in children with CHD.

References

1. Anderson JV, Woodruff PW, Bloom SR (1988) The effect of treatment of congestive heart failure on plasma atrial natriuretic peptide concentration: A longitudinal study. Br Heart J 59(2):207–211
2. Andersson S, Tikkanen I, Pesonen E, Meretoja O, Hynynen M, Fyhrquist F (1987) Atrial natriuretic peptide in patent ductus arteriosus. Pediatr Res 21(4):396–398
3. Andersson S, Tikkanen I, Pesonen E, Wallgren EJ, Fyhrquist F (1988) Atrial natriuretic peptide and atrial pressures in newborns with transposition of the great arteries. Acta Paediatr Scand 77(1):72–75
4. Bates ER, Shenker Y, Grekin RJ (1986) The relationship between plasma levels of immunoreactive atrial natriuretic hormone and hemodynamic function in man. Circulation 73:1155–1160
5. Eisenhauer T, Talartschik J, Scheler F (1986) Detection of fluid overload by plasma concentration of human atrial natriuretic peptide (h-ANP) in patients with renal failure. Klin Wochenschr 64 [Suppl VI]:68–72
6. Fyhrquist F, Tikkanen I (1988) Atrial natriuretic peptide in congestive heart failure. Am J Cardiol 62(2):20A–24A
7. Kikuchi K, Nishioka K, Ueda T, Shiomi M, Takahashi Y, Sugawara A, Nakao K, Imura H, Hori C, Mikawa H (1987) Relationship between plasma atrial natriuretic polypeptide concentration and hemodynamic measurements in children with congenital heart diseases. J Pediatr 111(3):335–342
8. Kikuchi K, Shiomi M, Morie K, Ohie T, Nakao K, Imura H, Mikawa H (1988) Plasma atrial natriuretic polypeptide concentration in healthy children from birth to adolescence. Acta Paediatr Scand 77(3):380–384
9. Lang RE, Unger T, Ganten D, Weil J, Bidlingmaier F, Dohlemann D (1985) Alpha atrial natriuretic peptide concentrations in plasma of children with congenital heart and pulmonary disease. Br Med J 291:1241
10. Matsubara H, Nishikawa M, Umeda Y, Taniguchi T, Iwasaka T, Kurimoto T, Yamane Y, Inada M (1987) The role of atrial pressure in secreting atrial natriuretic polypeptides. Am Heart J 113:1457–1462
11. Nakaoka H, Imataka K, Amano M, Fujii J, Ishibashi M, Yamaji T (1985) Plasma levels of atrial natriuretic factor in patients with congestive heart failure. N Engl J Med 313:892–893
12. Raine AEG, Erne P, Bürgisser E, Müller FB, Bolli P, Burkart F, Bühler FR (1986) Atrial natriuretic peptide and atrial pressure in patients with congestive heart failure. N Engl J Med 315:533–537
13. Rascher W, Seyberth HW (1987) Atrial natriuretic peptide and patent ductus arteriosus in preterm infants. Arch Dis Child 62(11): 1165–1167
14. Riegger AJG, Kromer EP, Kochsiek K (1985) Atrial natriuretic factor in severe congestive heart failure. Dtsch Med Wochenschr 110:1607–1610
15. Stewart JM, Seligman KP, Zeballos G, Romano A, Clarke BJ, Woolf PK, Norwood WJ, Gewitz MH (1987) Elevated atrial natriuretic peptide after the Fontan procedure. Circulation 76(3Pt2):77–82
16. Tulassay T, Seri I, Rascher W (1987) Atrial natriuretic peptide and extracellular volume contraction after birth. Acta Paediatr Scand 76:444–446
17. Uchiyama M, Satokata I, Aikawa T, Sakai K (1987) Plasma atrial natriuretic peptide in congenital heart disease. Acta Paediatr Scand 76(4):669–670
18. Weil J, Gerzer R, Strom T, Lang RE, Dohlemann C, Knorr D, Bidlingmaier F

(1987a) Increased plasma cyclic guanosine monophosphate concentrations in children with high levels of circulating atrial natriuretic peptide. Pediatrics 80(4):545–548
19. Weil J, Strom TM, Brangenberg R, Sebening W, Haufe M, Lang RE, Bidlingmaier F, Gerzer R (1987b) Plasma atrial natriuretic peptide levels in children with cardiac diseases: Correlation with c-GMP levels and haemodynamic parameters. Horm Res 28(1):64–70

Atrial Natriuretic Peptide and Atrial Size

A. Machraoui[1], J. Gude[1], B.-E. Braun[2], D. Jäger[1], B. Lemke[1], M. Krieg[2], and J. Barmeyer[1]

[1] Department of Cardiology and Angiology and [2] Institute of Clinical Chemistry and Laboratory Medicine, University Clinic Bergmannsheil Bochum, FRG

Key words: Atrial natriuretic peptide – Atrial size – Planimetrics – Echocardiography

Introduction

Enlarged plasma volume causes an increase of atrial size, and leads to a higher wall tension playing an important role in the secretion of ANP. Dependent on the compliance of the atrial myocardium different pressures may occur. Therefore it is likely that an atrial dilation – but not necessarily the increase of the atrial pressure – resulted in an increased ANP secretion.

The aim of this study was to examine the dependence between the atrial size and the ANP level in patients with chronic heart diseases.

Methods

The right atrial pressure (RAMP) and the pulmonary capillary wedged pressure (PCWP) were evaluated in 32 patients (age range from 44 to 85 years, mean age 58.2 years) with chronic heart diseases (Table 1). Blood samples were drawn from a peripheral vein and the pulmonary artery, plasma ANP was measured by radioimmunoassay without previous extraction. Immediately after the Swan-Ganz-catheterization the computed planimetric measurements of endsystolic areas of the right (RAA) and left atrium (LAA) were performed by 2D-echocardiography from the apical four chamber view. This was done by different examiners who did not know the evaluated pressures.

Results

The ANP level taken from the peripheral vein as well as the ANP level taken from the pulmonary artery correlated well with the RAA (Fig. 1). Higher ANP levels were found more frequently with low atrial pressures than with normal atrial sizes. There was no significant correlation between the atrial pressures and the atrial areas.

Discussion

The present results confirm the expected relation between the atrial size and the ANP secretion. Indeed not the atrial volume, but the atrial area was used to evaluate the atrial size. Nevertheless we were able to demonstrate that measurement of the atrial area is sufficient to estimate the atrial size. Correlation between ANP and right atrial area was better than between ANP and right atrial pressure. There was no correlation

Table 1. Heart diseases in the examined patients. n = number of patients

Heart diseases	n
coronary heart disease	20
dilated cardiomyopathy	5
acquired valvulopathy	4
hypertensive heart disease	1
pulmonary heart disease	2
total	32

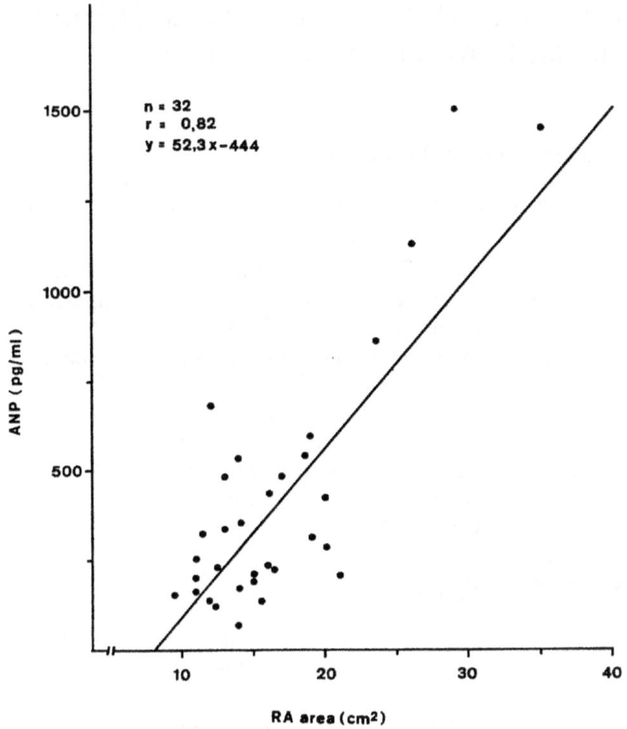

Fig. 1. Correlation between right atrial area (RA area) and ANP level

between the atrial area and the atrial pressure. In singular cases atrial pressure was low in spite of an increased ANP and an increased atrial area.

In animal experiments a good correlation was found between the ANP level and the left atrial area measured by echocardiography [4]. It was also reported about a good correlation between the atrial pressure and the ANP [1, 5].

Haass et al. [3] found a better correlation between the diameters of the right and left atrium and ANP than with atrial pressure (r = 0.60−0.71). But correlation coefficients were lower than those of this present study having used atrial areas.

In heart transplant recipients higher ANP levels than in volunteers were found in spite of normal atrial pressures [2]. We observed a similar phenomenon in a 50 year old patient who underwent a heart transplantation. This patient had enlarged right and left atrial areas (23.2 cm and 23.1 cm, respectively) with low right atrial and pulmonary capillary wedged pressure (1 mmHg and 10 mmHg, respectively) but with a very high ANP level (860 pg/ml). This fact confirms the assumption that atrial size is a more important factor for ANP secretion than the pressure.

References

1. Arendt RM, Ritter D, Gerbes AL, Stangl F, Bach P, Zachringer J (1985) Elevated plasma levels of atrial natriuretic factor (ANP) in hypertensive patients (abstract). Clin Exp Hypertension A8 (1):132
2. Chapman M, Lister P (1987) Raised concentrations of plasma atrial natriuretic peptides in cardiac transplant recipients. Br Med J 294:122
3. Haass M, Fischer TA, Lang RE, Schöring A, Dietz R (1987) Vorhofgröße und atriales natriuretisches Peptid. Z Kardiol 76:44
4. Moe GW, Howard RJ, Angus C, de Bold AJ, Armsbroug PW (1987) Pathophysiologic role of atrial size and pressure in the modulation of plasma natriuretic factor during evolving experimental heart failure. Circulation 76:IV−135
5. Punzengruber Ch, Hartter E, Weissel M, Burghuber OC, Ludvik B, Woloszczuk W (1987) Peripheral an right atrial plasma levels of atrial natriuretic peptids and their relation to atrial pressure. Z Kardiol 76:72−75

Neurohormonal and Hemodynamic Data in Patients with Dilated Cardiomyopathy Depending on Inotropic and Lusitropic Abnormalities

J. Dusleag, W. Klein, B. Eber, B. Rotman, and V. Weinrauch

Division of Cardiology, Department of Internal Medicine, University Hospital Graz, Graz, Austria

Key words: Dilated cardiomyopathy – Systolic and diastolic dysfunction – Neurohormonal abnormalities

Introduction

The term "congestive heart failure" which has been applied to a wide variety of diseases states, was once viewed as a single entity [1]. With the advances in our understanding of the coupling between the heart and circulation the distinction between inotropic respectively systolic and lusitropic respectively diastolic abnormalities has come to be of considerable clinical importance. Both the systolic and diastolic dysfunction can produce the hemodynamic abnormalities characteristic of congestive heart failure [2, 3].

In our current study we correlated neurohormonal and hemodynamic data in patients with dilated cardiomyopathy, depending on systolic and diastolic dysfunction.

Patients

Participants in this study were 19 patients with DCMP. Their mean age was 53 ± 2 years (range from 18 to 76). There were 18 men and 1 woman. Mean ejection fraction was 29% (range from 15–46%). All patients had some limitation in functional capacity class II to IV assessed by New York Heart Association classification. 3 patients were considered class II, 13 class III and 3 were class IV. The control group comprised 10 patients with comparable distribution of age and sex catheterised for a variety of clinical indications but in whom no evidence of cardiovascular disease was found.

Methods

After all medication was discontinued for at least 3 days, excluding digitalis, left and right heart catheterisation, left ventricular angiogram, coronary angiography and echocardiography were performed. Before administration of contrast medium and after each patient had been supine for at least 30 minutes, blood samples were withdrawn from the femoral vein for determination of plasma-ANP, plasma renin activity (PRA), angiotensin II (AT II), aldosterone (A), noradrenaline (NA) and vasopressin (V).

In distinguishing between systolic and diastolic dysfunction the patients were divided into 3 different groups depending on hemodynamic criteria (Table 1).

Table 1. Pathophysiological differentiation depending on hemodynamic criteria

	systolic dysfunction	diastolic dysfunction	combined systolic-diastolic dysfunction
CI	↓↓	normal / (↓)	↓↓
SVR	↑↑	normal / (↑)	↑↑
LVEDP	normal / (↑)	↑↑	↑↑
vasoconstrictor systems[a]	↑↑?	normal?	↑↑?
α-hANP[a]	normal?	↑↑?	↑↑?

[a] hypothesis

Abbreviations: CI = cardiac index; SVR = systemic vascular resistance; LVEDP = left ventricular end-diastolic pressure

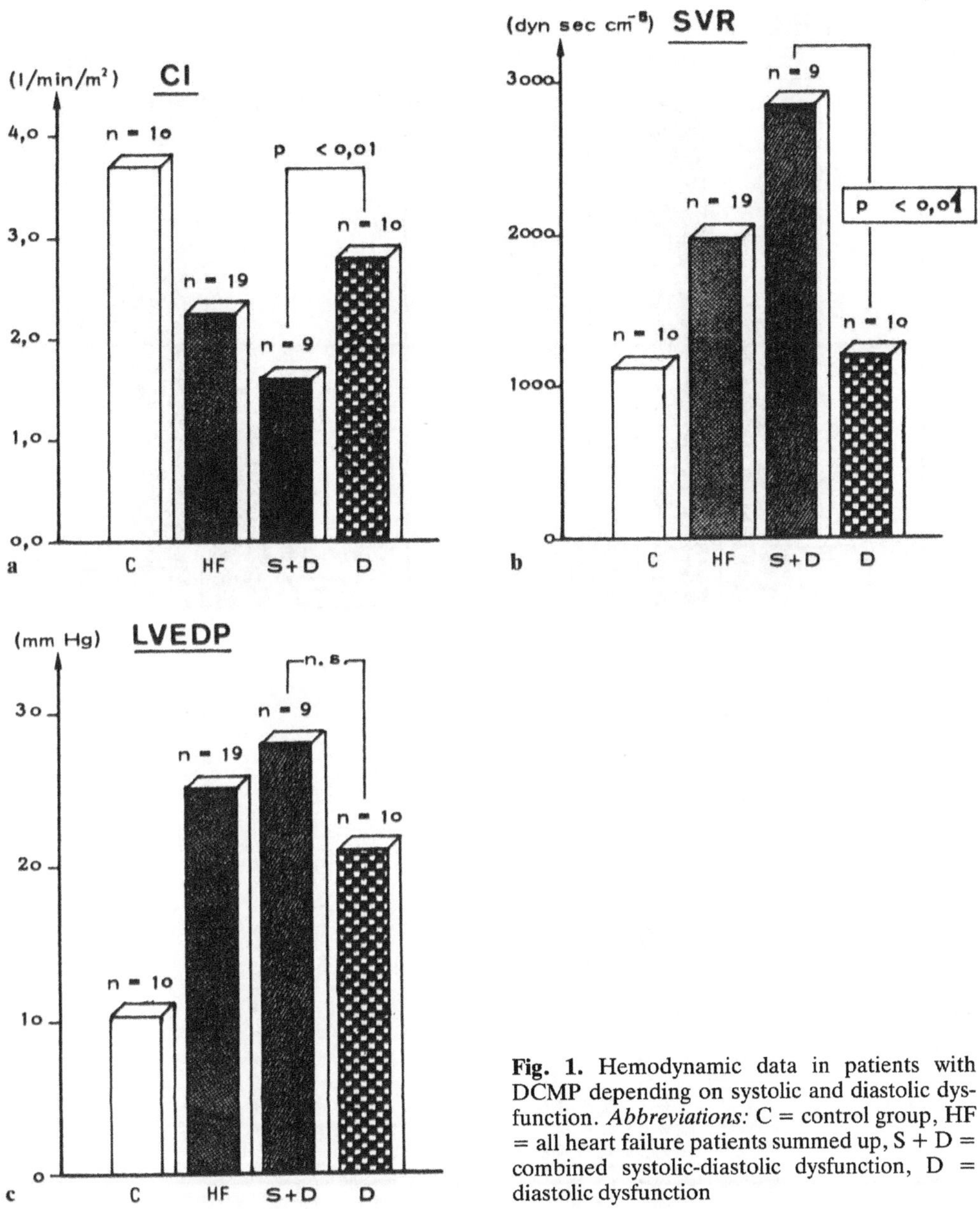

Fig. 1. Hemodynamic data in patients with DCMP depending on systolic and diastolic dysfunction. *Abbreviations:* C = control group, HF = all heart failure patients summed up, S + D = combined systolic-diastolic dysfunction, D = diastolic dysfunction

Statistical Analysis

The statistical significance of the difference was evaluated by the Student's t-Test. Coefficient of correlation was determined by linear regression analysis. Values were considered significant at $p < 0.05$.

Results

None of the heart failure patients showed the criteria of group I (pure systolic dysfunction = S), 10 patients were considered group II (diastolic dysfunction = D) and 9 patients were group III (combined systolic-diastolic dysfunction = S + D).

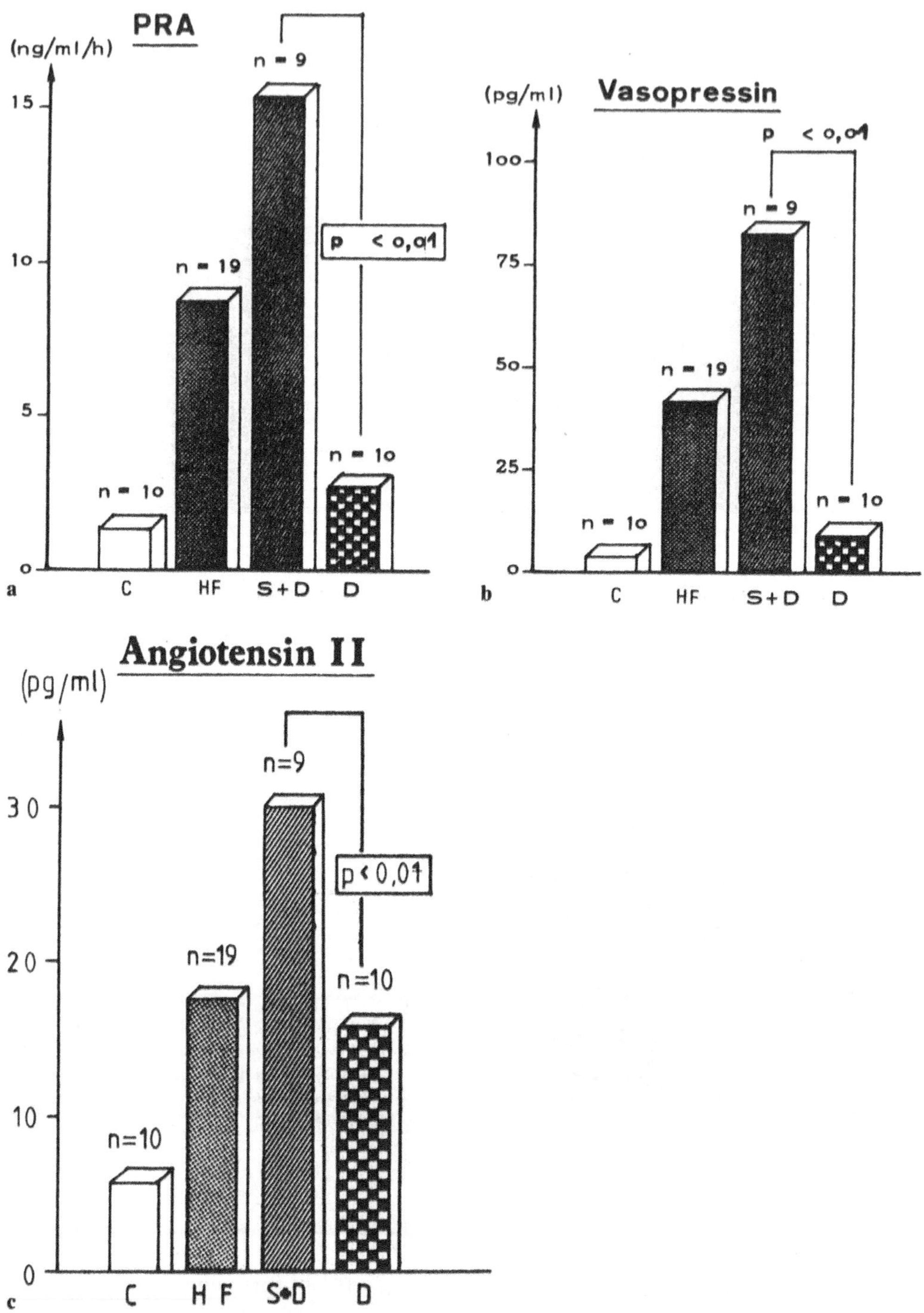
PRA
(ng/ml/h)
15
1o
5
o
n = 10
n = 19
n = 9
n = 1o
p < o,o1
a
C
HF
S+D
D
Vasopressin
(pg/ml)
100
75
50
25
o
n = 1o
n = 19
n = 9
n = 1o
p < o,o1
b
C
HF
S+D
D
Angiotensin II
(pg/ml)
30
20
10
0
n=10
n=19
n=9
n=10
p < 0,01
c
C
H F
S+D
D

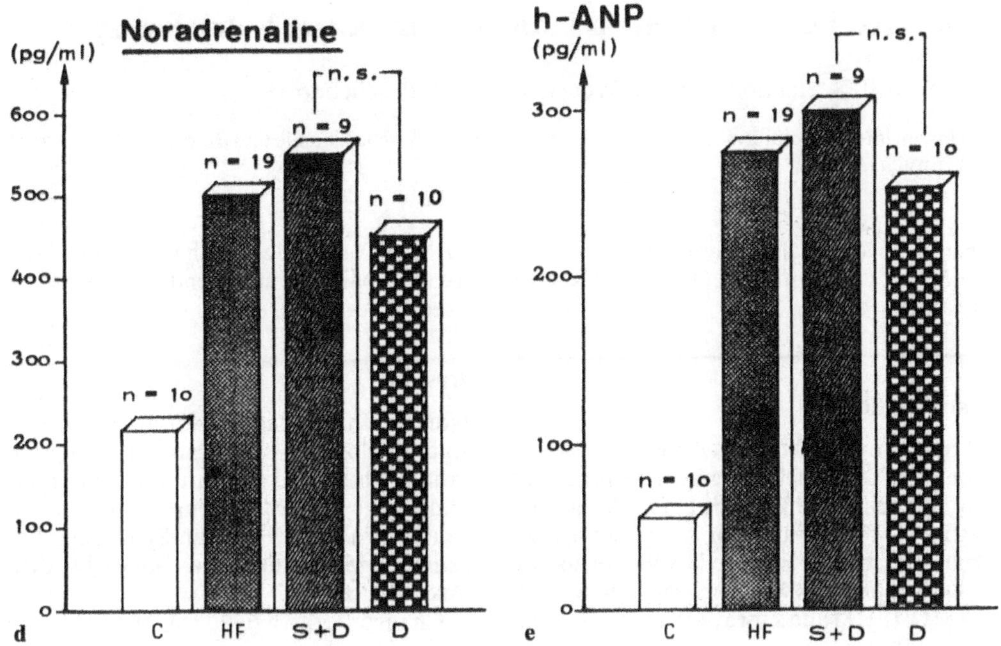

Fig. 2. Neurohormonal data in patients with DCMP depending on systolic and diastolic dysfunction

Conclusions

1. The determination of a "neurohormonal profile" consisting of alpha-ANP, plasma renin activity, angiotensin II, vasopressin and noradrenaline from the peripheral venous blood makes it possible to distinguish systolic from diastolic dysfunction in patients with dilated cardiomyopathy.
2. The vasoconstrictive hormones (plasma renin activity, angiotensin II, vasopressin) are significantly elevated in patients with predominant systolic dysfunction compared with the diastolic heart failure patients.
3. Alpha-ANP is significantly elevated in patients with impaired diastolic performance, whereas normal or just slightly elevated levels of the vasoconstrictive hormones are found.

References

1. Packer M (1988) Neurohormonal interactions and adaptations in congestive heart failure. Circulation 77:721
2. Poole-Wilson PA, Buller NP (1988) Causes of symptoms in chronic congestive heart failure and implications for treatment. Am J Cardiol 31A
3. Soufer R, Wohlgelernter D, Vita NA et al. (1985) Intact systolic left ventricular function in clinical congestive heart failure. Am J Cardiol 55:1032–1036

Elevated Levels of ANF in Patients with Mitral Valve Prolapse

F. Dienstl[1], S. Hauptlorenz[2], M. Wencker[1], and B. Puschendorf[2]

[1] Universitätsklinik für Innere Medizin, [2] Institut für medizinische Chemie und Biochemie, Universität Innsbruck, Austria

Key words: Atrial natriuretic factor (ANF) – Mitral valve prolapse (MVP) – Exercise testing

Introduction

Atrial natriuretic factor (ANF) is a recently found 28 aminoacid long peptide produced by the heart and stored in granula of both atria [1]. The stimulus for ANF release is atrial stretch [2]. Elevated ANF levels are found in patients with congestive heart failure (CHF) [3] and supraventricular arrhythmias [4].

We investigated patients with mitral valve prolapse (MVP). MVP is a frequent, mostly benign valvular malfunction. It is characterized by a systolic prolaps of one or both mitral leaflets into the lft atrium [5]. In many cases MVP is an accidental finding. Severe cases may be accompanied by mitral regurgitation. There is a high coincidence of MVP and connective tissue disorders such as Marfan-Syndrome. Some authors consider MVP to be a forme fruste of connective tissue disorders.

Methods

ANF plasma concentrations were measured in 10 patients (5 male, 5 female) with MVP and 12 healthy controls (6 male, 6 female). Blood was withdrawn at 0, 10, 14 and 20 o'clock of the same day. Additionally, all patients and 10 volunteers underwent standarized bicycle ergometric testing. ANF samples were collected before testing, after 5 min 50 W and after 5 min 100 W ergometric stress, after 10 and 20 min rest.

EDTA blood was seperated by centrifugation, and samples were frozen immediately. ANF was detected by a radioimmunoassay without prior extraction (EIKEN, Jpn.). Samples of one patient were analysed in the same assay. Results are given as mean ± SEM. For statistical analysis a two-sided t-Test for paired or independent samples was used.

Results

None of the 10 patients with MVP showed signs of clinically significant mitral regurgitation. The blood pressure was within normal range in both groups. One patient (male, 22a) had a Marfan-Syndrome. The remaining 9 patients had an isolated MVP of unknown orgin.

Changes of ANF during the day were noticed in all individuals but they follow no obvious pattern. Plasma ANF levels are significantly higher in patients with MVP compared to a group of healthy individuals (Fig. 1).

All patients and volunteers completed ergometric testing without discomfort. Again, we found significantly higher ANF levels in patients with MVP than in healthy persons. We found a slight but significant increase of ANF at the end of 5 min 100 W loading in the control group (57.3 ± 5.5 vs. 61.0 ± 9.6 pg/ml, n.s.). Patients with MVP showed a 23% increase of ANF (89.1 ± 9.2 to 109.5 ± 16.8 pg/ml, $p < 0.05$) between the two loading steps.

Discussion

Our data show that patients with MVP without signs of clinically significant mitral regurgitation or CHF have significantly elevated ANF levels. Also, patients with mVP show a significant increase in ANF under submaximal exercise testing whereas control values show little changes.

The reason for this result is still unclear.

One explanation for the increased ANF levels could be a discrete change in hemodynamics caused by the prolapsing mitral valve that cannot be detected by routine diagnostic methodes. Increased

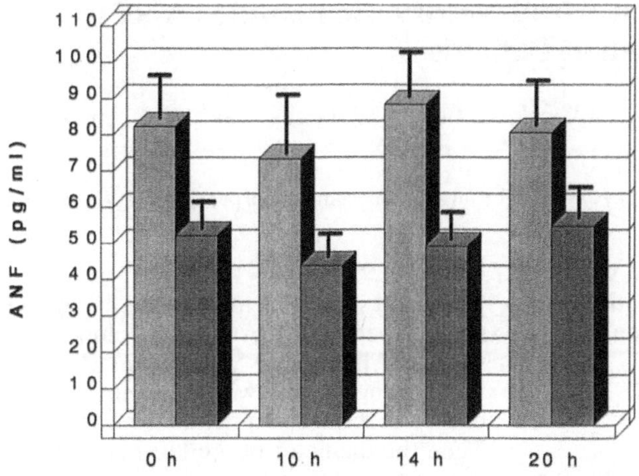

Fig. 1. Increased ANF levels ± SEM in 10 patients with MVP (light shade) compared to 12 healthy individuals (dark shade) at 0, 10, 14 and 20 o'clock

stretch in papillary muscle could also contribute to this finding. Connective tiussue disorders with an impaired skeleton of the heart could cause a higher susceptibility to atrial stretch than in healthy individuals. However, more histopathological and histochemical research will be needed to give a satisfactory explanation for this phenomenon.

This study adds another pathologic state to the list of diseases with increased ANF levels. Elevated ANF levels are no diagnosis but require further investigation to stecify the underlying cardiac disease.

Once more, ANF has proved to be a little specific but a very sensitive parameter in various cardiac diseases.

Once more, ANF has proved to be a little specific but a very sensitive parameter in various cardiac diseases.

References

1. Ballermann BJ, Brenner BM (1986) Role of atrial natriuretic peptides in body fluid homeostasis. Circ Res 58:619–630
2. Edwards BS, Zimmerman RS, Schwab TR, Heublein DM, Burnett JC (1988) Atrial stretch, not pressure, is the principal determinant controlling the acute release of atrial natriuretic factor. Circ Res 62:191
3. Pettersson A, Hedner J, Hedner T, Held P, Swedberg K, Towle AC (1986) Increased plasma levels of atrial natriuretic peptide with congestive heart failure. Eur Heart J 7:693
4. Hauptlorenz S, Wencker M, Lechleitner P, Dienstl F, Puschendorf B (1988) Atrial natriuretic factor (ANF) in various cardiac diseases. Fresenius Z Analyt Chem 330:414
5. Perloff JK, Child JS (1987) Clinical and epidemiologic issues in mitral valve prolapse: overview and perspective. Am Heart J 113:1324

Water Immersion Induced Atrial Natriuretic Peptide (ANP) Secretion in Heart Transplant Patients

F. Kokot[1], Z. Religa[3], S. Pasyk[2], A. Więcek[1], J. Frycz[2], W. Grzeszczak[1], A. Bochenek[3], and J. Dulawa[1]

[1]Department of Nephrology, [2]Cardiology and [3]Cardiosurgery, Silesian School of Medicine, Katowice, Poland

Key words: Heart transplant patients – ANP Secretion – Water immersion

Introduction

This paper aimed to study the intactness of ANP secretion in heart transplant patients and its relationship to renin (PRA), aldosterone (Ald) and vasopressin (AVP) secretion. ANP secretion was stimulated by central hypervolemia induced by head out water immersion (WI).

Material and Methods

6 male heart transplant patients (HTP) and 10 healthy subjects were examined. The mean age of the HTP was 43.3 ± 5.5 years and the mean time after heart transplantation 144.3 ± 25.8 days. As immunosuppressive therapy only cyclosporine A (mean dose 320 ± 38.6 mg/d) and azathioprine (mean dose 75 ± 17.5 mg/d) were used. At the time of the study the mean blood level of cyclosporine A was 538.7 ± 98.4 ng/ml and the mean plasma creatinine level 134.2 ± 13.2 μmol/l (means ± SEM). In all these patients no clinical signs of heart failure and rejection (confirmed by cardiac biopsy) were present. Heart transplantation was performed using the Colley and Shumway technique. The control group consisted of 10 male healthy subjects (mean age 36.9 ± 2.1 years) with a mean plasma creatinine level of 93.4 ± 2.4 μmol/l.

In all examined subjects the following experimental protocol was used.

After an overnight rest at 8 a.m. blood pressure (BP) and heart rate (HR) were assessed. Then blood samples were withdrawn for the estimation of ANP, PRA, Ald, AVP, creatinine, hemoglobin and the hematocrit value. Between 8 and 10 a.m. all examined subjects remained in a supine position ("bed rest"). At 10 a.m. blood pressure and heart rate were estimated, and blood samples were withdrawn for the estimation of the above mentioned parameters. Then the diameter of the left heart atrium was assessed using the Hewlett-Packard 77020 AC phased array system. After completion of this examination all subjects were exposed to head out water immersion (WI) in a bath tube for two hours using tap water of 35–36°C. After completion of WI all above mentioned parameters were assessed again. During water immersion all examined subjects remained in a semidecling position.

All endocrine parameters were assessed by radioimmunoassay [2]. ANP was estimated using ANP-antibodies kindly supplied by Dr. Gutkowska (Montreal). Methodological details of ANP are given in [3]. Alterations of the plasma volume induced by WI were assessed using the method of Greenleaf et al. [1]. Statistical evaluation of the results were performed using the "t" test of Student for paired and unpaired variables respectively.

Results

Results are presented in Table 1 and 2. No significant influence of bed rest on the estimated parameters was found. WI induced an increase of plasma volume (PV), which was of comparable magnitude in both examined groups. This increase of PV was accompanied by a significant suppression of PRA, Ald and AVP and an increase of plasma ANP. In HTP basal levels of plasma ANP were significantly elevated and the ANP response to central hypervolemia reduced. Also significantly elevated AVP plasma levels were found in HTP. These endocrine abnormalities in HTP seem to be

Table 1. Mean arterial blood pressure (MAP), heart rate (HR) diameter of the left atrium (LA) and change of plasma volume (ΔPV) in heart transplant patients (HTP) and healthy subjects. The atrial diameter was assessed only before and after 120 min of water immersion. The ΔPV concerns the difference between the −120 and 0′ values and the 0′ and 60′ and 120′ values respectively. Means ± SEM. The statistical significance concerns the difference between the values assessed at 0′ and 60′ or 120′ after WI respectively

	HTP				Healthy subjects			
	bed rest		WI		bed rest		WI	
	−120′	0′	60′	120′	−120′	0′	60′	120′
MAP mmHg	109.18 ±6.02	104.44 ±5.21	89.44[c] ±5.12	98.33[a] ±4.87	88.83 ±2.27	85.16 ±3.25	75.99[c] ±3.76	79.66[a] ±3.2
HR beats/min	83.33 ±5.69	88.67 ±3.23	99.33[a] ±9.43	98.67[a] ±9.00	71.20 ±2.73	68.4 ±2.67	80.60[a] ±3.72	80.80[a] ±3.46
LA (cm)	–	4.10 ±0.37	–	4.44 ±0.28	–	3.28 ±0.15	–	3.62[b] ±0.11
ΔPV %	–	1.64 ±0.8	9.95[c] ±2.83	9.57[c] ±1.0	–	0.1 ±0.63	6.4[c] ±0.80	10.9[c] ±1.98

[a] $p < 0.05$, [b] $p < 0.01$, [c] $p < 0.001$

Table 2. Plasma renin activity (PRA), plasma level of aldosterone (Ald), vasopressin (AVP) and atrial natriuretic peptide (ANP) in heart transplant patients (HTP, N = 6) and healthy subjects (N = 10) 120 minutes (−120) and immediately before (0′) water immersion (WI) and 60′ and 120 minutes after WI. Means ± SEM. The statistical significance concerns the difference between the values assessed at 0′ and 60′ and 120′ after WI respectively

	HTP				Healthy subjects			
	bed rest		WI		bed rest		WI	
	−120′	0′	60′	120′	−120′	0′	60′	120′
PRA ng/ml/h	2.15 ±0.33	2.20 ±0.35	1.14[a] ±0.26	0.96[a] ±0.27	2.78 ±0.18	2.67 ±0.21	1.60[a] ±0.15	1.52[a] ±0.16
Ald ng/dl	8.93 ±1.11	9.42 ±1.22	5.82[a] ±0.91	5.62[a] ±0.91	9.79 ±0.70	8.81 ±0.46	6.99[a] ±0.52	5.37[a] ±0.41
AVP pg/ml	5.63 ±0.82	6.18 ±0.92	3.78[a] ±0.84	3.05[a] ±0.68	2.11 ±0.16	2.07 ±0.11	1.18[a] ±0.13	1.12[a] ±0.20
ANP pg/ml	144.17 ±12.88	138.17 ±14.69	247.83[a] ±36.26	237.0[a] ±31.28	68.68 ±7.0	74.1 ±7.1	213.1[a] ±14.8	218.42[a] ±12.71

[a] $p < 0.001$

caused by latent failure of the transplanted heart. No straight correlation was found between plasma ANP and PRA, Ald and AVP under basal conditions and after WI both in HTP and normals.

Conclusion.

In HTP, ANP secretion is abnormal both under basal and stimulatory conditions and not straightly related to renin, aldosterone and vasopressin secretion.

References

1. Greenleaf JE, Covertino VA, Mangseth GL (1979) Plasma volume during stress: osmolality and red cell volume. J Appl Physiol 47: 1031–1038
2. Grzeszczak W, Kokot F, Duława J (1987) Effect of naloxone administration on endocrine abnormalities in chronic renal failure. Am J Nephrol 7:93–100
3. Kokot F, Grzeszczak W, Więcek A (1989) Water immersion induced alterations of atrial natriuretic peptide in patients with non-inflammatory acute renal failure. Nephrol Dial Transplant (In press)

Right Atrial Inversion Causes Increased ANF Secretion During Cardiopulmonary Bypass

M. Dahm, S. Nikolic, K. Owusu, D. Heublein, E. L. Yellin, J. Burnett Jr., and R. W. M. Frater

Department of Cardiothoracic Surgery, Albert Einstein College of Medicine, Bronx, NY and Mayo Clinic, Rochester, MN, USA

Key words: ANF – Cardiopulmonary bypass – Atrial inversion

Introduction

ANF is a polypeptide with important influence on blood pressure, cardiac output and sodium excretion. As the physiological stimulus for ANF release right atrial volume, i.e. right atrial distension has been demonstrated in animals [3, 4] and patients [5, 7]. Significant changes in ANF serum level have been reported during CPB [2]: after onset of CPB ANF level rises and stays elevated. During CPB RAP is very low or negative so that right atrial distension cannot account for this increase in secretion. Aim of this study was to determine if the inversion of the right atrium during CPB causes the increased release of ANF.

Methods

These experiments were performed in 7 dogs. Anaesthesia was induced with pentobarbital and maintained by isoflurane. The chest was opened through a sternotomy. Catheters were placed in IVC, SVC, RA and aorta to sample blood. Aortic and right atrial pressures were recorded simultaneously. Right heart bypass was established by extrapericardial canulation of SVC, IVC and pulmonary artery. RAP was controlled by variation of flow. An equilibration period was allowed before each sample. ANF was determined by radioimmunoassay and right atrial secretion (sRA = (RV) – (VC) calculated. The concentration in the venous blood was assumed (VC) = 0.75 (IVC) + 0.25 (SVC). This assumption was derived from flow measurement in two experiments.

Results

Data were analysed using linear regression for 34 hemodynamic states with RAP above zero and 8 with RAP below zero: Both, secretion and concentration in the RA correlated with RAP ($p < 0.01$, $p < 0.001$) for atrial pressures greater than zero. For negative pressures an inverse correlation was found ($p < 0.05$, $p < 0.01$).

Discussion

ANF concentration in the systemic circulation reveals an increase during cardiac surgery. This study was designed to evaluate the pathophysiological mechanism leading to increased circulating ANF during CPB. The results obtained suggest that atrial inversion increases right atrial ANF secretion. Trauma has been excluded by no touch policy and extrapericardial canulation.

From our results we conclude that normal control of ANF secretion by right atrial pressure is abolished during CPB. The unphysiological stimulus of atrial inversion as seen with RA pressures below zero causes high right atrial ANF production. These findings may be part of the pathophysiological mechanism causing the fall in vascular resistance with onset of CPB, since one of the physiological effects of ANF is the relaxation of muscle cells in the wall of some vessels [1] in vitro and in vivo [6].

References

1. Deth RC, Wong K, Fukozawa S, Roco R, Smart JL, Lynch CJ, Awad R (1982) Inhibition of rat aorta contractile response by natriuresis-inducing extract of rat atrium. Fed Proc 41:983
2. Dewar ML, Walsh G, Chiu RC-J, Kochamba K, Gutkowska J, Genest J, Cantin M (1986)

Atrial natriuretic factor: response to cardiac operation. J Thorac Cardiovasc Surg 96: 266–270
3. Kleinert HD, Maack T, Atlas SA, Jauszewicz A, Sealey JE, Laragh JH (1984) Atrial natriuretic factor inhibits angiotensin-, norepinephrine and potassium induced vascular contractility. Hypertension 6 [Suppl I]:I–143–147
4. Lang RE, Tholken H, Ganten D, Luft FC, Ruskoaho H, Unger T (1985) Atrial natriuretic factor – a circulating hormone stimulated by volume loading. Nature 314:264–266
5. Matsubara H, Nishihawa M, Umeda Y, Taniguchi T, Iwasaka T, Kurimoto T, Yamane Y, Inada M (1987) The role of atrial pressure in secreting atrial natriuretic polypeptides. Am Heart J 113(6):1457–1462
6. Richards AM, Nicholls MG, Ikram H, Webster MWI, Yandle TG, Espiner EA (1985) Renal, hemodynamic and hormonal effects of human alpha atrial natriuretic peptide in healthy volunteers. Lancet I:545–549
7. Rodeheffer RJ, Tanaka I, Imada T, Hollister AS, Robertson D, Inagami T (1986) Atrial pressure and secretion of atrial natriuretic factor into the human central circulation. JAAC 8 (1):18–26

Renal Resistance against Atrial Natriuretic Peptide in Congestive Heart Failure: Effect of ACE Inhibition

G. Wambach, U. Schittenhelm, M. Stimpel, and W. Kaufmann

Medizinische Klinik II der Universität Köln

Key words: ACE inhibition – ANP – Congestive heart failure – Enalapril – hANP

Introduction

Recent studies demonstrate elevated plasma levels of atrial natriuretic peptide both in experimental models of heart failure and in patients with congestive heart failure (Raine et al. 1986; Tsunoda et al. 1986). Despite elevated plasma ANP levels, retention of sodium and water occurs leading to increased plasma volume and edema. This is probably due to a reduction in the natriuretic potency of ANP in heart failure as shown by infusion of exogenous ANP both in experimental animal and man (Scriven and Burnett 1985; Cody et al. 1986; Koepke and DiBona 1987). The underlying mechanism, however, responsible for the renal resistance to ANP is unknown. Activation of the sodium retaining renin-angiotensin system is thought to account for the impaired renal action of ANP. We tested this hypothesis by compairing the renal effects of exogenous ANP in patients with congestive heart failure before and after blockade of the renin-angiotensin system by the ACE-inhibitor enalapril.

Patients, Protocol and Methods

10 patients with chronic heart failure (7 males, 3 females, aged 32–68 years) (grade III–IV, New York Heart Association) were included in the study. Congestive heart failure was secondary to coronary heart disease in three patients, to cardiomyopathy in six patients and to mitral valve stenosis in one patient. Patients were monitored on the intensive care unit on two consecutive days. Routine laboratory findings are outlined in table I. All patients were monitored by electrocardiogram. They had central venous catheter and an urinary bladder catheter. Previous medication (digoxin 0.2 mg/d in 9 patients, furosemide 60 mg/d in 4 patients, ISDN 60 mg/d in 5 patients) was stopped the evening before the infusion. On day one, patients received an in-

Table 1. Routine clinical and laboratory findings in patients with congestive heart failure

n (m/f)	20 (7/3)
age (y)	32–68
body weight (kg)	70.5 ± 4.8
s-Na^+ (meq/l)	131 ± 1.1
s–K^+ (meq/l)	4.7 ± 0.2
s-crea. (mg/dl)	1.5 ± 0.2

travenous infusion of 1–28 hANP (Fa. Bissendorf) (0.1 μg/kg/min) over a period of 30 minutes at 16:00. Systolic and diastolic blood pressure were recorded in supine position every 30 minutes from 90 minutes before the start of the infusion up to 90 minutes after the end of the infusion. Urine collections for periods of 30 minutes were performed starting at −90 minutes up to +120 minutes. Urine volume, urinary Na^+, K^+, creatinine, creatinine clearance and excretion of cyclic GMP were measured. Blood samples were drawn at the end of each period of 30 minutes for measurements of ANP, renin concentration, aldosterone and angiotensin I converting enzyme activity. On day two, the same protocol was performed after treatment with enalapril 2.5 mg p.o. every 8 hours for a total of 24 hours.

Plasma-ANP-levels were measured by radioimmunoassay after extraction as described earlier (Wambach et al. 1987). Plasma renin concentration was measured according to the method of Hummerich and Krause (1975). Serum aldosterone, ACE activity, cGMP were determined using commercially available kits (Serono Freiburg, Paesel Frankfurt, NEN Dreieich).

Results

During the control infusion of ANP, urinary volume increased from 28 ± 7 to 54 ± 9 ml/30 min and urinary sodium output from 2.5 ± 0.6 to 3.4 ± 1.1 mmol/30 min when 30 minutes periods before and during ANP infusion were compared (Fig. 1).

Treatment with enalapril (3 × 2.5 mg p.o.) resulted in a reduction in plasma ACE activity from 84.7 ± 16.9 to 2.13 ± 0.86 U/l before and from 88.2 ± 16.0 to 2.52 ± 0.82 U/l immediately after the ANP infusion. Not unexpectedly, systolic and diastolic blood pressure were reduced after enalapril. The effect of ANP infusion on arterial blood pressure however was not different during the control period and after

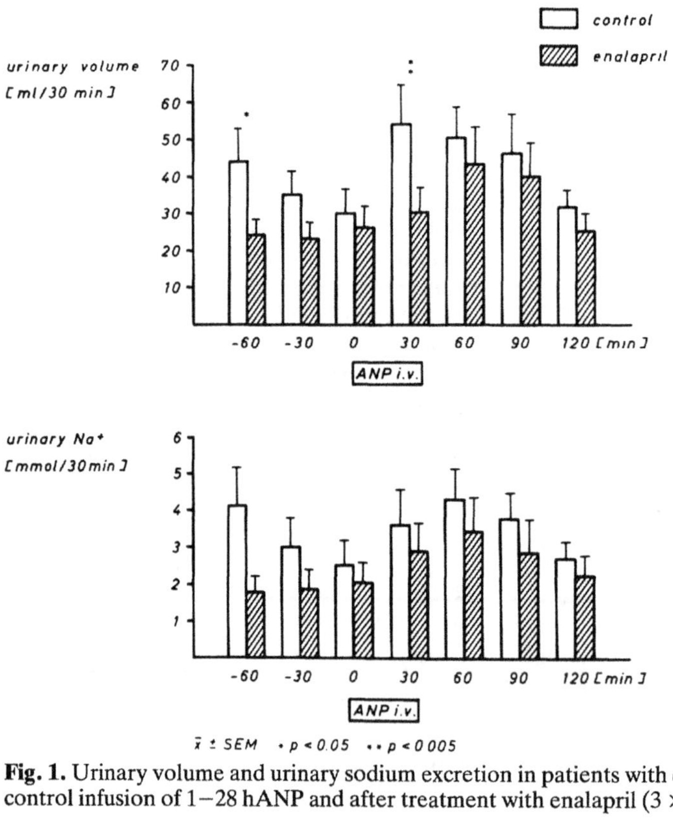

Fig. 1. Urinary volume and urinary sodium excretion in patients with congestive heart failure during a control infusion of 1–28 hANP and after treatment with enalapril (3 × 2.5 mg p.o.)

ACE inhibition. Urinary volume and urinary sodium output before, during and after ANP infusion were slightly reduced after ACE inhibition. Urinary creatinine excretion and creatinine clearance were not different during the control infusion and after ACE inhibition.

The effect of ANP infusion on plasma renin concentration and serum aldosterone was also studied in patients with CHF both after placebo and after enalapril treatment. Despite high basal levels for plasma renin and aldosterone, no significant reduction in aldosterone and renin was observed after the infusion of ANP. ACE inhibition by enalapril was followed by a rise in renin and suppression in aldosterone. Again, ANP infusion did not alter renin and aldosterone concentrations.

Discussion

Several attempts were made to explain the obvious inability of the atrial natriuretic peptide to control fluid retention in heart failure. An incomplete processing of ANP precursor was thought to result in higher immunoreactivity with reduced diuretic activity in patients with cardiac disease (Arendt 1986). However, Yamaji et al. analyzed circulating ANP in patients with heart failure by reverse phase chromatography (Yamaji et al. 1986). The majority of the peptide was found to be α-ANP with small amount of γ-ANP. Therefore, incomplete processing of ANP precursor does not explain the reduced activity of the hormone system in heart failure. Furthermore, elevated plasma levels and urinary excretion of the second messenger cGMP as shown in the present study and by others suggest a biological action on the target tissues for ANP in heart failure patients (Gerzer 1987).

However, the biological effect of ANP is obviously blunted in experimental and clinical heart failure: a reduced natriuresis after infusion of ANP was demonstrated in two different dog models of heart failure and in patients (Freeman et al. 1985; Cody et al. 1986; Riegger et al. 1987).

The renal resistance to ANP could be the result of the activation of the renin-angiotensin-system.

According to studies in experimental animals, A II and ANP seem to act like physiological antagonists. In the adrenal cortex, ANP inhibits the secretion of aldosterone when stimulated by A II (Campbell et al. 1985). In arterial vessels, ANP reduces the vasoconstriction induced by A II (Proctor and Bealer 1987). When administered into the brain, ANP reduces the stimulation of thirst, salt appetite and hormone release induced by A II (Nakaoka et al. 1986). It was therefore reasonable to assume an antagonism of both systems at the level of the kidney in heart failure. The results of the present study, however, do not support the notion that an activation of the renin-angiotensin system is responsible for the renal resistance to exogenous ANP since blockade of the renin system does not improve the natriuretic effect of an ANP infusion.

References

Arendt RM, Gerbes AL, Ritter D, Stangl E (1986) Molecular weight heterogenity of plasma ANF in cardiovascular disease. Klin Wochenschr 64 [Suppl III]:97–102

Campbell WB, Currie MG, Needleman P (1985) Inhibition of aldosterone biosynthesis by atriopeptins in rat adrenal cells. Circ Res 57:113–118

Cody RJ, Atlas SA et al. (1986) Atrial natriuretic factor in normal subjects and heart failure patients. Plasma levels and renal, hormonal, and haemodynamic responses to peptide infusion. J Clin Invest 78 (5):1362–1374

Freeman RH, Davis JO, Vari RC (1985) Renal response to atrial natriuretic factor in conscious dogs with caval constriction. Am J Physiol 248:R495–R500

Gerzer R, Heim JM, Schütze B, Weil J (1987) Cellular mechanisms of action of ANP. Klin Wochenschr 65 [Suppl VIII]:103–109

Hummerich W, Krause D (1975) Improvement of renin determination in human plasma using a commonly available renin standard in a radioimmunological method. Klin Wochenschr 53:559–569

Koepke JP, DiBona GF (1987) Blunted natriuresis to atrial natriuretic peptide in chronic sodium-retaining disorders. Am J Physiol 252:F865–F871

Nakaoka H, Imataka K, Amano M, Fujii J, Ishibashi M, Yamaji T (1986) Plasma levels of atrial natriuretic factor in patients with congestive heart failure. New Engl J Med 313 (14): 892–893

Proctor KG, Bealer SL (1987) Selective antagonism of hormone induced vasoconstriction by synthetic atrial natriuretic factor in the rat microcirculation. Circ Res 61 (1):42–47

Raine AEG, Erne P, Bürgisser E, Müller FB, Bolli P, Burkart F, Bühler FR (1986) Atrial natriuretic peptide and atrial pressure in patients with congestive heart failure. New Engl J Med 315:533–537

Riegger AJG, Kromer EP, Kochsiek K (1985) Der natriuretische Vorhoffaktor bei schwerer kongestiver Herzinsuffizienz. Dt Med Wochenschr 42:1607–1610

Scriven TA, Burnett JC Jr (1985) Effects of synthetic atrial natriuretic peptide on renal function and renin release in acute experimental heart failure. Circulation 72:892–897

Tsunoda K, Hodsman GP, Sumithran E, Johnston CI (1986) Atrial natriuretic peptide in chronic heart failure in the rat: a correlation with ventricular dysfunction. Circ Res 59:256–261

Wambach G, Götz S, Suckau G, Bönner G, Kaufmann W (1987) Plasma levels of atrial natriuretic peptide are raised in essential hypertension during low and high sodium intake. Klin Wochenschr 65:232–237

Yamaji T, Ishibashi M, Takaku F, Nakaoka H, Imataka K, Kitahara Y, Fujii J (1986) Nature of atrial natriuretic peptide in plasma from patients with congestive heart failure. Lancet I:402–403

Atrial Natriuretic Peptide in Patients with Essential Hypertension: Effects on Systemic and Renal Hemodynamics and Renal Excretory Function

H. G. Predel, O. Schulte-Vels, K. Glänzer, C. Geller, H. Meyer-Lehnert, and H. J. Kramer

Medizinische Poliklinik, University of Bonn, FRG

Key words: Atrial natriuretic peptide – Essential hypertension – Hemodynamics – Renal function

Introduction

Human atrial natriuretic peptide 1–28 (α-hANP) processed and secreted by myoendocrine cells located in the heart atria have been demonstrated to possess strong diuretic, natriuretic and vasodilatory properties [3, 17]. Furthermore, ANP modulates the activity of neural and hormonal systems involved in the regulation of arterial blood pressure (BP) and extracellular fluid volume (ECFV), e.g. of the adrenergic nervous and the renin-angiotensin aldosterone systems [15, 19]. This profile of biological actions suggests that ANP may play a role in at least some forms of essential hypertension in which chronic retention of sodium with subsequent ECFV expansion and an increase in total peripheral vascular resistance (TPR) are frequently observed.

However, the data published so far on a potential role of ANP in arterial hypertension are equivocal. While elevated plasma concentrations of α-hANP have been measured regularly in patients with severe hypertension, in mild to moderate hypertension plasma levels of α-hANP are frequently found within normal limits [2, 5, 15, 31]. In addition, the question is still open, whether increased α-hANP plasma levels in hypertensive patients represent a mechanism attenuating the rise in BP or whether they are merely an epiphenomenon of elevated BP.

The effects of i.v. infusion of exogenous α-hANP in men were studied by various investigators. Using relatively high doses they demonstrated antihypertensive, diuretic and natriuretic effects of ANP which were more pronounced in hypertensive than in normotensive subjects, but detailed information on the changes in systemic and renal hemodynamics during α-hANP infusion of smaller doses of α-hANP is lacking [26, 32].

Therefore, the purpose of the present study was to investigate the effects of low dose α-hANP-infusion over a period of 60 minutes in six patients with established essential hypertension (H) and in six healthy normotensive control subjects (C). Simultaneous measurements of systemic and renal hemodynamics and of renal excretory function as well as of the activity of specific neurohormonal systems were performed.

Patients and Methods

Study Design

Six male patients aged 37.6 ± 4.1 years with essential hypertension (H) and six normotensive age-matched healthy control subjects (C) aged 34.8 ± 5.2 years were included in this study. Systolic and diastolic BP in untreated patients was 154 ± 5/109 ± 4 mmHg and in C 117 ± 1/72 ± 2 mmHg. All subjects had given their informed written consent according to the declaration of Helsinki. Their body weight and height averaged 87.8 ± 4.0 kg and 178 ± 0.3 cm in hypertensive patients and 78.0 ± 4.4 kg and 180 ± 3.6 cm in C, respectively. To exclude secondary forms of hypertension and overt cardiac, hepatic or renal disease physical examination, including fundoscopy, complete hematologic and blood chemistry status, urine analysis, electrocardiogram and chest x-ray were performed in hypertensive patients and in C. Renal function, evaluated as endogenous creatinine clearance, was normal.

Antihypertensive drugs or other pharmacons were discontinued 72 h prior to the study. Their carbohydrate restricted diet had a normal sodium content. Fluid intake was unrestricted. Control subjects received a diet with similar protein and sodium content and had a similar fluid intake as the patients on the day prior to the study. The 24 h sodium and potassium excretion was 164 ± 18 and 85 ± 13 mmol in patients with H and 173 ± 19 and 86 ± 15 mmol in C, respectively.

The following protocol was performed in an identical manner in patients with H and in C: After an overnight fast all subjects received 15 ml per kg body weight tap water.

Plastic cannulas were inserted into both antecubital veins. One port was used for infusion of inulin and p-aminohippuric acid (PAH), the contralateral port was used for infusion of α-hANP [1−28] kindly provided by Drs. M. Bornemann and H. Küppers, Schwarz Pharma, Monheim, West-Germany. All subjects were in supine position one hour before the start of the study and remained in supine position throughout the experiment except for urine voiding at the end of each collection period after blood sampling and hemodynamic measurements had been performed.

Two control periods preceded the 1 h ANP-infusion, which was followed by two post-infusion periods, each period lasting 30 minutes. A priming dose of inulin and PAH was administered at 8.00 h followed by a continuous infusion of inulin and PAH in 0.9% saline at a rate of 5.55 ml/min. 100 μg α-hANP dissolved in 250 ml 0.9% NaCl was administered intravenously at a rate of 24 ng/min/kg body weight over a period of 60 minutes, using a calibrated infusion pump (Braun Melsungen, West-Germany). The infusion rate was 4.17 ml/min.

In a separate experiment the effects of 250 ml 0.9% NaCl alone, when infused in an identical manner, were studied. During or after the infusion of α-hANP no side-effects or adverse reactions were observed.

Urine was collected every 30 minutes by spontaneous voiding in upright position after hemodynamic parameters had been measured. Blood pressure (BP) and heart rate (HR) were measured at 10 minute intervals. Stroke volume (SV) was determined at the end of each 30 minute urine collection period but at 10 minute intervals during the α-hANP infusion period. Venous blood was drawn at the end of the first control clearance period, after 30 minutes and at the end of α-hANP infusion, and at the end of the second post-infusion clearance period.

Methods

BP was measured sphygmomanometrically. Stroke volume (SV) was determined by the cardiac impedance method using a Minnesota Impedance Cardiograph (Diefenbach, Frankfurt, West-Germany). Heart rate (HR) was monitored continuously by ECG. Cardiac output (CO) was calculated automatically from mean values of each 10 measurements of SV. Total peripheral vascular resistance (TPR) was calculated from mean arterial pressure (MAP) and CO: TPR = MAP/CO. GFR and effective RPF were estimated from inulin and PAH clearances [6]. Renal vascular resistance (RVR) was calculated from MAP and renal blood flow (RBF): RVR = MAP/RBF; RBF = RPF/(1-hematocrit).

For determination of α-hANP plasma concentrations by radioimmunoassay 5 ml of blood samples were collected into chilled siliconized glass tubes containing 500 µl EDTA and were centrifuged at 4 °C for five minutes at 1.700 g. Plasma α-hANP was extracted according to Kohno et al. [14]. Radioimmunoassay was performed as previously described [24] using an antibody against synthetic α-hANP and 125 I-α-hANP purchased from Peninsula Laboratories (St. Helens, UK). The effective range of the standard curve for α-hANP was between 0.5 and 50 pmol per assay tube.

Cyclic guanosine monophosphate (cGMP), vasopressin, aldosterone plasma concentrations and plasma renin activity (PRA) were measured by radioimmunoassay according to methods previously described [8, 10, 28, 29]. Urine catecholamine concentrations were determined fluorimetrically [16]. Plasma and urine concentrations of sodium and protassium were determined by flame photometry, and serum and urine creatinine concentrations were determined according to a conventional autoanalyzer method.

Statistical analysis was performed with Wilcoxon's signed rank test and when appropriate with Mann-Whitney U-test. A p value < 0.05 was considered as statistically significant. Data are given as means ± S.E.M.

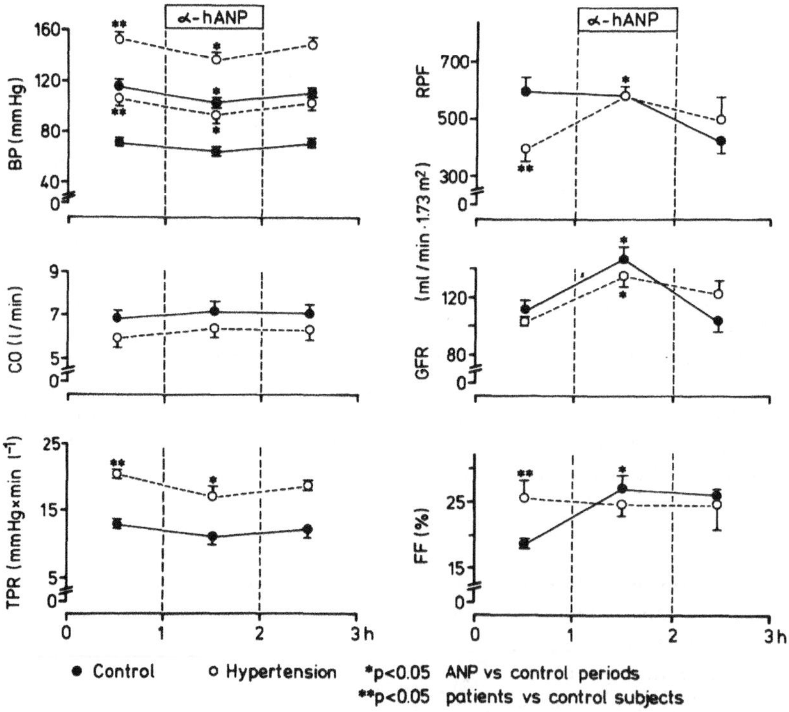

Fig. 1. Mean systolic and diastolic blood pressure (BP), cardiac output (CO), total peripheral resistance (TPR), renal plasma flow (RPF) glomerular filtration rate (GFR) and filtration fraction (FF) before, during, and after infusion of α-hANP

Results

Plasma α-hANP Concentrations and Renal Function before ANP-Infusion

Mean *Plasma α-hANP concentrations* under basal conditions were 30.9 ± 4.5 in hypertensive patients and 14.0 ± 1.7 pmo/l in C. Plasma levels of *cGMP* averaged 5.0 ± 1.0 pmol/ml in hypertensive and 3.8 ± 0.5 pmol/ml in control subjects.

Supine systolic and diastolic BP before ANP-infusion averaged 154.1 ± 5.1/109.1 ± 3.9 mmHg in hypertensive patients and 117.3 ± 1.4/72.0 ± 1.9 mmHg in C, respectively (Fig. 1). Mean arterial pressure (MAP) is shown in table 1. Heart rate *(HR)* averaged 69.0 ± 3.4 beats/min in hypertensive patients as compared to 59.6 ± 3.4 beats/min in C. Cardiac output *(CO)* was lower in hypertensive patients than in controls (Table 1; Fig. 1). Total peripheral vascular resistance *(TPR)* was significantly higher in hypertensive patients (Table 1, Fig. 1).

Baseline urine flow during the second preinfusion control period averaged 2.6 ± 0.2 ml/min in hypertensive patients as compared to 3.2 ± 1.2 ml/min in C. *Baseline urinary sodium and potassium excretion with* 312 ± 28 and 85 ± 12 μmol/min was slightly but not significantly higher in hypertensive patients than in C with 279 ± 86 and 104 ± 31 μmol/min, respectively (Fig. 2).

Baseline Renal Hemodynamics

Under control conditions *GFR* did not significantly differ between hypertensive patients and control subjects. *RPF* was significantly lower in the hypertensive patients and therefore, *FF* was significantly higher than in C (Table 1; Fig. 1). Also renal vascular resistance *(RVR)* was significantly higher ($p < 0.05$) in patients (0.19 ± 0.03 mmHg × min × ml^{-1}) than in C (0.09 ± 0.009 mmHg × min × ml^{-1}).

Baseline Hormonal Concentrations

PRA and plasma aldosterone concentrations were similar in hypertensive patients and in control subjects averaging 0.77 ± 0.29 ng/ml/h and 133.8 ± 29.1 pg/ml and 0.62 ± 0.14 ng/ml/h and 138.3 ± 17.9 pg/ml, respectively. *Vasopressin plasma concentrations* averaged 1.5 ± 0.4 pg/ml in hypertensive patients and 1.3 ± 0.4 pg/ml in control subjects. *Urinary excretion of adrenaline, noradrenaline and dopamine* was 0.07 ± 0.02, 0.21 ± 0.08 and 0.59 ± 0.11 μg/min in hypertensive patients and 0.04 ± 0.01, 0.17 ± 0.04 and 0.90 ± 0.05 μg/min in controls, respectively.

Effects of α-hANP Infusion

I.v. infusion of α-hANP resulted in a significant ($p < 0.05$) rise in plasma α-hANP concentrations averaging 124.9 ± 25.0 pmol/l in hypertensive patients and 88.5 ± 8.3 pmol/l in C (n.s.), respectively. The rise in plasma α-hANP levels was accompanied by a similar increase in plasma cGMP plasma concentration in hypertensive patients to 14.4 ± 1.0 pmol/l and to 17.8 ± 1.6 pmol/l, in C, respectively ($p < 0.05$).

Systemic Hemodynamic Responses to α-hANP Infusion

With α-hANP infusion systolic and diastolic BP significantly decreased in hypertensive patients to 138.5 ± 7.4 and 94.1 ± 4.2 mmHg. In C systolic BP also decreased significantly to 105.7 ± 1.4 mmHg ($p < 0.05$), whereas diastolic BP only slightly decreased to 64.8 ± 2.6 mmHg (Fig. 1). MAP was, thus, significantly reduced by ANP in hypertensive and in control subjects (Table 1).

HR remained unaffected in hypertensive patients (72.3 ± 5.0 beats/min) and in C (62.8 ± 2.9 beats/min). Initially CO rose slightly but insignificantly in both hypertensive and control subjects. It returned within the first 15 minutes to pre-infusion values in both groups despite continuous α-hANP-infusion. TPR significantly ($p < 0.05$) declined in hypertensive patients in contrast to a moderate decline in C (Table 1; Fig. 1).

Renal Responses to α-hANP Infusion

Maximal effects of ANP occurred 30 and 60 min after start of α-hANP-infusion. Urine flow increased by 515% to 16.0 ± 2.0 ml/min in hypertensive patients and by 163% to

Table 1. Effects of α-hANP Infusion on Systemic and Renal Hemodynamics in Patients with Essential Hypertension and in six control subjects

	MAP (mmHg)	CO (l/min)	TPR (mmHg · min/l^{-1})	GFR (ml/min/1.73 m^2)	RPF	FF (%)
Patients						
before ANP	123.5 ± 5.6[a]	6.1 ± 0.3	20.6 ± 1.2[b]	105 ± 12	407 ± 67[b]	25.8 ± 2.0[b]
during ANP	107.6 ± 5.1[a]	6.5 ± 0.4	16.4 ± 1.4[a]	139 ± 10[a]	559 ± 89[a]	25.5 ± 3.4
Controls						
before ANP	88.1 ± 2.4	6.8 ± 0.3	13.3 ± 0.8	111 ± 6	595 ± 53	18.9 ± 0.9
during ANP	78.8 ± 1.6[a]	7.2 ± 0.5	11.3 ± 0.9	147 ± 11[a]	578 ± 24	26.8 ± 3.0[a]

[a] ANP vs. control periods: $p < 0.05$
[b] patients vs. control subjects: $p < 0.05$
MAP = mean arterial pressure; CO = cardiac output; TPR = total peripheral resistance; GFT = glomerular filtration rate; RPF = renal plasma flow; FF = filtration fraction

8.4 ± 1.7 ml/min in C; sodium excretion rose by 399% to 1559 ± 288 μmol/min in hypertensive patients and by 115% to 601 ± 154 μmol/min in C ($p < 0.05$). Potassium excretion significantly increased in hypertensive patients by 79% to 152 ± 18 μmol/min ($p < 0.05$), but only by 15% to 120 ± 16 μmol/min in C. Urine flow and sodium excretion remained above pre-infusion levels during the 60 min post-infusion period (Fig. 2). GFR significantly rose by 32% in hypertensive patients and by 32% in C ($p < 0.05$). RPF increased significantly by 37% in hypertensive patients ($p < 0.05$), but remained unaltered in C. Thus, FF also remained unaltered in patients, whereas it increased by 42% in control subjects ($p < 0.05$; Table 1; Fig. 1) RVR significantly decreased to 0.12 ± 0.02 mmHg × min × ml^{-1} in hypertensive patients ($p < 0.05$) but only moderately to 0.09 ± 0.01 mmHg × min × ml^{-1} in C (n.s.)

Hormonal Repsonses to α-hANP Infusion

PRA decreased slightly in hypertensive patients 0.53 ± 0.16 ng/ml/h (n.s.) but significantly in C to 0.32 ± 0.11 ng/ml/h ($p < 0.05$).

Plasma aldosterone concentrations significantly decreased to 69.0 ± 7.6 pg/ml and to 101.8 ± 8.9 pg/ml in hypertensive and in control subjects, respectively. Vasopressin plasma concentrations remained unaltered in hypertensive patients and in control subjects (1.4 ± 0.2 and 1.5 ± 0.3 pg/ml, respectively). Urinary excretion of adrenaline, noradrenaline and dopamine was 0.05 ± 0.02 (n.s.), 0.07 ± 0.01 ($p < 0.05$) and 0.20 ± 0.04 (n.s.) μg/min in hypertensive patients and 0.02 ± 0.01 (n.s.), 0.04 ± 0.01 ($p < 0.05$) and 0.30 ± 0.05 (n.s.) in C, respectively.

The infusion of vehicle alone (saline without α-hANP) did not affect any of the above parameters.

Discussion

In the present study basal α-hANP plasma concentrations were significantly higher in hypertensive patients than in the normotensive control group, whereas cGMP plasma concentrations were similar in both groups. This finding may point to a blunted biological activity of ANP in hypertensive subjects possibly due to receptor down-regulation or to the presence of biologically inactive precursor forms of ANP [1, 15, 24].

I. v. infusion of exogenous α-hANP at a rate of 24 ng/min/kg caused a 6-fold increase of α-hANP plasma levels in control subjects as compared to a 3.5-fold rise in hypertensive patients. Nevertheless, the maximum plasma concentrations reached during the infusion were not significantly different between both groups and were within the range of plasma concentrations which are found under physiological and pathophysiological conditions. They were accompanied by a parallel rise in plasma cGMP concentrations. Maximal systemic and renal hemodynamic changes were observed during the initial 30 minutes of ANP infusion and maximal renal excretory effects occurred between 30 and 60 minutes after the start of ANP infusion. Return to basal values occurred within 30 minutes after cessation of ANP infusion, which agrees with the short plasma half-life of circulating α-hANP [9, 21]. BP decreased significantly in hypertensive patients and in controls but the decrease was more pronounced in hypertensive patients. The following mechanisms for ANP-induced reduction in BP may be considered: *First,* ANP may have caused direct vasorelaxation, which was found to be positively correlated with vascular preconstriction [25]. Since in the present study basal TPR was significantly higher in our hypertensive patients than in C, the more pronounced fall in TPR in these patients is in good agreement with this concept. A decrease in cardiac output was not observed in our subjects during ANP-infusion.

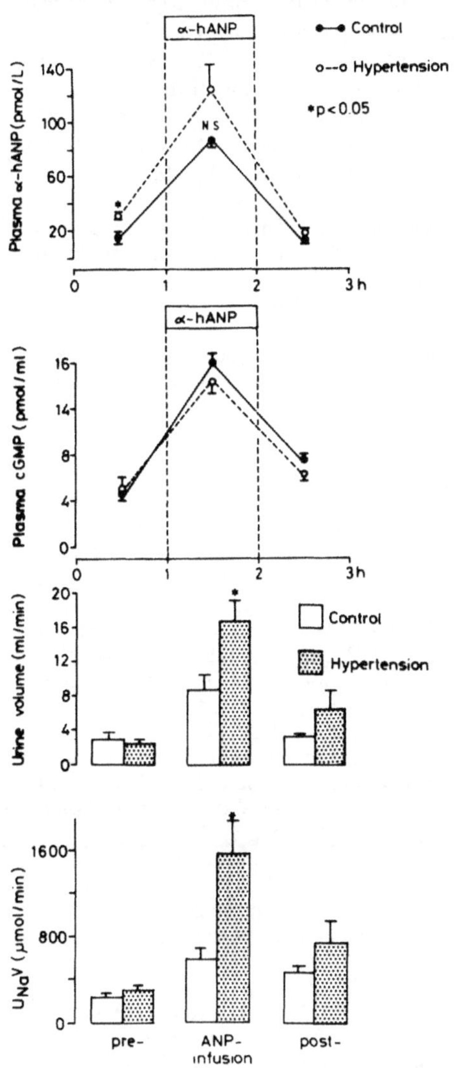

Fig. 2. Mean ANP and cGMP plasma concentrations, mean urine volume and urine sodium excretion before, during, and after α-hANP infusion.

Second, inhibition of enhanced sympathoadrenal activity and modification of the baroreceptor sensitivity may have contributed to the fall in BP. Thus, heart rate during ANP infusion remained unaltered. This points to a blunted baroreceptor response to BP reduction in the presence of ANP in patients with essential hypertension, who may already exhibit a decrease in baroreceptor sensitivity or it may be related to a direct inhibition by ANP of the sympathetic nervous system activity, which seems to be more pronounced in patients with essential hypertension than in normotensive subjects.

Third, the hypotensive effect of ANP may be related to a reduction of circulating blood volume which presumably resulted from the diuresis and natriuresis as well as from a shift of fluid volume from the intra- into the extravascular space induced by ANP. This latter phenomenon is supported by a small but significant rise in hematocrit which cannot be explained only on the basis of urinary fluid loss.

A significant diuresis and natriuresis during the infusion of α-hANP were observed in both hypertensive and in normotensive subjects but were significantly more pronounced in hypertensive patients. This may have been due to different responses of renal hemodynamics in hypertensive patients as compared to C. Thus, a significant increase in RPF and decrease in renal vascular resistance was observed only in hypertensive patients possibly related to an elevated basal tone of their renal vasculature. Under control conditions our patients revealed a significant reduction in RPF in the presence of normal GFR. In addition, a redistribution of kidney perfusion towards the renal medulla must be considered, which may result in medullary wash-out and has been postulated to represent one of the natriuretic mechanisms of ANP [19].

Furthermore, despite the greater fall in BP during α-hANP infusion in hypertensive patients, their BP still remained higher than in control subjects, therefore, resulting in a higher glomerular perfusion pressure. Finally, a more pronounced direct tubular effect of ANP in our hypertensive patients cannot be excluded.

Basal PRA and plasma aldosterone concentrations were similar in hypertensive patients and in control subjects. Infusion of ANP suppressed PRA in both groups, reaching statistical significance ($p < 0.05$) only in control subjects. On the other hand plasma aldosterone concentrations decreased significantly in both the hypertensive patients and in control subjects suggesting a direct inhibitory effect of ANP on adrenal aldosterone secretion. In contrast, in both groups of subjects ANP-infusion did not significantly affect plasma concentrations of vasopressin. These findings are in accordance with previous experiments [22, 23]. Urinary adrenaline and noradrenaline excretion, which was only slightly higher in hypertensive patients during the control period, was reduced in hypertensive patients and in control subjects during α-hANP infusion.

In summary, we have shown that low-dose i.v. administration of synthetic α-hANP results in a significant BP reduction accompanied by a marked increase in GFR, diuresis and natriuresis in normotensive and in hypertensive subjects. The effects on BP and on renal excretory function were significantly more pronounced in hypertensive patients than in controls and an increase in RPF associated with a decrease in renal vascular resistance was only observed in hypertensive patients. Blood pressure reduction by ANP may have been related first, to a direct vasorelaxant action, second. to intravascular volume contraction induced by ANP and third, to a reduction in sympathetic nervous activity and an inhibition of baroreceptor sensitivity.

The more pronounced effect of ANP on renal excretory function in our hypertensive patients probably resulted first, from direct hemodynamic effects of ANP, i.e. intrarenal vasodilation and intrarenal redistribution of blood flow as well as higher glomerular perfusion pressure and, second, possibly from an enhanced direct or indirect tubular action of ANP.

The apparently higher sensitivity of the renal vasculature to circulating ANP can not be explained by differing basal PRA, plasma concentration of vasopressin or catecholamine secretion but may reflect a higher sensitivity of renal ANP receptors. Alternatively, the higher renal vascular resistance in the presence of normal pressor hormone activities points to an enhanced receptor sensitivity towards these vasoactive hormones. Further studies are required to elucidate a potential difference in sensitivity of renal receptors to ANP and other circulating hormones between normotensive and hypertensive subjects.

Acknowledgments: This study was supported in part by grants from the Ministerium für Wissenschaft und Forschung des Landes Nordrhein-Westfalen, FRG (FA-8871 and IV A6-402-046-87).

The authors gratefully acknowledge the excellent technical assistance of Mrs. A. Bäcker and Mrs. H. Stelkens.

References

1. Arendt RM, Gerbes AL, Ritter D, Stangl E (1986) Molecular weight heterogeneity of plasma-ANF in cardiovascular disease. Klin Wochenschr 64 [Suppl VI]:97–102
2. Arendt RM, Ritter D, Gerbes AL, Stangl E, Bach P, Zaehringer J (1985) Elevated plasma levels of alpha atrial natriuretic factor in hypertensive patients (Abstract). Clin Exp Hypertension A8(1):132
3. Atlas SA, Laragh JH (1986) Atrial natriuretic peptide: a new factor in hormonal control of blood pressure and electrolyte homeostasis. Ann Rev Med 37:397–414
4. DeBold AJ, Borenstein HB, Veress AT, Sonnenberg H (1981) A rapid and potent natriuretic response to intravenous injection of atrial myocardial extract in rats. Life Sci 28:89–94
5. Larochelle P, Cusson JR, Gutkowska J, Schiffrin EL, Hamet P, Kuchel O, Genest J, Cantin M (1987) Plasma atrial natriuretic factor concentrations in essential and renovascular hypertension. Br Med J 294:1249–1252
6. Earle DP, Berliner RW (1946) A simplified clinical procedure for measurement of glomerular filtration rate and renal plasma

flow. Proceedings of the Society for Experimental Biology and Medicine 62, pp 262–269
7. Edwards BS, Schwab TR, Zimmermann RS, Heublein DM, Jiang NS, Burnett JC (1986) Cardiovascular, renal, and endocrine response to atrial natriuretic peptide in angiotensin II mediated hypertension. Circ Res 59:663–667
8. Glaenzer K, Prüßing B, Duesing R, Kramer HJ (1982) Hemodynamic and hormonal responses to 8-Arginine-Vasopressin in healthy man: effects of indomethacin. Klin Wochenschr 60:1234–1239
9. Gnaedinger MP, Lang RE, Hasler L, Uehlinger DE, Shaw S, Weidmann P (1986) Plasma kinetics of synthetic alpha-human atrial natriuretic peptide in man. Min Electrol Metab 12:371–374
10. Haber E, Koermer T, Page LB, Kliman B, Purnode A (1960) Application of a radioimmmunoassay for angiotensin I to the physiologic measurements of plasma renin activity in normal human subjects. J Clin Endocrinol Metab 29:1349–1355
11. Janssen WMT, deJong PE, van der Hem GK, et al. (1986) Effect of human atrial natriuretic peptide on blood pressure after sodium depletion in essential hypertension. Br Med J 293:351–353
12. Katsube N, Schwartz D, Needleman P (1986) Atriopeptin turnover: quantitative relationship between in vivo changes in plasma levels and atrial content. J Pharmacol Exp Ther 239:474–479
13. Kihara M, Nakayama K, Nakao K, Sugawara A et al. (1985) Accelerated natriuresis induced by synthetic atrial natriuretic polypeptide in spontaneously hypertensive rats. Clin Exp Theor Pract A7:539–551
14. Kohno M, Takaori K, Matsuura T, Murakawa K, Kanayama Y, Takeda T (1986) Atrial natriuretic polypeptide in atria and plasma in experimental hyperthyroidism and hypothyroidism. Biochem Biophys Res Commun 134:178–183
15. Kramer HJ (1988) Atrial Natriuretic Hormones. Gen Pharmac 19:747–753
16. Kramer HJ, Stinnesbeck B, Klautke G, Kipnowski J, Klingmueller D, Glaenzer K, Duesing R (1985) Interaction of renal prostaglandins with the renin-angiotensin and renal adrenergic nervous system in healthy subjects during dietary changes in sodium intake. Clin Sci 68:387–393
17. Lappe RW, Todt JA, Wendt RL (1987) Effects of atrial natriuretic factor on the vasoconstrictor actions of the renin-angiotensin system in conscious rats. Circ Res 61: 134–140
18. Larochelle P, Cusson JR, Gutkowska J, Schiffrin EL, Hamet P, Kuchel O, Genest J, Cantin M (1987) Plasma atrial natriuretic factor concentrations in essential and renovascular hypertension. Br Med J 294:1249–1252
19. Maack TM, Kleinert HD (1986) Renal and cardiovascular effects of atrial natriuretic factor. Biochem Pharmacol 35:2057–2064
20. Matsubara H, Yukihisa U, Yamane Y, Nishikawa M, Taniguchi T, Inada M (1987) Role of atrial natriuretic polypeptides for exaggerated natriuresis in essential hypertension. Am J Cardiol 60:708–714
21. Nakao K, Sugawara A, Morii N, Sakamoto M, Yamata T, Imura H (1986) The pharmacokinetics of alpha-human atrial natriuretic polypeptide in healthy subjects. Eur J Clin Pharmacol 31:101–103
22. Naruse M, Obana K, Naruse K, Yamaguchi H, Demura H, Inagami T, Shizume K (1987) Atrial natriuretic polypeptide inhibits cortisol secretion as well as aldosterone secretion in vitro from human adrenal tissue. J Clin Endocrinol Metab 64:10–16
23. Ogawa K, Arnolda LF, Woodcock EA, Hiwatari M, Johnston CI (1987) Lack of effect of atrial natriuretic peptide on vasopressin release. Clin Sci 72:525–530
24. Predel HG, Kipnowski J, Meyer-Lehnert H, Arendt RM, Kramer HJ (1989) Human atrial natriuretic peptide in non-dialyzed patients with chronic renal failure. Clin Nephrol 31:150–155
25. Proctor KG, Bealer SL (1987) Selective antagonism of hormone-induced vasoconstriction by atrial natriuretic factor in the rat microcirculation. Circ Res 61:42–49
26. Richards AM, Nicholls MG, Espiner EA, Ikram H, Yandle TG, Joyce SL, Cullens MM (1985) Effects of alpha-human atrial natriuretic peptide in essential hypertension. Hypertension 7:812–817
27. Sagnella GA, Markandu ND, Shore AC, MacGregor GA (1986) Raised circulating levels of atrial natriuretic peptide in essential hypertension. Lancet I:179–181
28. Steiner AL (1974) In: Hardman JG, O'Malley BW (eds) Methods of Enzymology, Vol 38. Academic Press, New York, p 96
29. Vetter W, Vetter H, Siegenthaler W (1973) Radioimmunoassay for aldosterone without chromatography: 2. Determination of plasma aldosterone. Acta Endocrinol 74:558–567
30. Volpe M, Sosa E, Mueller FB, Camargo MJF, Glorioso N, Laragh JH, Maack T, Atlas SA (1986) Differing hemodynamic responses to atrial natriuretic factor in two models of hypertension. Am J Physiol 250:871–878

31. Wambach G, Goetz S, Suckau G, Boenner G, Kaufmann W (1987) Plasma levels of atrial natriuretic peptide are raised in essential hypertension during low and high sodium intake. Klin Wochenschr 65:232–237

32. Weidmann P, Gnaedinger MP, Zisweiler HR, et al. (1986) Cardiovascular, endocrine and renal effects of atrial natriuretic peptide in essential hypertension. J Hypertension 4 [Suppl 2]:71–83

Atrial Natriuretic Peptide in Pulmonary Embolism

T. T. van Loenhout[1], A. C. I. T. L. Tan[2], H. S. Tan[1], P. W. C. Kloppenborg[3], and Th. J. Benraad[3]

[1] Department of Medicine, Canisius Wilhelmina Hospital, Nijmegen, the Netherlands
[2] Department of Experimental and Chemical Endocrinology
[3] Division of Clinical Endocrinology, Department of Medicine, University of Nijmegen, Nijmegen, the Netherlands

Key words: ANP – Pulmonary embolism

Atrial Natriuretic Peptide (ANP) is secreted from the heart in response to increased atrial pressure and diameter [1]. One can therefore expect elevated plasma levels of ANP in patients with acute obstruction of the pulmonary bloodflow as in pulmonary embolism. We hypothesized that during dissolution of the embolus, ANP levels would decrease.

Therefore we followed ANP levels in 12 patients with proven pulmonary embolism. Diagnosis was made on the basis of acute dyspnoea, chest pain attached to the respiration and a marked obstruction of the blood flow on technetium scintigraphy. In addition, 5 patients with peripheral venous thrombosis were followed. As peripheral venous thrombosis is not associated with increased atrial pressures, we expected no change in ANP levels in these patients. Furthermore the plasma renin activity (PRA) and the aldosterone levels were measured to study the interrelationships between these three hormones.

Both groups received the same therapy, consisting of heparin during the first 7 days, followed by oral anticoagulants. Blood samples were collected daily (at 8 a.m.) from all patients (supine position) for up to 11 days after admission. After prior extraction of the plasma on Seppak C-18 cartridges, ANP was measured in a non-equilibrium assay using a highly specific antibody raised in sheep and a well defined monoiodotyrosyl tracer [2]. Sensitivity of the assay was 4 pg/ml plasma, recovery averaged 96%. Intra- and interassay coefficients of variation were 8.6 and 11.6% respectively. Normal values ranged from 8 to 77 pg/ml (mean $\pm$ SD = 34 $\pm$ 15, n = 61).

For each patient the Spearman correlation coefficient (c.c.) was calculated. After normalisation the mean and the 95% confidence interval (95% C.I.) of the normalized c.c. were calculated.

Although initial values of ANP varied widely, the subsidence of clinical signs and symptoms of pulmonary embolism was attended with consistent changes in both plasma ANP and PRA levels. ANP significantly decreased during treatment (mean c.c. -0.68, $p < 0.01$, 95% C.I.: -0.30 to -1.0), while concomitantly the plasma renin activity rose (mean c.c. $+0.68$, $p < 0.01$, 95% C.I.: $+0.10$ to $+1.0$) (Fig. 1). In the patients with peripheral venous thrombosis no consistent changes were detected, neither in ANP nor in PRA. No consistent change in plasma aldosterone was observed in either group of patients.

Acute pulmonary embolism can increase the pressure on the right side of heart [3] and thereby provide a stimulus to the secretion

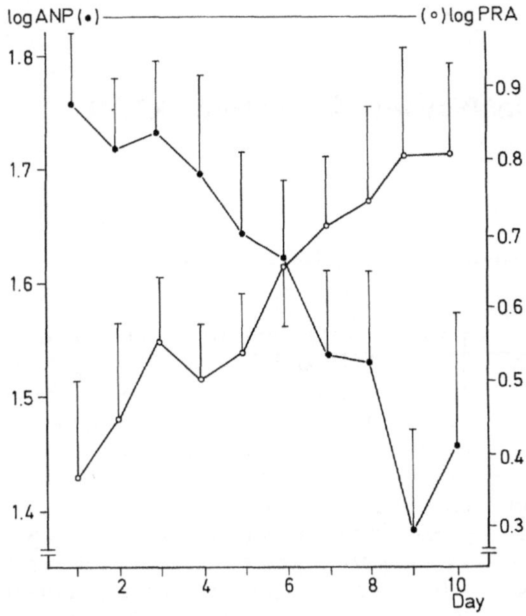

Fig. 1. Reciprocal changes in ANP (pg/ml) and PRA (nmol/l/h) levels during treatment of pulmonary embolism. Bars denote mean ± SEM

of ANP. We hypothesized that the dissolution of a pulmonary embolus will generally lead to restitution of normal intra-cardiac pressures and thereby to normal values of ANP. The decrease of ANP during treatment of pulmonary embolism confirms this hypothesis, and the observed absence of a similar decrease in a few patients with peripheral venous thrombosis is in agreement with it.

Therefore, we propose that measurements of ANP-levels could be of value in assessing the decline of pulmonary blood flow obstruction in patients with pulmonary embolism.

References

1. Raine AEG, Erne P, Burgisser E et al. (1986) Atrial natriuretic peptide and atrial pressure in patients with congestive heart failure. N Engl J Med 315:533–537
2. Rosmalen FMA, Tan ACITL, Tan HS, Benraad ThJ (1987) A sensitive radioimmunoassay of atrial natriuretic peptide in human plasma, using a tracer with an immobilized glycouril agent. Clin Chim Acta 165:331–340
3. McIntyre KM, Sasahara AA (1971) The hemodynamic response to pulmonary embolism in patients without prior cardiopulmonary disease. Am J Cardiol 28:289–294

A Cross-Sectional Study of Atrial Natriuretic Peptide (ANP) in Renal Transplant Recipients

C. J. Doorenbos and P. van Brummelen

Department of Nephrology and Hypertension, University Hospital Leiden, The Netherlands

Key words: – Age factors – Atrial natriuretic peptide – Blood pressure – Kidney transplantation

Introduction

The sodium- and volume-homeostasis in renal transplant recipients is maintained despite their use of prednisone for immunosuppression and despite denervation of the transplant. So far the role of ANP in this condition is unknown. Therefore we measured plasma ANP levels in these patients and investigated the relation of the results with relevant clinical parameters.

Patients and Methods

56 patients, 32 males and 24 females, age 18 to 66 years with a stable renal function, were studied 3 weeks to 16 1/2 years after transplantation. Immunosuppression consisted of prednisone combined with cyclosporine, azathioprine or both. 43 patients were on antihypertensive treatment. Plasma ANP was measured with a radioimmunoassay after Sep-Pak C-18 extraction [1]. Statistical analysis was done by multiple regression analysis. Because of a non-normal distribution log ANP was used for calculations. Student's unpaired t-test was used to assess the influence of immunosuppressive and antihypertensive therapy.

Results

The mean values (± SD) for blood pressure were 143 ± 23 mmHg systolic and 87 ± 12 mmHg diastolic. The creatinine clearance was 54 ± 23 ml/min and the urinary sodium excretion was 152 ± 68 mmol/24 h. The plasma levels of ANP ranged between 1 and 941 pg/ml, median 15, mean 85 pg/ml. A positive correlation was found between plasma ANP and both age of the patients ($r = 0.436$, $p < 0.001$) and systolic blood pressure ($r = 0.438$, $p < 0.001$), but not with diastolic blood pressure ($r = 0.233$, n.s.). Plasma ANP correlated negatively with creatinine clearance ($r = -0.490$, $p < 0.001$) and with sodium intake based upon 24 hours urinary excretion ($r = -0.401$, $p < 0.01$). There was no significant effect of immunosuppresive or antihypertensive therapy on the plasma level of ANP except that users of diuretics had higher ANP levels ($p < 0.001$). They were older ($p < 0.02$), and had a lower sodium intake ($p < 0.002$) and creatinine clearance ($p < 0.001$).

Discussion

We found that plasma ANP correlated positively with both age and systolic blood pressure, similar to normal subjects [2]. The creatinine clearance was negatively correlated with plasma ANP, probably due to both hypervolaemia and diminished ANP clearance [3]. The negative correlation between plasma ANP and urinary sodium excretion was surprising, since normal subjects had higher ANP levels at a higher sodium intake [4]. However, our patients with a lower sodium intake had a worse renal function (creatinine clearance correlated with sodium excretion: $r = 0.634$, $p < 0.001$), and possibly their sodium intake was not restricted sufficiently to prevent hypervolaemia.

Unexpectedly, users of diuretics had higher plasma ANP levels. This may be due to the fact that these patients were older and had a worse renal function. However, hydrochlorothiazide has been reported to raise plasma ANP levels in hypertensives [5], suggesting a direct effect of diuretics on plasma ANP levels. In conclusion, the present study indicates, that in renal transplant recipients the influence of age, systolic blood pressure and renal function on plasma ANP levels is preserved despite renal denervation and immunosuppression.

References

1. Doorenbos CJ, Daha MR, Van Brummelen P (1987) Radioimmunoassay for determination of atrial natriuretic peptide in human plasma. Pharm Weekblad Scientific Ed 9:189
2. Sagnella GA, Markandu HD, Shore AC, MacGregor GA (1986) Raised circulating levels of atrial natriuretic peptides in essential hypertension. Lancet I:179–181
3. Saxenhofer H, Gnaedinger MP, Weidmann P, et al. (1987) Plasma levels and dialysance of atrial natriuretic peptide in terminal renal failure. Kidney Int 32:554–561
4. Shenker Y, Sider RS, Ostafin EA, Grekin RJ (1985) Plasma levels of immunoreactive atrial natriuretic factor in healthy subjects and in patients with edema. J Clin Invest 76:1684–1687
5. Chalmers JP, Wing LMH, West MJ, et al. (1986) Effects of enalapril and hydrochlorothiazide on blood pressure, renin-angiotensin system, and atrial natriuretic factor in essential hypertension: a double blind factorial cross-over study. Austr New Zealand J Med 16:475–480

ANP and Pregnancy

Artrial Natriuretic Peptide Concentrations in Preeclampsia

F. Casper[1], R. Seufert[1], and R. E. Lang[2]

[1] Department of Obstetrics and Gynecology, University of Mainz, FRG
[2] German Institute for High Blood Pressure Research, University of Heidelberg, FRG

Key words: Pregnancy induced hypertension – Preeclampsia

Introduction

During pregnancy various humoral and functional mechanisms were recognized, that regulate the water and electrolyte household. In preeclampsia, increased water-sodium retention results from a variety of pathophysiological changes in the endocrinological system. There are also organ-specific changes, such as renal clearance reduction up to 30% in comparison to normal pregnancy. For many years, physiologists expected to find additional cardial mechanisms that influence homeostasis. In 1981, de Bold [3] identified ANP a new humoral factor that leads to increased water and sodium excretion. The influence of ANP in preeclampsia has been the subject of controversial discussion.

Patients and Methods

For the past year we have been performing a prospective matched – pair study on preeclamptic women and pregnant women with normal blood pressure. Mean age (26 years), parity and week of gestation were similar in both groups. Patients were diagnosed as preeclamptic and classified according to the criteria of the American College of Obstetricians and Gynecologists [4]. In the normotensive group clinical cardiological examination and ECG ruled out cardial diseases. None of these were taking medications other than iron or vitamin supplements. Observation period was between the 34th and 39th week's gestation. Blood samples were drawn from a peripheral vein and kept in chilled EDTA plastic tubes until separation of plasma by centrifugation at 4 °C. After centrifugation each sample was stored at −78 °C. Plasma ANP concentrations were determined by a radioimmunoassay. This test was performed using an antibody generated in NZW rabbits immunized with alpha-h ANP coupled to bovine thyroglobulin [9, 10].

Results

In the normotensive group plasma concentration was 15.3 ∓ 3.57 (SEM) pg/ml, in the hypertensive group 45.5 ∓ 7.62 (SEM) pg/ml. One week after delivery plasma concentration was almost simular in both collectives: normotensive = 16.2 ∓ 1.75 (SEM) and hypertensive = 17.8 ∓ 5.11 (SEM) pg/ml.

Figure 1 shows the average concentration of plasma ANP in weekly intervals. Levels are measured 3 weeks before delivery and one week post partum. ANP/hematocrit ratio proved to be significant, while correlation was higher in the normotensive group (preeclampsia: $r = 0.69$; normotensive: $r = 0.74$; $p < 0.05$).

Discussion

The physiological adjustments in normal pregnancy include an increase in plasma volume, renal plasma flow, glomerular filtration rate and a decrease in total peripheral resistance. As atrial natriuretic peptide (ANP) is involved in the control of plasma volume most studies confirmed that concentrations are increased during pregnancy [2, 8]. Cowan [1] even reported of two subsets of patients with preeclampsia who could be identified on the basis of ANP levels alone

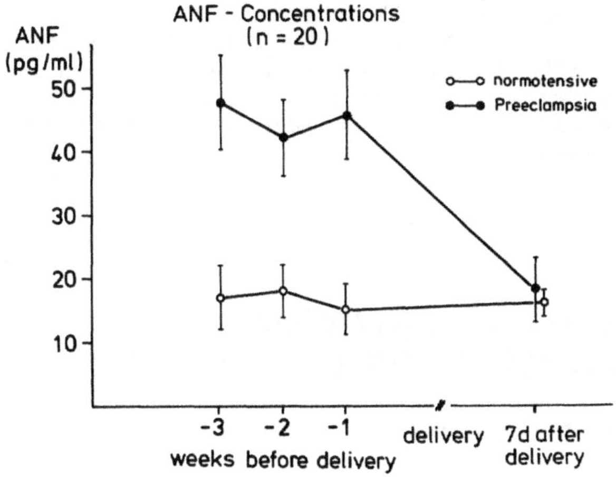

Fig. 1. Plasma ANP-levels in preeclamptic and normotensive pregnant women in weekly intervals

before the clinical parameters occurred. In contrary to the above results Rutherford [6] reported no significant rise in plasma ANP throughout the second and third trimester. In contrast, pregnancies complicated by preeclampsia are associated with a reduction of plasma volume and central venous pressure [8]. Nevertheless our results showed increased concentration of ANP. In one woman with preeclampsia, who presented with severe blood pressure rise and markly intravascular volume depletion ANP levels were found which were nearly threefold in contrast to average levels in the preeclamptic group. According to our results Niesert [5] found a positive correlation between the increase of plasma ANP in normotensive pregnant women and the increase in diastolic blood pressure after infusion of angiotensin II. Within several days after delivery women with pregnancy induced hypertension presented with normal blood pressure. Post partum similar ANP levels in women with normotensive and hypertensive blood pressure during pregnancy were observed [7]. Factors that regulate ANP secretion during pregnancy and the reasons for increased values in preeclampsia are still unclear. The aim of our prospective study is to identify further pathophysiological parameters, in particular prostaglandines, and to determine the value of ANP in this clinical entity.

References

1. Cowan BD, Martin JN, Tucker JM, Martin RW, Morrison JC, Kikokawa T, Mukhergèe AB (1988) High plasma concentrations of human atrial natriuretic polypeptide in women with pregnancy – induced hypertension. Proceedings ISSHP, Montreal, p 45
2. Cusson JR, Gutkowska J, Rey E, Mickon N, Boucher M, Larochelle P (1985) Plasma concentration of atrial natriuretic factor in normal pregnancy. N Engl J Med 313: 1230–1231
3. De Bold AJ, Borenstein HB, Veress AT, Sonnenberg H (1981) A rapid and potent natriuretic response to intravenous injection of atrial myocardial extract in rats. Life Sci 28:89–94
4. Eastmann J, Bell ST, Dieckmann WJ (1952) Definition and classification of toxaemias brought up to date. American Committee on Maternal Welfare, Chicago
5. Niesert S, Günter HH, Kaulhausen H (1987) Atrial natriuretic peptidide during pregnancy. Lancet II:404–405
6. Rutherford AJ, Anderson JV, Elder MG, Bloom SR (1987) Release of atrial natriuretic peptide during pregnancy and immediate puerperium. Lancet I:928–929
7. Steegers EA, Tan AC, Coumans HJ, Benraad TJ, Groeneveld EA, Jongsma HW, Hein PR (1988) Atrial natriuretic peptide, aldosterone, plasma renin activity and diuresis in puerperium. Proceedings JSSHP, Montreal, p 46
8. Thomsen JK, Storen TL, Thambsborg G, De Nully M, Bodker B, Skouby S (1987) Atrial

natriuretic peptide concentrations in pre-eclampsia. Br Med J 294:1508–1510
9. Weidmann P, Hasler L, Gnädinger MP, Lang RE, Uehlinger DE, Shaw S, Rascher W, Renbi FC (1986) Blood levels and renal effects of atrial natriuretic peptide in normal man. J Clin Invest 77:734–742
10. Weil J, Bidlingmaier F, Döhlemann C, Kühnle V, Strom T, Lang RE (1986) Comparison of plasma atrial natriuretic peptide levels in healthy children from birth to adolescence and in children with cardiac diseases. Pediatr Res 20:1328–1331

Renal and Hormonal Reactions During Water Imnmersion in Healthy Pregnant Women and Patients with EPH-Gestosis

W. Schnizer[1], M. Mesrogli[2], A. L. Gerbes[3], R. M. Arendt[4], H. Knorr[1], P. Schöps[1], M. Waßmann[2], and J. Schneider[2]

[1] Institute of Medical Balneology and Climatology, University of Munich, FRG
[2] Department of OB/GYN, University of Hannover, FRG
[3] Department of Medicine II, Klinikum Großhadern, University of Munich, FRG
[4] Department of Medicine I, Klinikum Großhadern, University of Munich, FRG

Key words: Atrial natriuretic factor – Water immersion – EPH-gestosis – Renal excretion – Renin – Aldosterone

Introduction

Head-out water immersion (WI) increases central venous and atrial volume by shifting blood from peripheral vessels to the intrathoracic venous bed. Because of stimulation of central low pressure and volume receptoprs there is an influence in hemodynamic and renal regulations. Thus thermoneutral WI results in a progressive diuresis, natriuresis and kaliuresis; concerning hormonal reactions WI leads to a decrease of antidiuretic hormone (ADH), renin and aldosterone in the blood (for Rev. see [4]). Furthermore it could be demonstrated in a previous study, that WI stimulates atrial natriuretic factor (ANF) in man [5] and thus seems to be a useful mean to study the physiological role of ANF in acute volume regulation.

In pregnancy there are changes in the control of extracellular water and electrolyte homeostasis and therefore it may be of interest to look at the responses of healthy pregnant women and patients with EPH-gestosis in a standardized water bath, regarding renal functions, plasma volume, renin, aldosterone and especially the atrial natriuretic factor.

Methods

Experiments were done with 27 women (group I [n = 13]: no pathological symptoms; group II [n = 14]: EPH-gestosis) after obtaining their informed consent. At the time of the studies the women were pregnant between the 28th and the 38th week. Furthermore a group (n = 9) of healthy non-pregnant women were investigated concerning ANF. The subjects were on an ordinary diet; alcohol, tobacco, tea and coffee were forbidden at the day of the experiment. The procedure consisted of a 40 min control period, followed by a 40 min bath (35 °C) and a 40 min recovery period. Blood samples drawn from a brachial vein by means of a butterfly needle were analysed for ANF (radio-immuno-assay with XAD-extracted plasma [1]), plasma renin activity (PRA) and aldosterone (commercial kits). Urine samples were collected after every period for determinations of urine output, sodium and potassium (flame photometry), creatinine (Jaffe reaction) and osmolality (freezing point depression). Changes of the hematocrit allowed the calculation of changes in the plasma volume. If necessary patients received medication. Data are given as means and standard errors of the mean.

Results

As can be seen in Fig. 1, WI significantly increased ANF plasma levels in all three groups. After 40 minutes there was an increase of about 50–70%. In the recovery period the hormone decreased with tendency to baseline levels. Neither basal nor stimulated values showed statistical differences between the groups. Only three pregnant women didn't respond.

WI was followed by a significant decrease in PRA and aldosterone. The drop in plasma levels was similar in the groups. No relationship between these hormonal changes and ANF could be found.

There were distinct effects of WI concerning renal excretion. Urinary flow rate was enhanced to 3 or 4 times of controls. Mean values of sodium and potassium excretion were increased, too. The gestosis-group showed lower basal values for sodium and significantly higher excretion rates after WI compared to the healthy pregnant women. Correspondingly there was an increase in fractionated excretions. In all groups WI resulted in increased osmotic and free water clearance. Creatinine clearance reached significantly higher values only in the gestosis group. During WI rises of plasma volume of about 8 or 9% could be demonstrated.

Discussion

A striking change in hemodynamics occurs in women during pregnancy and some 900 mmol sodium progressively accumulates and total body water increases by 6 to 8 liters, distributed amongst the fetus, the placenta and enlarged maternal blood and interstitial fluid volumes. Abnormalities of sodium and water balance are thought to be connected with diseases such as pre-eclampsia. On the other side pregnancies complicated by pre-eclampsia are associated with a reduction of plasma volume and central venous pressure. Furthermore the renin-aldosterone axis is involved in circulatory regulation and water and electrolyte balance.

Some authors demonstrated an elevation of plasma ANF levels during normal pregnancy and much higher levels in patients suffering from EPH-gestosis [2, 7, 8, 10]. Higher ANF levels in normal pregnancy were thought to be a consequence of the increased blood volume. Other results suggest that plasma ANF levels are normal in women during uncomplicated pregnancy [6, 3]. In our studies the basal values didn't show any significant differences between the groups.

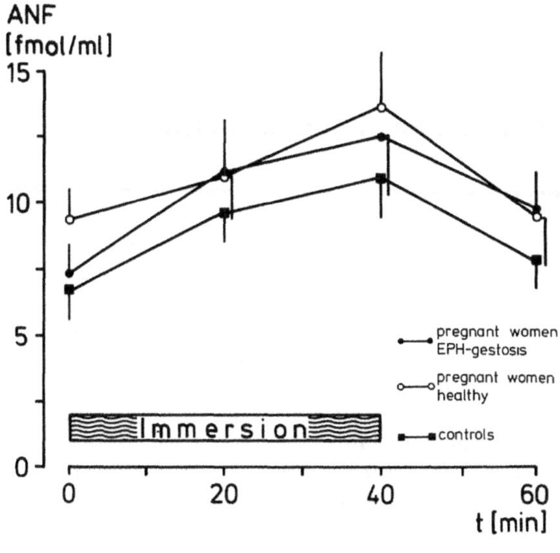

Fig. 1. Behaviour of plasma ANF during and after thermoneutral water immersion in healthy pregnant women, patients with EPH-gestosis and non-pregnant controls

There is the question if the trigger mechanisms of ANF secretion are less sensitive to central blood volume changes in pregnancy and uncomplicated pregnancy. Results from investigations with the WI model published Doniec-Ulman et al. [3] are consistent with this hypothesis. They documented a less stimulation rate for ANF in healthy pregnant women and women with moderate EPH-gestosis as compared to non-pregnant controls. Contrary to this we found comparable values of stimulated ANF during WI in all groups. We didn't observe any changes in the slope of the ANF-increases. That might not indicate a desensitisation of ANF secretion. Also an intact ANF-system seems to be necessary to normalize the water and electrolyte balance in the postnatal period [9]. However, statements about the WI-induced maximum concentrations of ANF cannot be given by our studies. Renin and aldosterone showed the decrease which is known in immersion physiology.

References

1. Arendt RM, Gerbes AL, Ritter D, Stangl E (1986) Molecular weight heterogeneity of plasma-ANF in cardiovascular disease. Klin Wochenschr 6 [Suppl VI]:97–102
2. Cusson JR, Gutkowska J, Rey E, Michon N, Boucher M, Larochelle P (1985) Plasma concentration of atrial natriuretic factor in normal pregnancy. N Engl J Med 313: 1230–1231
3. Doniec-Ulman I, Kokot F, Wambach G, Drab M (1987) Water immersion-induced endocrine alterations in women with EPH gestosis. Clin Nephrol 28:51–55
4. Epstein M (1978) Renal effects of head-out water immersion in man: implications for an understanding of volume homeostasis. Physiol Rev 58:529–581
5. Gerbes AL, Arendt RM, Schnizer W, Silz S, Jüngst D, Zähringer J, Paumgartner G (1986) Regulation of atrial natriuretic factor release in man: effect of water immersion. Klin Wochenschr 64:666–667
6. Hirai N, Yanaihara T, Nakayama T, Ishibashi M, Yamaji T (1988) Plasma levels of atrial natriuretic peptide during normal pregnancy and in pregnancy complicated by hypertension. Am J Obstet Gynecol 159: 27–31
7. Miyamoto S, Shimokawa H, Sumioki H, Tuono A, Nakano H (1988) Circadian rhythm of plasma atrial natriuretic peptide, aldosterone and blood pressure during the third trimester in normal and preeclamptic pregnancies. Am J Obstet Gynecol 158: 393–399
8. Otsuki Y, Okamoto E, Iwata I, Nishino E, Mitsuda N, Mori M, Takagi T, Sugita N, Tanizawa O (1987) Changes of concentration of human atrial natriuretic peptide in normal pregnancy and toxaemia. J Endocrin 114: 325–328
9. Rutherford AJ, Anderson JV, Elder MG, Bloom SR (1987) Release of atrial natriuretic peptide during pregnancy and immediate puerperium. Lancet I:928–929
10. Thomsen JK, Storm TL, Thamsborg G, de Nully M, Bodker B, Skouby S (1987) Atrial natriuretic peptide concentrations in preeclampsia. Br Med J 294:1508–1510

Atrial Natriuretisches Peptid vor und nach der Entbindung

H. H. Günter, G. Toboll, and St. Niesert

Frauenklinik der Medizinischen Hochschule Hannover im Krankenhaus Oststadt, FRG

Summary. In 12 women the ANP-concentration was determined before and after the delivery. The results were compared with the ANP levels of non pregnant women. A significant difference was shown between the ANP concentration of pregnant (94.4 ± 49.6 pg/ml) and non pregnant women (42.2 ± 20.4 pg/ml; $p < 0.001$). Post partum a significant decrease was observed (67.3 ± 34.4 pg/ml; $p < 0.05$). The changes of the ANP concentration after delivery could be responsible for the diuresis and weight loss post partum.

Kew yords: Human Atrial Natriuretic Peptide – Pregnancy – Delivery

Einleitung

Während der Schwangerschaft kommt es zu einem Anstieg der Herzfrequenz, der Gesamtblutmenge und des Herzzeitvolumens, andererseits nimmt die Angiotensin-Sensibilität ab. Studien über Konzentrationsveränderungen des ANP während der Schwangerschaft im Wochenbett kommen zum Teil zu widersprüchlichen Ergebnissen. In dieser Studie sollten die ANP-Konzentrationen unmittelbar vor und nach der Entbindung sowie die ANP-Spiegel im Nabelschnurblut ermittelt werden.

Material und Methode

Bei 12 Frauen wurde die ANP-Konzentration vor der Geburt und am ersten Tag des Wochenbetts untersucht und mit derjenigen von vierzehn nicht schwangeren Frauen verglichen. Ebenfalls wurde der ANP-Spiegel im venösen (n = 12) und arteriellen (n = 5) Nabelschnurblut bestimmt. Alle Patientinnen waren normoton, hatten keine ernsten Vor- und Nebenerkrankungen und nahmen, abgesehen von Eisen- und Vitamin-Präparaten, keine Medikamente zu sich. Die Patientinnen wurden zwischen der 38. und 42. SSW entbunden (10 Spontangeburten, zwei Kaiserschnitte). Das mittlere Geburtsgewicht der Kinder betrug 3572 ± 520 g. Die Blutabnahme erfolgte in 5 ml EDTA-Röhrchen, die den Proteinase-Inhibitor Aprotinin enthielten (1000 KIU/ml). Nach dem Zentrifugieren und Pipettieren der Proben wurden sie bei einer Temperatur von −26 °C bis zur Analyse gelagert. Die Bestimmung des ANP erfolgte mit einem direkten Radioimmunoassay (IBL GmbH Hamburg). Die statistischen Analysen wurden mittels Wilcoxon-Test durchgeführt.

Ergebnisse

Der präpartale ANP-Wert lag hochsignifikant ($p < 0{,}001$) über demjenigen der nicht schwangeren Frauen (94,4 ± 49,6 pg/ml gegenüber 42,2 ± 20,4 pg/ml) und gleichfalls signifikant ($p < 0{,}05$) über der postpartalen ANP-Konzentration (67,3 ± 34,4 pg/ml; x ± SD). Eine Korrelation zwischen mütterlichen ANP-Werten und dem mütterlichen Gewicht zum Zeitpunkt der Geburt und zur Gewichtszunahme während der Schwangerschaft bestand nicht. Ebenfalls ließ sich keine Korrelation zum systolischen und diastolischen Blutdruck sowie zur mütterlichen Plasma-Natrium- und Plasma-Kreatinin-Konzentration nachweisen.

In der Nabelschnurarterie (n = 5) konnte mit 68,2 ± 47,9 pg/ml ANP ein höherer Wert ermittelt werden als in der Nabelvene mit 44,4 ± 36,1 pg/ml.

Diskussion

In den bisher publizierten Voruntersuchungen werden für den Schwangerschaftsverlauf abnehmende [1], unveränderte [4] und auch ansteigende [3] ANP-Konzentrationen im mütterlichen Blut angegeben.

Steegers [5] und Rutherford [4] fanden einen Anstieg am 3. bis 5. postpartalen Tag. Rutherford begründete seine Ergebnisse mit der zu diesem Zeitpunkt zu beobachtenden Diurese. Gregoire [2] beschrieb eine signifikante Erhöhung des ANP-Spiegels im Schwangerschaftsverlauf, aber auch nach der Gravidität beobachtete er bis zum 90. Tag post partum einen weiteren Anstieg. Im Gegensatz zu diesen Arbeitsgruppen konnten wir eine signifikante Verminderung des ANP im Wochenbett feststellen. Unsere Ergebnisse könnten damit erklärt werden, daß der bereits nach der Geburt rapide einsetzende Abfall der Natrium- und Wasser-retinierenden Schwangerschaftshormone (z.B. Progesteron) zu einer Diurese führt und die niedrige ANP-Konzentration lediglich eine Reaktion auf diese physiologischen Vorgänge darstellt.

Bei der Untersuchung des Nabelschnurblutes wurden in dieser Studie in der Nabelarterie höhere ANP-Konzentrationen als in der Nabelvene festgestellt. Ähnliche Ergebnisse werden in der Literatur berichtet [3]. Ob es sich hierbei um einen Metabolismus des ANP in der Plazenta oder um einen Übertritt des kindlichen ANP in den mütterlichen Kreislauf handelt, ist nicht geklärt.

References

1. Andoh A, Tamura H, Igarashi M, Ichihawa S, Miyata A, Kaugawa K, Matsuo H (1986) Atrial natriuretic peptide and the renin-aldos-

terone system in normal pregnancy. 5th Congress Society for Study of Hypertension in Pregnancy, Nottingham
2. Gregoire I, El Esper N, Fournier A, Fievet P, Wesleel PF, De Bold A, Favre H (1988) Sequential study of plasma atrial natriuretic factor and urinary dopamine in normotensive pregnant women before and after delivery. 6th Congress Society for Study of Hypertension in Pregnancy, Montreal, p 2
3. Otsuki Y, Okamoto E, Iwata I, Nishino E, Mitsuda N, Mori M, Takagi I, Sugita N, Tanizawa O (1987) Changes in concentration of human atrial natriuretic peptide in normal pregnancy and toxaemia. J Endocr 114:325–328
4. Rutherford AJ, Anderson JV, Elder MO, Bloom SR (1987) Release of atrial natriuretic peptide during pregnancy and immediate puerperium. Lancet I:928–929
5. Steegers E, Tan A, Coumans H, Benraad T, Goeneveld E, Jongsma H, Hein P (1988) Atrial natriuretic peptide, aldosterone-plasma-renin-activity and diuresis in puerperium. 6th Congress Society for Study of Hypertension in Pregnancy, Montreal, p 22

ANP and Ca-Antagonists

Calcium-Calmodulinantagonists Influence Release of Cardiodilatin/ANP from Atrial Cardiocytes

K. Addicks, W. G. Forssmann, H. Henkel, U. Holthausen, V. Menz, G. Rippegather, and D. Ziskoven

Department of Anatomy, Universities of Cologne and Heidelberg, FRG

Key words: Calcium-calmodulin-antagonists – Cardiodilatin – ANP – Atrial cardiocytes

Introduction

Calcium influx induces not only contraction of cardiocytes, but seems also to be necessary for the storage and release of Cardiodilatin/ANP from atrial cardiocytes. Calciumantagonists like Verapamil, and Calcium-Clamodulinantagonists like Fendiline influence calcium influx and coupling to calmodulin in the cell, and facilitate chronotropy, inotropy and vasodilatation. Calciumantagonists influence as well secretion of endocrine glands. These observations prompted us to examine wether Verpamil and Fendiline induce changes in CDD/ANP content of atrial cardiocytes and release.

Methods

Following isolated perfusion of rat hearts according to v. Langendorff with Krebs-Henseleit solution for 20 min., Verapamil, Fendiline or BAY-K8644 were added to the perfusion solution for further 20 min.

For ultrastructural observations atrial myocardium was immediately removed and fixed with glutaraldehyde (3.5%). To demonstrate the intracellular content of calcium a calcium precipitation according to Poenie and Epel (1987) was applied.

Right atrial myocardium was prepared for immunohistochemical staining to demonstrate CDD/ANP in the tissue. Measurement of CDD/ANP was performed from effluate and tissue using a specific radioimmunoassay for CDD/ANP.

Results

Under the condition of the isolated cardiac perfusion stimuli for secretion of atrial peptides like atrial extension are excluded.

Following administration of Calciumantagonists like Verapamil or Calcium-Calmodulin-antagonists like Fendiline the atrial granula-containing perinuclear area enlarges. The same effect is observed ultrastructurally influenced by administration of Claciumagonists like BAY-K8644. The diameter of vesicles grows up under influence of Verapamil and Fendiline and demonstrates the blockade of secretion of atrial peptides, whilsts administration of BAY-K8644 raises up the amount of the small vesicles as well as of the larger ones. These observations give already the hint that BAY-K8644 accelerates the turn over of Cardiodilatin/ANP synthesis and secretion in atrial myocytes.

The immunohistochemical analysis confirm the ultrastructural observations. Influenced by Calciumantagonists like Verapamil or Calcium-Calmodulinantagonists like Fendiline a blockade of secretion leads to the increase of CDD/ANP in the tissue (analysed histochemically and biochemically), but decreases CDD/ANP in the effluate. Calciumagonists like BAY-K8644 induce an increase of CDD/ANP in the tissue and in contrast to the applied Clacium-Calmodulin-antagonists to an increase of CDD/ANP in the effluate.

References

Addicks K, Lenz U, Lehmann D, Dammrau R (1987) Der Effekt von Kalzium- und Calmodulinantagonisten auf den Katecholamingehalt kardialer Nervenfasern. In: Autonome Innervation des Herzens, Steinkopff, Darmstadt, S 109–115

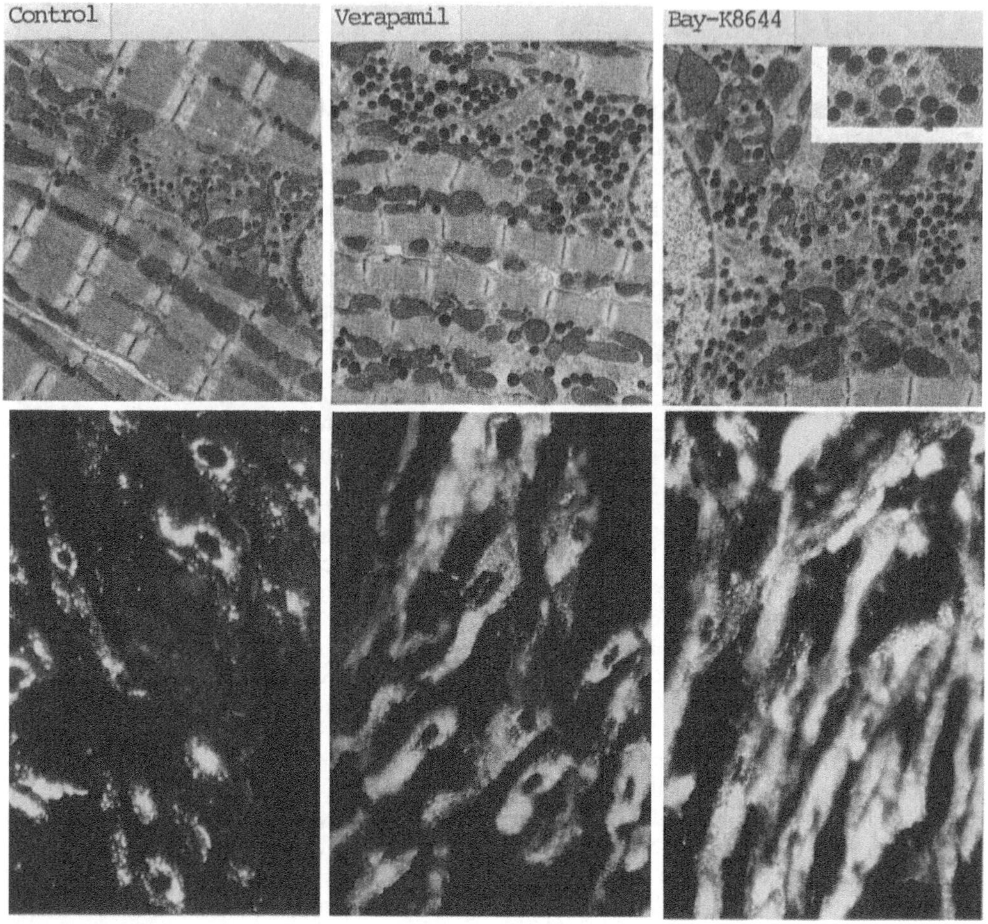

Fig. 1. Content of Cardiodilatin/ANP in effluate expressed in %

Time of perfusion	Control	Verapamil	Fendiline	BayK-8544
1 min.	100,0%	100,0%	100,0%	100,0%
3 min.	88,5	81,4	85,1	130,4
5 min.	85,2	83,7	84,3	130,9
15 min.	79,0	72,2	75,3	119,9
19 min.	85,0	40,4	57,3	102,1

Content of Cardiodilatin/ANP in right atrial myocardium in ng/g protein:

Control	Verapamil	Fendiline	BayK-8644
570 ± 96	1116 ± 43	1202 ± 87	1224,1 ± 488

Calcium-Calmodulin Antagonists Influence Content of Catecholamines in Cardiac Sympathetic Axons and Adrenal Medulla

K. Addicks, V. Menz, U. Holthausen, D. Ziskoven, C. Pikhard, W. Schänzer, and W. Rück

Department of Anatomy, University of Cologne, Department of Biochemistry, DSHS, Cologne and R&D Thiemann, Waltrop, FRG

Key words: Calcium-calmodulin-antagonists – Catecholamines – Cardiac sympathetic axons – Adrenal medulla

Introduction

The transmitter release from nerve endings depends on the presence of extracellular calcium and is influenced by administration of Calcium-Calmodulin Antagonists. An ideal object to study the calcium influence onto sympathetic nerve activity is the model of the isolated perfused heart.

Material and Methods

Hearts were taken in order to perfuse them isolated 3, 5, or 40 minutes according to v. Langendorff. We added Verapamil, Fendiline, Trifluorperazine, BAY-K8644 (1×10^{-6} molar) to the solvent. Thereafter the hearts were shockfrozen with a liquid nitrogen cooled Wollenberg clamp. The total catecholamine content of the right ventricle was analysed in using gaschromatographic masspectroscopy (GC/MS). Making precise assertion about state of function from sympathetic axons, we examined histochemically the intraaxonal catecholamine content by fluorescence microscopy with a picture-analysing system. The area of fluorescing nerve fibers expressed in percent of total screen is a measure of quantity for axonal stored catecholamines.

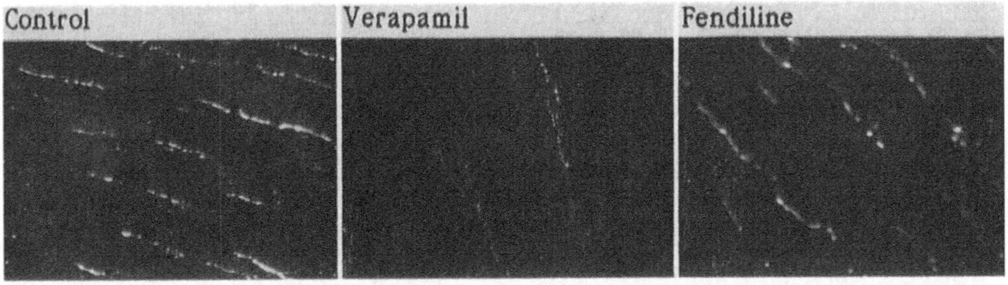

Fig. 1. Amount of fluorescing adrenergic nerve fibres:

	Control NACL	Verapamil 10^{-6}mol	Fendiline 10^{-6}mol
% of fluorescing fibers	1.14 ± 0.09% n = 9	0.47 ± 0.01% n = 6	0.83 ± 0.08% n = 5
noradrenaline in myocardium	705 ± 125 ng/g n = 13	526 ± 170 ng/g n = 15	522 ± 143 ng/g n = 15
noradrenaline in adrenal medulla	327 ± 72 μg/g n = 9	413 ± 38 μg/g n = 7	430 ± 96 μg/g n = 8
adrenaline in adrenal medulla	1303 ± 149 μg/g n = 9	1426 ± 147 μg/g n = 7	1427 ± 124 μg/g n = 8

n

Results

40 min. isolated perfusion without an addition of Ca^{++} antagonists does not reduce the amount of fluorescing sympathetic nerve fibres in the ventricular myocardium. After adding calciumantagonists like Verapamil, Calcium-Calmodulin antagonists like Fendiline and Calmodulin antagonists like Trifluorperazine a reduction of fluorescing catecholamines in the sympathetic nerve fibres is established. In contrast adding a calcium agonist to the perfusion solution the intraaxonal catecholamine content increases. Because catecholamines are relatively steady in the intracellular compartment the change of fluorescence is explained as change between intraaxonal and extraaxonal compartments. In analogy to this there is an increase of fluorescence in the background after adding calciumantagonists. The result is explained by membrane stabilisating effects of calciumantagonists and an inhibition of the membrane flow processes. For norepinephrine there is a reuptake of 80% after release. It follows that the reuptake is more inhibited by calciumantagonists than release. The calciumantagonist inhibits reuptake more than release. The data exhibit that the content of catecholamines in sympathetic nerves and in adrenal medulla is influenced by Verapamil or Fendiline in a compensatory manner. Corresponding to the concentration of applied Verapamil or Fendiline ($10^{-8}-10^{-5}$ mol) the amount of intraaxonal catecholamines decreases and the catecholamine content of adrenal medulla increases. Concentrations above 10^{-5} mol the membrane stabilizing effects of Verapamil but not of Fendiline stop the changes of content of catecholamines.

References

1. Addicks K, Lenz U, Lehmann D, Dammrau R (1987) Der Effekt von Kalzium- und Calmodulinantagonisten auf den Katecholamingehalt kardialer Nervenfasern. In: Autonome Innervation des Herzens. Steinkopff, Darmstadt, S 109–115

Beeinflußt Nifedipin die Sekretion von Atrialem Natriuretischem Peptid (ANP) während Wasserimmersion?

H. Meyer-Lehnert, C. Till, H.-G. Predel, and H. J. Kramer

Medizinische Universitäts-Poliklinik, Bonn, FRG

Are Nifedipine-Induced Alterations of Renal Excretory Function During Water Imersion Releated to Atrial Natriuretic Peptide (ANP)?

Summary. It is well known that calcium channel blockers affect renal hemodynamics and renal excretory function. On the other hand, it has been proposed that secretion of ANP may involve calcium (Ca)-dependent mechanisms. We investigated the effect of nifedipine (N) on renal function and ANP secretion during 2 hr head-out water immersion in six healthy volunteers (24 ± 2 yrs). The protocol was repeated with HWI alone and after N without HWI. Plasma ANP (fmol/ml) was stimulated by 1 hr HWI alone (27.30 ± 4.41 vs 7.75 ± 1.53, $p < 0.01$). N alone increased ANP at 1 hr (29.55 ± 5.90, $p < 0.01$ vs baseline). With HWI plus N, increase of ANP was higher than with HWI alone (46.0 ± 10.90 vs 27.30 ± 4.41, $p < 0.01$). Urinary cGMP (nmol/min) was increased with N alone (4.47 ± 0.51 vs 1.91 ± 0.37, $p < 0.01$), but there was no synergistic effect with HWI. Urine volume (ml/min) increased during HWI (3.08 ± 0.86 vs 1.91 ± 0.37) and with N alone (3.56 ± 0.33, $p < 0.01$ vs baseline). The effect of HWI plus N on urine volume was partially additive (6.93 ± 1.82, $p < 0.01$ vs HWI). Urinary sodium excretion (μmol/

min) was also enhanced by N alone (497 ± 87 vs 133 ± 27 baseline, $p < 0.05$) and the effect of N plus HWI was again partially additive when compared with HWI alone (870 ± 83 vs 255 ± 38, $p < 0.05$). N alone did not affect blood pressure, but during HWI, blood pressue was lower with N as compared to HWI alone (126 ± 2/71 ± 2 vs 136 ± 6/86 ± 2 mmHg, $p < 0.05$). The present data confirm HWI as a potent stimulus for ANP secretion. There appears to be an association of N-induced changes in renal excretory function with alterations of ANP secretion; N and HWI appear to have a partially additive effect. From the present study, however, there is no evidence for a specific effect of N on Ca-dependent mechanisms in ANP release.
Key words: Head-out water immersion – Atrial peptides – Calcium channel blockers

Einleitung

Über den Freisetzungsmechanismus von atrialen natriuretischen Peptiden (ANP) aus Cardiozyten ist bisher wenig bekannt. Es gibt Hinweise dafür, daß die ANP-Sekretion zumindest partiell von einem transmembranösen Calciumeinstrom abhängig ist (Nakamura et al. 1987) und daß Phospholipid-abhängige Mechanismen eine Rolle spielen (Sonnenberg und Veress 1984).

Untersuchungen über die Wirkung von Calciumantagonisten auf die ANP-Freisetzung beim Menschen haben zu offenbar widersprüchlichen Ergebnissen geführt. So wurde berichtet, daß Nifedipin bei gesunden Probanden und bei Hypertonikern zu einem Anstieg der Plasma-ANP führte (Shima et al. 1987). Andere Autoren dagegen beobachteten eine Suppression der ANP-Sekretion durch Verapamil (Haufe et al. 1987).

In der vorliegenden Studie sollte die Wirkung des Calciumantagonisten Nifedipin auf die durch Wasserimmersion stimulierte Freisetzung von endogenem ANP untersucht werden.

Methoden

Bei sechs gesunden Probanden (Alter 24 ± 2 Jahre) wurde eine Wasserimmersion von zwei Stunden mit jeweils einer einstündigen Basal- und einer einstündigen Erholungsphase durchgeführt. Nach 48 Stunden wurde die Wasserimmersion nach oraler Gabe von 10 mg Nifedipin wiederholt. Ferner erfolgte eine Gabe von Nifedipin ohne Immersion. Plasma-ANP-Spiegel, Urinausscheidung von ANP und cGMP im Plasma und im Urin wurden während der Basalphase, nach 30, 60 und 120 Minuten unter Immersion und während der Erholungsphase bestimmt. Plasma-ANP wurde nach der Methode von Kohno et al. (1986) extrahiert. Der ANP-Radioimmunoassay (RIA) wurde mit einem Antikörper gegen α-hANP und mit ^{125}J-α-hANP von Peninsula (St. Helens, UK) durchgeführt. cGMP wurde im Plasma und im Urin mit einem RIA-Kit von DRG (Marburg, FRG) bestimmt.

Ergebnisse

Abb. 1 zeigt den Verlauf der Plasma ANP-Konzentrationen in den drei Versuchsgruppen. Wasserimmersion stimulierte die Plasma-ANP-Spiegel nach 30, 60 und 120 Minuten; der höchste Wert wurde bereits nach 30 Minuten erreicht. Die Gabe von Nifedipin allein ging ebenfalls mit einer Erhöhung von ANP einher. Die Gabe von Nifedipin mit anschließender Immersion führte gegenüber der alleinigen Immersion nach 60 und 120 Minuten zu signifikant höheren ANP-Spiegeln.

Plasma-cGMP stieg unter Immersion (15,6 ± 1,1 vs 29,6 ± 2,4 pmol/ml, basal vs 60 min, $p < 0{,}01$), nach Gabe von Nifedipin jedoch nicht. Nifedipin hatte auch keinen Einfluß auf den durch Immersion induzierten cGMP-Anstieg (25,0 ± 1,9 pmol/ml).

Die Urinausscheidung von cGMP wurde durch Immersion allein nicht beeinflußt. Die Gabe von Nifedipin dagegen war von einer Erhöhung der cGMP-Ausscheidung begleitet (0,7 ± 0,1 nmol/min basal vs 4,5 ± 0,5 nmol/min nach 30 min, $p < 0{,}01$). Nifedipingabe mit anschließender Immersion führte nicht zu einer weiteren Erhöhung der cGMP-Ausscheidung.

Diskussion

Neben der bekannten Stimulation der ANP-Sekretion durch Wasserimmersion

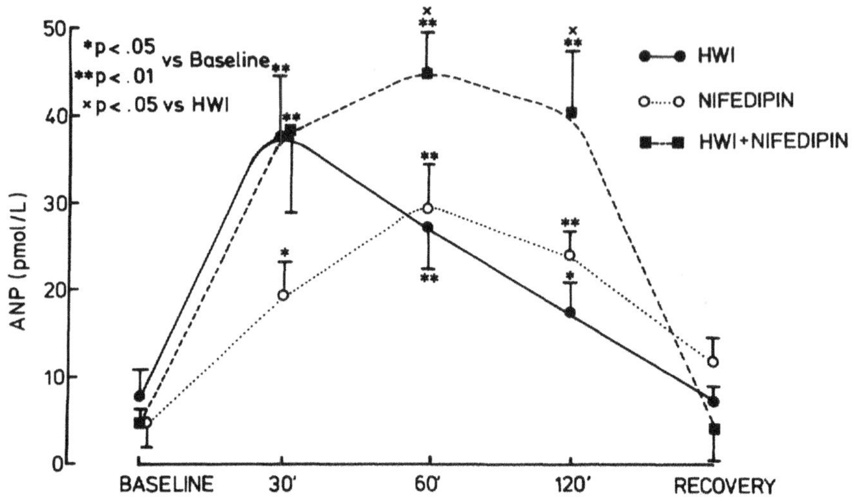

Abb. 1. Plasma ANP-Spiegel während Wasserimmersion (head-out water immersion, HWI), unter Nifedipin und während Wasserimmersion bei gleichzeitiger Nifedipingabe. (Baseline: einstündige Basalphase vor Immersion, Recovery: einstündige Erholungsphase nach Immersion)

(Müller et al. 1986) zeigten die vorliegenden Untersuchungen auch eine stimulierende Wirkung von Nifedipin auf die Plasma-ANP-Spiegel. Diese Befunde sind mit denen anderer Autoren vereinbar (Shima et al. 1987, Rapelli et al. 1987). Unsere Ergebnisse sprechen nicht für einen inhibitorischen Effekt von Nifedipin auf die ANP-Freisetzung, sondern vielmehr für eine protrahierte ANP-Freisetzung in Gegenwart des Calciumantagonisten während der Wasserimmersion.

Der durch Nifedipin induzierte Anstieg des Plama-ANP war nicht mit einem Anstieg des Plasma-cGMP, jedoch mit einer vermehrten Urinausscheidung von cGMP verbunden. Dies könnte auf einer unspezifischen Stimulation der renalen cGMP-Produktion und/oder -Exkretion beruhen. Diese Befunde bedürfen weiterer Klärung.

Unsere Ergebnisse deuten darauf hin, daß Wasserimmersion und die Gabe des Calciumantagonisten Nifedipin einen partiell additiven Effekt auf die Stimulation der ANP-Sekretion haben. Die Untersuchungen ergaben keinen Hinweis für einen direkten Effekt von Nifedipin auf calciumabhängige Mechanismen der ANP-Sekretion. Es ist möglich, daß die Wirkung von Nifedipin auf einer Veränderung der Hämodynamik des zentralen Blutvolumens beruht. In vitro-Studien an isolierten Cardiozyten könnten zu einer Klärung dieses Problems beitragen.

References

Haufe MC, Weil J, Ernst JE, Gerzer R, Theisen K (1987) Secretion of atrial natriuretic factor (ANF) is suppressed by verapamil and unaffected by atenolol in man. Circulation 76 [Suppl IV]:270 (Abs.)

Kohno M, Takaori K, Matsuura T, Murakawa K, Kanayama Y, Takeda T (1986) Atrial natriuretic polypeptide in atria and plasma in experimental hyperthyreodism and hypothyreodism. Biochem Biophys Res Commun 134:178–183

Müller FB, Erne P, Raine AEG, Bolli P, Linder L, Resink TJ, Cottier C, Bühler FR (1986) Atrial antipressor natriuretic peptide: release mechanisms and vascular actions in man. J Hypertension 4 [Suppl 2]:S109–S114

Nakamura N, Takeshita A, Hirooka Y, Imaizumi T, Nakamura M (1987) Mechanisms that mediate release of atrial natriuretic factor (ANF) during stretch. Circulation 76 [Suppl IV]:270 (Abs.)

Rapelli A, Dessi-Fulgheri P, Madeddu P, Glorioso N (1987) Studies on the natriuretic effect of nifedipine in hypertensive patients: increase in levels of plasma atrial natriuretic factor without

participation of the renal kallikrein-kinin system. J Hypertension 5 [Suppl 4]:S61–S65
Shima J, Ogihara T, Hara H, Iinuma K, Kumahara Y (1987) Effects of calcium antagonists on the secretion of atrial natriuretic peptide in normal volunteers. Curr Therap Res 42: 115–121
Sonnenberg H, Veress AT (1984) Cellular mechanism of release of atrial natriuretic factor. Biochem Biophys Res Commun 124:443–449

No Effects of Calcium Channel Blockers on the Secretion of Human Atrial Natriuretic Peptide: Studies with Nifedipine, Gallopamil and Flunarizine

L. Duntas, F. S. Keck, J. Rosenthal, U. Loos, and E. F. Pfeiffer

Abteilung Innere Medizin I, Medizinische Klinik und Poliklinik Universität Ulm, FRG

Key words: Calcium channel blockers – ANP

The secretion of atrial natriuretic peptide (ANP) is depended mainly by volume loading and atrial stretch. Different humoral factors such as acetylcholine, epinephrine, calcium and sodium ions stimulate the release of ANP [1, 2]. Medicaments which can alter the intracellular Ca^{++} may influence the secretion of ANP. It was the aim of this study to determine influences of selective and non selective calcium channel blockers on the secretion of human ANP.

Methods

Fifteen healthy subjects, aged 26–54 years (36 ± 11 mean ± SD) were studied. The subjects were randomised as follow: 1) Five subjects (Gr-1) received 10 mg Nifedipine (Adalat, Bayer AG, Leverkusen, FRG) sublingually. 2) Five subjects (Gr-2) received 50 mg Gallopamil p.o. (Procorum, Fa. Minden GmbH, FRG) and 3) Five subjects (Gr-3) received 5 mg Flunarazine p.o. (Sibelium, Jansen, Neuss, FRG). Blood samples were drawn, for measurements of plasma concentrations of ANP and total catecholamines (tCatx), at 0, 5, 20, and 30 min. for Gr-1 and at 0, 10, 30, and 60 min. for Gr-2 and Gr-3. Blood pression and heart frequency were monitored throughout the whole study. ANP was determined by a direkt RIA (Fa. IBL – Hamburg, FRG, normal range: 30–80 pg/ml). Catecholamines were determined also by means of a RIA-Kit (DRG, Marburg, FRG, normal range: 0–1200 pg/ml).

Results

All values are presented as mean ± SD. We could not observe any significant rise of plasma concentrations of ANP in any of studied groups. The levels of ANP were fluctuated between 33 ± 8 and 58 ± 10 pg/ml always within the normal range (Fig. 1). The highest ANP level (64 pg/ml) was documented 5 min. after nifedipine intake but still without statistical significance. The levels of total catecholamines were found between 647 and 914 pg/ml, also in normal range (Fig. 2). Blood pressure did not change significantly during the study. In contrary, heart rate was increased significantly ($p < 0.005$) thirty min. after sublingual administration of nifedipine (Table 1).

Statistical analysis was performed by Student's t-test.

Discussion

This study shows that acute administration of different calcium channel blockers failed to affect the secretion of atrial natriuretic peptide. The intake of nifedipine, one of the most potent dihydropyridines compounds, caused 30 min. after administration a significant increase of heart frequency. No significant reduction in blood pressure was ob-

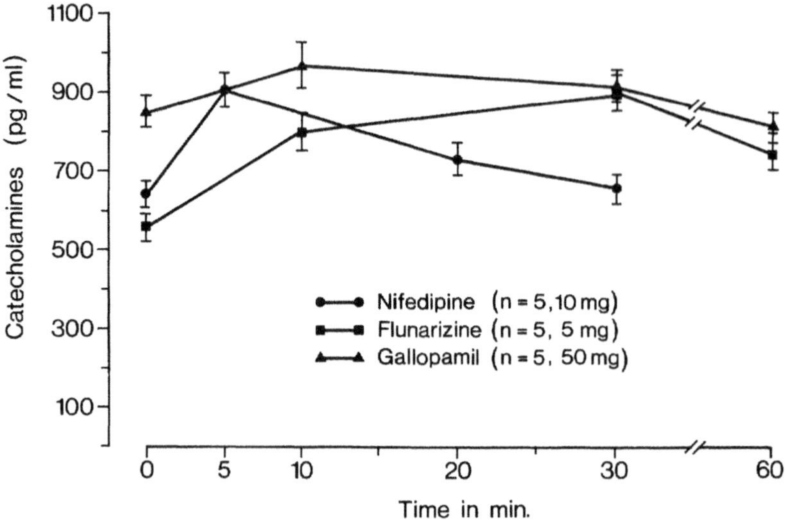

Fig. 1. Plasma ANP levels after sublingual administration of nifedipine and oral administration of gallopamil and flunarizine. The values are presented as mean ± SD

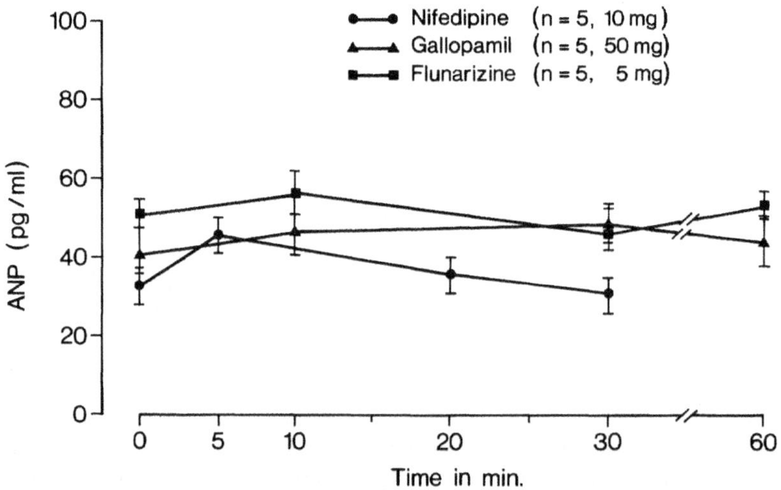

Fig. 2. Plasma catecholamines after sublingual administration of nifedipine and oral administration of gallopamil and flunarizine. The values are presented as mean ± SD

Table 1. Changes in heart rate after intake of nifedipine (10 mg), gallopamil (50 mg) and flunarizine (5 mg) in 15 healthy subjects. Data are expressed as mean ± SD

	Time in min					
	0	5	10	20	30	60
Nifedipine (10 mg)	64 ± 7	71 ± 5	68 ± 5	72 ± 6	78 ± 7[a]	–
Gallopamil (50 mg)	60 ± 6	–	64 ± 7	68 ± 6	60 ± 5	62 ± 7
Flunarizine (5 mg)	61 ± 7	–	66 ± 4	62 ± 5	60 ± 6	66 ± 7

[a] = $p < 0.005$

served. The increase of heart rate can be explained partly by the negative inotropic effect of the drug and partly by the reflex sympathetic drive due to baroreceptor stimulation. The levels of total catecholamines remained in normal range and this may indicate that after nifedipine administration, the stimulation of sympathetic nervous system is not prominent in volunteers compared to patients with coronary artery disease or patients pretreated with B-receptor antagonists [3]. Shima et al. [4] reported recently that nifedipine (10 mg) and diltiazem (60 mg) may increase circulating ANP levels.

Unfortunately, these authors did not measure the catecholamines to see if there is a time correlation between the peak of ANP and plasma catecholamines.

In our study, also the administration of gallopamil and flunarizine failed to change the ANP concentrations. These results are in agreement with those of Saito et al. [5] who reported that a calcium agonist facilitate the secretion of atrial natriuretic peptide from isolated perfused rat hearts. Thus, it seems that acute administration of calcium channel blockers do not affect the ANP secretion. The negative inotropism of some calcium antagonists, such as nifedipine, at least in halthy volunteers seems to be not strong enough to influence the circulating ANP levels.

References

1. Arjamma O, Vuolteenaho O (1985) Sodium ion stimulates the release of atrial natriuretic polypeptides (ANP) from rat brain. Biochem Biophys Res Commun 132:375
2. Eskay R, Zukowska-Grojec Z et al. (1986) Circulating atrial natriuretic peptide in conscious rats: Regulation of release by multiple factors. Science 232:321–639
3. Joshi PI, Dadal JJ et al. (1981) Nifedipine and left ventricular function in beta-blocked patients. Br Heart J 45:457–459
4. Saito Y, Nakao K et al. (1986) Bay K 8644, a voltagesensitive calcium channel agonist, facilitates secretion of atrial natriuretic polypeptide from isolated perfused rat hearts. Biochem Biophys Res Commun 138: 1170–1176
5. Shima J, Ogihara T et al. (1987) Effects of calcium antagonists on the secretion of atrial natriuretic peptide in normal volunteers. Curr Ther Res 42:115–123

Effect of Nifedipine on Plasma ANP-Levels and Pulmonary Hemodynamics in Patients with Pulmonary Hypertension During Exercise

G. Wambach, U. Schröder, M. Stimpel, G. Bönner, and W. Kaufmann

Medizinische Klinik II der Universität Köln, FRG

Key words: Nifedipine – Plasma ANP-levels – Pulmonary hemodynamics – Pulmonary hypertension

Introduction

Calcium ions seem to be intimately involved in the secretion of atrial natriuretic peptide: in isolated atrial tissue, ANP release was stimulated by the addition of calcium and calcium agonists. In contrast, calcium antagonists were found to inhibit ANP release under the same conditions (Ruskoaho et al. 1986). In fact, calcium entry blockers were found to modulate ANP plasma levels in vivo both in experimental animal and in patients with arterial hypertension (Stasch et al. 1988). It remains however unclear, whether calcium antagonists modulate ANP secretion by a direct effect on the atrial tissue or by their effects on arterial and venous circulation. We investigated the impact of acutely administered nifedipine on ANP plasma levels and pulmonary hemodynamics both at rest and during exercise in order to differentiate these mechanisms.

Patients, Protocol and Methods

A total of 22 patients (18 male, 4 female, aged 55 ± 4 years) were included. For diagnostic purpose, a Swan-Ganz-catheter was placed into the pulmonary artery via the vena femoralis. 10 ml of blood were drawn from the A. pulmonalis for measurements of ANP both at rest and during exercise (50 Watt on a bicycle for 5 minutes). Systemic arterial blood pressure and pressures in the right atrium, right ventricle, pulmonary artery and pulmonary wedge pressure were recorded both at rest and during exercise. In addition, cardiac output was measured by thermodilution threefold at rest and again threefold at the end of the 5 minutes exercise. Cardiac index and total peripheral resistance were calculated. Thereafter, 20 mg nifedipine were administered orally and the hemodynamic measurements as well as blood sampling for ANP were repeated 60 minutes later both at rest and after exercise. Venous blood samples were drawn for measurements of nifedipine plasma levels at time 0 and at 60 minutes. ANP plasma levels were determined in a radioimmunological method after extraction of the plasma with SEP-PAK C 18 cartridges (Wambach 1988).

Nifedipine plasma levels were measured by gaschromatography after extraction with toluol according to the method of Menke et al. (1988).

Results

During control exercise, systolic arterial blood pressure, mean pulmonary artery pressure, cardiac index and total peripheral resistance increased significantly (Table 1). The hemodynamic changes were paralleled by a rise in plasma ANP levels from 171.2 ± 32.0 pg/ml to 350.0 ± 62.1 pg/ml. Treatment with nifedipine 20 mg p.o. resulted in plasma nifedipine levels of 66.4 ± 7.0 measured 60 minutes after the ingestion of the tablets. Following nifedipine administration baseline levels for systolic and diastolic blood pressure, pulmonary artery pressure and total peripheral resistance declined compared to control values whereas heart rate and stroke volume increased significantly. Baseline plasma ANP levels, however, remained unaltered. During exercise systemic blood pressure, pulmonary artery pressure and total peripheral resistance were significantly lowered following nifedi-

Table 1. Hemodynamic effects of nifedipine at rest (a) and during exercise (b): correlation with plasma ANP levels

	control		nifedipine	
	a	b	a	b
HMV (L/min)	6.67 ± 0.40	11.61 ± 0.77	7.69 ± 0.50	12.35 ± 0.77
CI (L/min × m^2)	3.49 ± 0.21	6.04 ± 0.36	4.03 ± 0.27	6.46 ± 0.40
SVI (ml × min^{-1}/m^2)	46.24 ± 1.93	58.33 ± 3.61	49.43 ± 2.72	57.24 ± 2.97
TPR (mmHg/min^{-1} × L)	204.5 ± 13.7	283.8 ± 23.5	188.8 ± 16.6	199.0 ± 18.5
RR (mmHg) syst.	149.0 ± 4.3	174.9 ± 4.6	128.4 ± 3.8	164.7 ± 4.7
diast.	91.6 ± 2.3	94.9 ± 2.8	78.6 ± 2.7	87.2 ± 3.2
mean	109.6 ± 2.8	118.3 ± 3.2	95.6 ± 3.6	111.8 ± 3.5
PA (mmHg) syst.	26.23 ± 1.28	58.86 ± 2.57	28.05 ± 1.51	49.41 ± 2.97
diast.	8.68 ± 0.66	18.00 ± 1.54	8.50 ± 0.49	10.55 ± 0.88
mean	15.7 ± 0.70	37.36 ± 1.72	16.32 ± 0.80	27.14 ± 1.33
		p < 0.001 (b vs. b)		
ANP (pg/ml)	171.2 ± 32.0	350.0 ± 62.1	158.7 ± 28.0	237.3 ± 33.8
	n.s. (a vs. a)			

n = 22; x̄ ± SEM

pine compared to control. Again, the rise in plasma ANP during exercise was reduced to 237.3 ± 33.8 pg/ml compared to the first control exercise test.

Discussion

Dynamic exercise is a potent stimulus for ANP secretion in man. This is shown in the present study confirming a number of earlier reports (Hartter et al. 1987; Petzl et al. 1987; Nishikimi et al. 1986). Acute administration of nifedipine did not alter baseline levels of plasma ANP in our study, however, the rise in plasma ANP induced by exercise was significantly reduced following nifedipine administration. The diminished stimulation of ANP plasma levels by exercise was observed together with a reduction in blood pressure, pulmonary artery pressure and total peripheral resistance during exercise after nifedipine administration compared to the control test. These results are in agreement with the concept that nifedipine lowers exercise induced ANP release via its effect on arteriolar resistance and systemic and pulmonary blood pressure in patients with exercise induced pulmonary hypertension.

Similar observations were made in patients with essential hypertension after acute administration of nisoldipine (Akioka et al. 1987). ANP levels at rest were not altered by this new calcium channel blocker. However, rise in ANP during exercise was lowered by nisoldipine paralleled with a reduction in systemic arterial blood pressure and in pulmonary artery wedge pressure.

References

Akioka K, Kohno M, Nishikimi T, Teragaki M, Yasuda M, Oku H, Takeuchi K, Takeda T (1987) Influence of nisoldipine on hemodynamics and atrial natriuretic polypeptides at exercise loading in hypertensive patients. In: Hugenholtz PG, Meyer J (eds) Nisoldipine 1987. Springer, Berlin Heidelberg New York

Hartter E, Petzl DU, Osterode W, Böhm H, Woloszcuk W (1987) Verhalten von hANP bei Ergometerbelastung von Gesunden und Herzpatienten: Möglichkeiten einer diagnostischen Wertigkeit. In: Kreye VAW, Bussmann WD (Hrsg) ANP und das kardiovaskuläre System. Steinkopff, Darmstadt, S 159–168

Menke G, Kausch M, Rietbrock N (1988) Eine Modelluntersuchung zur Bioäquivalenz von gelöstem Nifedipin aus Weichgelatinekapseln. Arzneim-Forsch/Drug Res 38 (I):300

Petzl DH, Hartter E, Osterode W, Böhm H, Woloszcuk W (1987) Atrial natriuretic peptide release due to physical exercise in healthy persons and in cardiac patients. Klin Wochenschr 65:194–196

Nishikimi K, Kolmo M, Matsuura T (1986) Effect of exercise on circulating atrial natriuretic polypeptide in valvular heart disease. Am J Cardiol 58:1119–1120

Ruskoaho H, Toth M, Ganten D, Unger T, Lang RE (1986) The phorbol ester induced atrial natriuretic peptide secretion is stimulated by forskolin and Bay K 8644 and inhibited by 8-bromo-cGMP. Biochem Biophys Res Commun 139:266–274

Stasch JP, Kazda S, Hirth C (1987) The different effects of a calcium antagonist and a sodium-retaining vasodilator on blood pressure, cardiac hypertrophy and atrial natriuretic peptides in adult spontaneously hypertensive rats. J Hypertension 5 [Suppl 5]:S211–S213

Stasch JP, Kazda S, Hirth C (1987) Role of nisoldipine on blood pressure, cardiac hypertrophy, and atrial natriuretic peptides in spontaneously hypertensive rats. Hypertension 10/3:303–307

Wambach G (1988) Radioimmunologische Bestimmung des humanen atrialen natriuretischen Peptids – Vergleich von Verfahren mit und ohne Plasmaextraktion. Cor Vas 4: 173–177

Influence of Captopril and Nitrendipine on ANF – Renin – Aldosterone Relationships During Low and High Salt Diet

S. Degenhardt, J. Quellenberg, C. Görzgen, and G. Wambach

Medizinische Klinik II der Universität – Poliklinik – Köln, FRG

Key words: Captopril – Nitrendipine – ANF – Renin – Aldosterone – Salt diet

Introduction

The influence of antihypertensive therapy upon the regulation of atrial natriuretic factor in perhypertensive subjects has not been elucidated so far. We investigated the relationship between atrial natriuretic factor and the renin-angiotensin-aldosterone system in young male athletes with exercise induced hypertension.

Patients and Methods

12 otherwise healthy normotensive male athletes (age 17–29 years) with exercise induced hypertension (RRsys 200 mmHg at (200 – age) Watt) were restricted to a controlled low salt diet (50 mmol NaCl/d) for 14 days. Blood for determinations of atrial natriuretic factor (ANF), plasma renin concentration (PRC) and aldosterone was drawn on day 10 after 75 minutes of supine rest and again 75 minutes after an oral dose of captopril 25 mg (C). The same procedure was conducted on day 13 when nitrendipine 10 mg (N) was given. After a washout period of 14 days the subjects were put on a high salt diet (250 mmol NaCl/d) for another 14 days. On days 10 and 13 the investigations were repeated as described while saline was infused (6.6 ml NaCl 1.5%/min). Statistics: t-statistics, paired observations, 2-tailed, $p < 0.05$, multivariate regression analysis.

Results

Resting blood pressures were not different during either part of the study.

Hormone values were (mean ± SEM):

ANF: Baseline ANF values were higher under salt loading conditions only before C but not before N ($p = 0.27$). No changes occured after the administration of C or N on the low salt diet. On the high salt diet ANF increased after C and N.

Renin: Baseline renin values were higher during the low salt diet. On the low salt diet renin increased after C while no change occured after N. On the high salt diet renin slightly decreased after N.

Aldosterone: Baseline aldosterone was higher during the low salt diet. On the low salt diet aldosterone fell after C. On the high salt diet the decrease of aldosterone after C was less but significant. Decreases of aldosterone after N on either diet failed to achieve significance.

		Blood pressures (mmHg, mean ± SEM n = 12)		
		systolic	diastolic	MAP
low salt diet	before C	130 ± 2.9	84 ± 1.8	99 ± 2.0
	after C	129 ± 3.8	79 ± 2.2	95 ± 2.5
	before N	128 ± 2.7	79 ± 1.7	96 ± 1.5
	after N	131 ± 3.3	80 ± 2.6	98 ± 3.2
high salt diet	before C	134 ± 2.4	82 ± 2.0	99 ± 1.7
	after C	131 ± 2.7	81 ± 3.2	98 ± 2.8
	before N	133 ± 3.6	79 ± 2.6	97 ± 2.4
	after N	136 ± 4.0	80 ± 2.3	99 ± 2.4

Resting blood pressures were not different during either part of the study.
Hormone values were (mean ± SEM):

Hormone values were (mean ± SEM n = 12):

		ANF (pg/ml)	Renin (μU/ml)	Aldosterone (pg/ml)
low	before C	26.3 ± 3.1	29.6 ± 3.7	213.8 ± 30.4
salt	after C	25.4 ± 4.2	119.2 ± 32.0	122.2 ± 18.8
diet	before N	34.0 ± 5.4	35.3 ± 9.6	176.6 ± 46.7
	after N	29.2 ± 3.9	34.2 ± 11.2	150.7 ± 37.1
		n = 11		
high	before C	37.8 ± 4.8	9.2 ± 1.7	59.5 ± 10.6
salt	after C	62.2 ± 11.2	11.0 ± 3.0	41.9 ± 9.0
diet	before N	38.3 ± 7.1	8.2 ± 0.8	46.9 ± 12.8
	after N	53.1 ± 11.0	6.2 ± 0.8	38.5 ± 9.7

Multivariate regression analysis showed a strongly negative correlation between ANF and aldosterone on the low salt diet (before C), which fell below significance during the high salt diet. On high salt ANF was inversely correlated with renin after N administration but not at baseline. Renin and aldosterone were positively correlated during low salt at baseline and after N, but not after C. On high salt any correlation between renin and aldosterone was lost.

Discussion

As expected baseline values of renin and aldosterone were high and ANF was low during salt restriction. The inverse correlation of ANF and aldosterone conforms with previous findings of a direct suppressor action of ANF on angiotensin II- and ACTH-induced aldosterone release by adrenal glomerulosa cells [1]. Under salt loading conditions baseline ANF was higher and renin and aldosterone were suppressed.

There was no detectable influence of captopril or nitrendipine on ANF values during sodium restriction. This could be due to the already very low baseline levels of ANF. Captopril alleviates the workload of the heart by reducing afterload and preload and mildly attenuates sympathetic nervous outflow. These features antagonize atrial stretch and stimulation of the sympathetic nervous system, both stimuli of ANF secretion.

After nitrendipine on the high salt diet ANF rose when baseline values were already high whereas no change could be found when baseline values were low. Natriuresis and diuresis after oral administration of calcium antagonists are well recognized phenomena [2, 3]. An increase of natriuresis coincides with a contraction of plasma volume, which should exert an inhibitory influence on ANF release from the atria. The observed increase of ANF plasma levels supports earlier findings that ANF plays a part in the natriuresis after calcium-antagonist administration [4]. We cannot exclude, however, that saline infusion mediated the rise of ANF levels in this setting. If a steady state was not achieved at 75 minutes a further increment of the subjects thoracic blood volumes at 150 minutes of infusion could have accounted for the increase of ANF secretion.

Conclusion

Our observations confirm that the regulation of atrial natriuretic factor is functionally opposed by the renin-angiotensin system. No abnormalities were detected in the prehypertensive subjects studied. As the number of observations was small and the hypotheses tested were many the regulation of atrial natriuretic factor during antihypertensive therapy deserves further study.

References

1. Atarashi K, Franco-Saenz R, Mulrow PJ, Snajdar RM, Rapp JP (1984) Inhibition of aldosterone production by atrial natriuretic factor. J Hypertension 2 [Suppl 3]:293–295

2. Ene MD, Williamson PJ, Roberts CJC, Waddell G (1985) The natriuresis following oral administration of calcium antagonists – nifedipine and nitrendipine. Br J Pharmacol 19:423–427
3. Fukui K, Tamaki T, Yamamoto A, Shoji T, Fujisawa Y, Iwao H (1987) Salidiuretic actions of the calcium antagonist nitrendipine in dogs. Naunyn Schmiedebergs Arch Pharmacol 336:572–577
4. Rappelli A, Dessi-Fulgheri P, Madeddu P, Glorioso N (1987) Studies on the natriuretic effect of nifedipine in hypertensive patients: increase in levels of plasma atrial natriuretic factor without participation of the renal kallikrein-kinin system. J Hypertension 5 [Suppl 4]:S61–S65

The Heart in Acromegaly

Human Atrial Natriuretic Peptide in Active Acromegaly: Effects on Hormonal, Metabolic, Hemodynamic, and Renal Parameters

E. Jungmann, U. Schirmer, T. Haak, E.-H. Scheuermann, and K. Schöffling

Department of Endocrinology, Center of Internal Medicine, Johann Wolfgang Goethe-University, Frankfurt am Main 70, FRG

Key words: Human atrial natriuretic peptide – Acromegaly – Kidney function – Insulin secretion – Carbohydrate metabolism

Introduction

Patients with active acromegaly are characterized by increased plasma volume, sodium retention, increased renal plasma flow and increased glomerular filtration rate [2] as well as hyperinsulinemia and insulin resistance [1]. Moreover, prevalence of hypertension is increased in active acromegaly [4]. Therefore, it appeared worthy of examination whether effects of human atrial natriuretic peptide (human ANF – (99–126), hANP) or any impairment of hANP action might contribute to the pathophysiology of active acromegaly.

Methods

After giving informed consent, 20 subjects voluntarily participated in our study (9 women, 11 men, aged 25–71 years). 11 patients had active acromegaly (somatomedin C, 3.1 ± 0.4 U/ml). 9 matched subjects with neurosurgically cured acromegaly and 2 of the patients being restudied after successful transsphenoidal operation served as controls (somatomedin C, 0.7 ± 0.2 U/ml, $p < 0.01$ vs. active acromegaly). 100 µg hANP (Bissendorf Peptide, Wedemark) or placebo were given as i.v. bolus injections according to a double-blind, randomized, placebo-controlled trial design.

Results

At base-line, patients differed from controls only in elevated creatinine clearance (197 ± 14 vs. 150 ± 14 ml/min, $p < 0.05$). Base-line hANP levels were similar, the prevalence of hANP levels above age-adjusted normal range being 56% in both groups.

In response to hANP, creatinine clearance and blood glucose concentrations remained unchanged. All other findings are summarized in Fig. 1. When calculated as percentage changes from respective base-line values, the responses of natriuresis and chloride excretion were increased in active acromegaly (ΔUNaV, +213 ± 54 vs. +80 ± 15% in controls, $p < 0.01$, ΔUClV, +134 ± 46 vs. +55 ± 13%, $p < 0.05$).

Discussion

There is no evidence for an essential role of hANP in the pathomechanisms of growth hormone excess: Neither was there an impairment of hANP action nor was the hANP system capable of compensating for growth hormone action in kidney or vasculature in active acromegaly. Increased renal responses to hANP in active acromegaly resemble findings in essential hypertension [6]. In pharmacological as well as in physiological [3] dosage hANP increases insulin levels by inhibiting insulin degradation. Insulin secretion is unaffected by hANP [5]. Whereas it remains to be established whether increased hANP levels contribute to the phenomenon of insulin resistance in essential hypertension, insulin resistance in active acromegaly is not due to hANP action.

References

1. Althoff PH, Schmidt K, Hofmeister-Wagner WD, Knigge H, Rosak C, Jungmann E, Schöffling K (1987) Glukosetoleranz unter

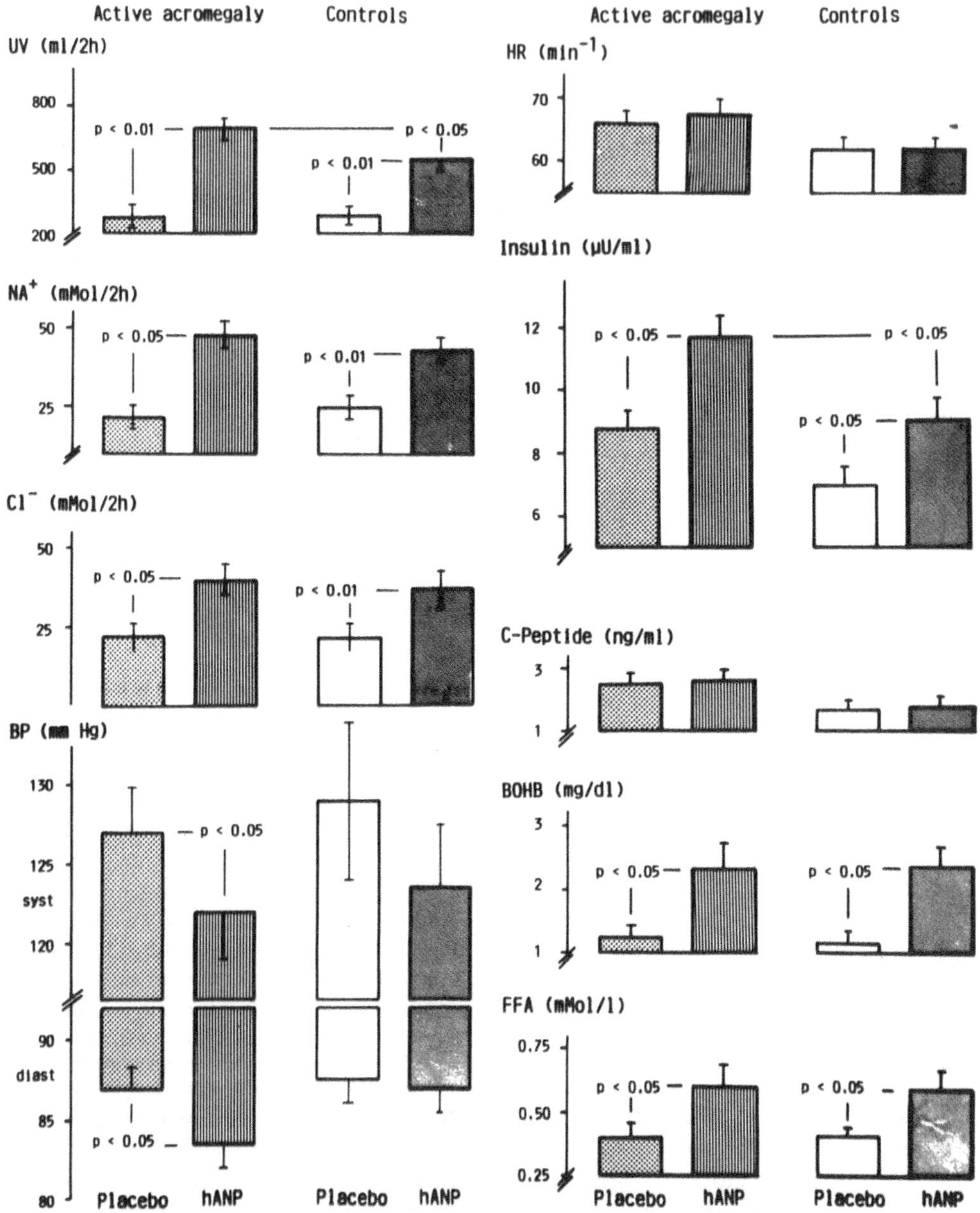

Fig. 1. Summary of hANP action in active acromegaly. Haemodynamic, hormonal and metabolic parameters are given as average ($\bar{x} \pm$ SEM) of all values obtained after the injections of hANP or placebo. Subjects with neurosurgically cured acromegaly served as controls (Abbreviations: UV, urinary volume, Na^+, urinary sodium excretion, Cl^-, urinary chloride excretion, BP, blood pressure, HR, heart rate, BOHB, Beta-Hydroxybutyrate, FFA, free fatty acids)

verschiedenen Pharmakotherapien der Akromegalie – differente Einflüsse von Bromocriptin und einem Somatostatin-Analogon. Akt Endokr Stoffw 8:193
2. Falkhed T, Sjögren B (1964) Extracellular fluid volume and renal function in pituitary insufficiency and acromegaly. Acta Endocrinol 46:80–88
3. Haak T, Jungmann E, Hannappel B, Schöffling K (1988) Zur Wirkung des humanen atrialen natriuretischen Peptides auf die Glucosetoleranz bei gesunden Probanden. Coll endocrinol südwestdtsch Arbeitsgruppen, Mainz
4. Hayward RP, Emanuel RW, Nabarro JDN (1986) Acromegalic heart disease: Influence of treatment of the acromegaly on the heart. Quart J Med 237:41–58
5. Kühn M, Ammon HPT, Verspohl EJ (1988) Atrial natriuretic peptide acts via specific receptors on cGMP system of rat abstract islets without affecting insulin release. Diabetologia 31:511A
6. Richards AM, Nicholls MG, Espiner EA, Ikram H, Yandle TG, Joyce SL, Cullens MM (1985) Effects of alpha-human atrial natriuretic peptide in essential hypertension. Hypertension 7:812–817

Human Atrial Natriuretic Peptide (hANP): Its Action on Renal Function and the Excretion of Membrane Marker Proteins of the Proximal Tubule in Patients with Active and Inactive Acromegaly

J. E. Scherberich[1], E. Jungmann[2], G. Hintz[1], U. Schirmer[2], and W. Schoeppe[1]

[1] Departments of Nephrology and [2] Endocrinology, Center of Internal Medicine, Johann Wolfgang Goethe-University, Frankfurt am Main, FRG

Key words: h-ANP (99-126) – Acromegaly – Kidney function – Tubular marker proteins

Introduction

Despite detailed evaluation of binding sites of ANP in the human kidney [1], the renal mechanism of action of ANP remains unclear [3]. Obviously, under the influence of ANP, various parts of the nephron exhibit different metabolic responses and hormone susceptibility [2, 3, 10]. Glomerular as well as the proximal and distal tubular functions are modulated by ANP [2, 6, 10].

Since renal hANP action was impaired in hyperfiltrating, uncomplicated type-1-diabetes mellitus [6], we were interested to study possible pathophysiologically relevant renal involvement of ANP in patients with acromegaly [2, 4, 5]. The effect of bolus injection of ANP on glomerular filtration rate, urine volume, electrolytes, excretion of tubular marker enzymes and other parameters was assessed in controls and patients with active and cured acromegaly.

Abbreviations: hANP = human atrial natriuretic peptide; GH = growth hormone; GGT = γ-glutranspeptidase; β-NAG = β-N-acetylglucosaminidase; AP = alkaline phosphatase; AMP = ala-(leu-,glyc-)aminopeptidase; Cl_{cr} = creatinine clearance; SDS-PAGE = Na-dedecylsulfate-polyacrylamide (gradient)gel electrophoresis; n.s. = not significant

Patients and Methods

A double-blind, placebo-controlled study was performed in 18 patients (9 female, 9 male, 37–67 years), where 10/18 (6 female, 4 male) suffered from active acromegaly (somatomedin C $\bar{x}$: 3 U/ml; GH $\bar{x}$: 10.2 bg/ml); 8 patients (3 female, 5 male) in whom acromegaly had been cured served as controls (somatomedin C < 1. U/ml; GHJ < 1.4 ng/ml). Both groups receiving either 100 μg hANP or placebo in random order had been fully informed of the nature of the study before giving their consent [5]. Blood and urine specimens were obtained before and after hANP i.v. bolus injection, and clinical and laboratory parameters were determined as described in detail previously [5, 6, 7–9].

Results and Discussion

In patients with active acromegaly, Cl_{cr}, which was significantly higher as compared to the controls ($2p < 0.05$), did not change after hANP injection among the both groups (207 ± 92 ml/min/1.73 m^2 vs. 166 ± 43 ml/min/1.73 m^2). In all patients studied Cl_{cr} was positively correlated with serum GH concentrations (Rs: 0.45, 2p: 0.05). Plasma renin activity (PRA) in active acromegaly and controls was not significantly different and unchanged after hANP injection: PRA (active acromegaly): 1.18 ± 0.93 ng AI/ml/h; inactive acromegaly, PRA: 0.90 ± 0.47 ng AI/ml/h. After hANP injection urine volumes increased within 120 min as follows:

– active acromegaly: after hANP from 247 ± 113 ml to 621 ± 176 ml; placebo n.s.
– inactive acromegaly: after hANP from 253 ± 207 ml to 498 ± 197 ml; placebo n.s.

In addition, Na^+ and Cl^- excretion in urine was significantly enhanced after hANP, and was more pronounced in patients with active acromegaly [5]. Furthermore, hANP was capable of rising urinary brush border membrane GGT, AP and lysosomal β-NAG activity (enzyme creatinine index; U/$mmol_{cr}$) in active acromegaly, but failed to do so in the controls (Fig. 1).

Rise of enzymuria was correlated with the increase in Na^+ and Cl^- excretion. ANP has been recognized to inhibit the luminal Na^+ entry in the inner medullary collecting duct cells [10]. No changes were observed in the excretion patterns of serum proteins as assessed by SDS-PAGE.

Our results indicate that hANP exerts a marked effect on the turnover and shedding of tubular marker proteins in patients with

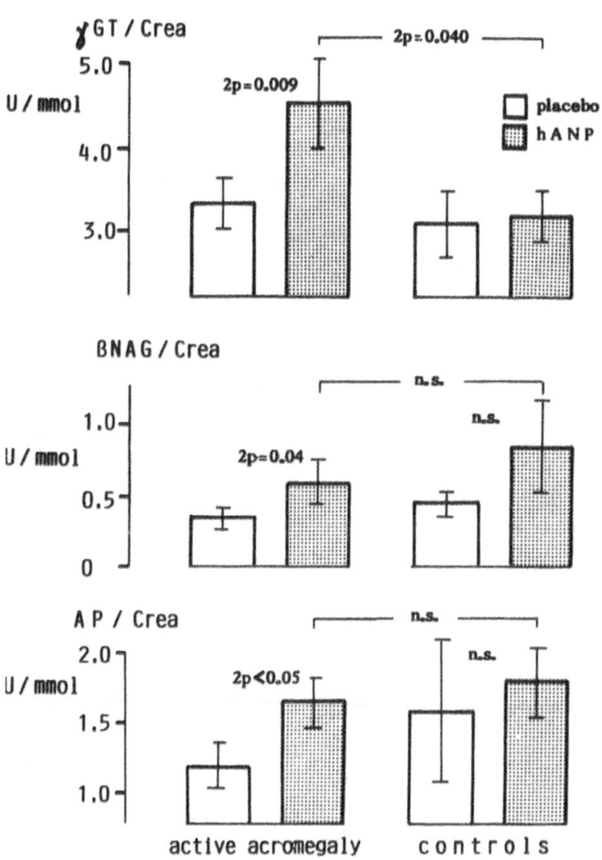

Fig. 1. The effect of 100 μg hANP i.v. bolus injection on urinary excretion of tubular membrane gamma-glutamyl-transpeptidase (GT), alkaline phosphatase (AP) and lysosomal N-acetyl β-D-glucosaminidase (βNAG) in patients with active acromegaly vs. controls. Elimination of tubular indicator proteins is expressed as enzyme creatinine ration (U/mmol creatinine)

active acromegaly. The glomerular (GFR) and tubular action (Na^+, Cl^-, AP, GGT, βNAG) in response to an increased metabolic stress (hANP bolus injection) is not impaired in patients with GH excess.

References

1. Brucksch A, Gröne HJ, Talartschik J, Fuchs E (1988) Binding sites of atrial natriuretic peptide in human renal tissue – quantification by in vitro receptor autoradiography. Klin Wochenschr 66:303–307
2. Dworkin LD, Brenner BM (1982) Hormonal influences on glomerular function. Contr Nephrol 33:1–13
3. Forssmann WG, Heidland A, Lang RE (eds) (1986) I. Workshop on cardiac hormones "potential role in health and disease". Klin Wochenschr 64 [Suppl VI]
4. Hirschberg R, Kopple J (1987) Effects of growth hormone on GFR and renal plasma flow in man. Kidney Int 32 [Suppl 2]:21–24
5. Jungmann E, Schirmer U, Scheuermann E, Zeuzem S, Schöffling K (1989) Renal action of human atrial natriuretic peptide in active acromegaly. In: Kaufmann W, Wambach G (eds) Endocrinology of the heart, pp 247–249
6. Jungmann E, Walter-Schräder MC, Haak T, Fassbinder W, Wambach G, Althoff PH, Schöffling K (1988) Impaired renal responsiveness to human atrial natriuretic peptide (hANP) in normotensive patients with diabetes mellitus. Klin Wochenschr 66:527–532
7. Kugler P, Wolf G, Scherberich JE (1985) Histochemical demonstration of peptidases in the human kidney. Histochemistry 83: 337–341
8. Scherberich JE, Gauhl C, Heinert G, Mondorf W, Schoeppe W (1984) Characterization and clinical significance of membrane bound proteases from human kidney cortex. Adv Exp Med Biol 167:179–184
9. Scherberich JE, Mondorf W, Falkenberg FW, Pierard D, Schoeppe W (1984) Monitoring drug nephrotoxicity: quantitative estimation of human kidney brush border antigens in urine as a specific marker of tubular damage. Contr Nephrol 42:81–92
10. Zeidel ML, Kikeri D, Silva P, Burrowes M, Brenner BM (1988) Atrial natriuretic peptides inhibit conductive sodium uptake by rabbit inner medullary collecting duct cells. J Clin Invest 82:1067–1074

Heart Size Reduction in Acromegalic Patientes Treated with the Long-Acting Somatostatin-Analogue SMS 201-995 (Somatostatin®)

P.-H. Althoff, K. Schmidt, D. Rübesam, A. G. Harris, E. Jungmann, and K. Schöffling

Department of Endocrinology, Center of Internal Medicine, J. W. Goethe-University, Frankfurt, FRG

Key words: Acromegaly – Pharmacotherapy – Somatostatin – Heart size reduction

---

Introduction and Aims of the Study

Cardiomegaly by hypertrophy of the heart in acromegalic patients – prevalence 85% in our patients with acromegaly [1] – is often complicated by complex arrhythmias and gradual cardiac-insufficiency [1, 3, 8]. The aim of the study was to evaluate the extend of heart size reduction in acromegalic patients under longterm-treatment with the long-acting somatostatin-analgoue SMS 201-995 (Sandostatin®, Sandoz) [2, 5, 7]. All patients had been treated before SMS 201-995 therapy by neurosurgery and/or radiation and medical treatment with bromocriptine (Pravidel®), so that hypersomatotropism before SMS 201-995 therapy was only moderate (s. Table 1a).

Methods

The heart size of 7 acromegalic patients was assessed by the reproducable roentgenological heartvolume determination [6] in the modification of Hopf [4], kidney and spleen size were measured by ultrasound (Sonoline SL; 3,5 MHz sector array and 5 MHz linear

Table 1a. Growth hormone secretion and somatomedine-C levels in acromegalics before and under treatment with SMS 201995

pat.-No.	before SMS GHb (ng/ml)	GHoGTT (ng/ml)	Sm-C (U/ml)	mean of 1.–9. month GHb (ng/ml)	GHoGTT (ng/ml)	Sm-C (U/ml)	SMS/die (μg)
1	6.5	4.9	4.5	1.6	1.8	1.5	422
2	5.7	8.4	8.8	2.5	2.1	2.7	200
3	19.4	19.4	3.7	2.2	1.7	3.1	200
4	2.9	2.6	5	5.4	1.7	3.9	128
5	27.5	19.9	6	9.2	6.4	4.6	267
6	25.1	20.1	4.4	3.1	1.5	2.5	244
7	32.9	30.7	4.2	24.5	1.3	2.2	200
mean	17.1	15.1	5.2	6.9	2.4	2.9	237.3
SD	11.2	9.4	1.6	7.6	1.7	1.0	85.5
SEM	4.2	3.5	0.6	2.9	0.6	0.4	32.3

Table 1b. Heartvolume before and after 6 month of treatment with SMS 201-995 in acromegalics

pat.-No.	heartvolume before SMS (ml/1.73 cmBSA	heartvolume after SMS (ml/1.73 cmBSA)	delta heartvolume (ml)	delta heartvolume (%)
1	1012	825	186	18
2	843	733	110	13
3	1096	931	165	15
4	722	693	29	4
5	946	788	158	17
6	833	811	23	3
7	848	863	− 14	− 2
mean	900	806	94	10
SD	116	73	74	7

array) before and under 6 months of SMS-treatment with 100 to 1500 μg/day of the somatostatin-analogue SMS 201-995 (SMS; Sandostatin®).

Serum somatomedin-C (SM-C) assay: Commercial RIA SM-C kit from IRE Medgenix, Fleurus, Belgium.

Results

Under 6 months of treatment with 100 to 1500 μg/day SMS 201-995 the mean GH-level was significantly reduced from 17.1 ± 11.0 ng/ml to 6.9 ± 7.6 ng/ml ($p < 0.01$[1]) and mean serum somatomedin-C (SM-C) levels were reduced from 5.2 ± 1.6 U/ml to 2.9 ± 1.0 U/ml ($p < 0.01$[1]) (s. Table 1a). Normalization of GH in basal state (<5 ng/ml) and following an oral glucose load (<2 ng/ml) and of SM-C (<1.9 U/ml in man; <2.2 U/ml in woman) was achieved by 3 patients.

The mean radiologic heartvolume before treatment was 900 ± 116 ml/1,73 m^2 BSA (normal values for women: 450–690 ml/1.73 m^2 BSA; for man: 450–790 ml/1.73 m^2). After treatment with SMS the mean heartvolume showed a significant reduction to 806 ± 73 ml/1.73 m^2 BSA; ($p < 0.05$[2]) (Table 1b). Besides marked reduction in size of the heart there was a marked reduction in size of spleen (width: 5.4 ± 1.2 cm vs. 4.9 ± 0.7 cm; anterior margin: 11.3 ± 2.3 cm vs. 10.6 ± 2.0 cm; $p < 0.05$[2]) and the kidney (length: 11.3 ± 0.5 cm vs. 11.0 ± 0.8 cm; width: 5.0 ± 0.6 cm vs. 4.6 ± 0.4 cm) noted under treatment with SMS.

[1] One sided Wilcoxon-test for paired differences

[2] Two sided Wilcoxon-test for paired differences

Discussion of Results and Conclusion

Long-term SMS 201-995 (Sandostatin®, Sandoz, Basel) therapy, not only controls GH-hypersecretion and clinical symptoms such as hyperhidrosis, soft tissue swelling, but also significantly reduces heart size. The effect is not organspecific, as other organs like the spleen and the kidneys show also a reduction of their size under treatment with SMS [7]. The effect is probably due to the pharmacological inhibition of growth hormone- and somatomedin-C-levels by SMS [2, 5].

References

1. Althoff P-H (1978) Die Akromegalie – Untersuchungen zur Pathophysiologie der Wachstumshormonsekretion und zur Pharmakotherapie mit Somatostatin und Bromocriptin. Habilitationsschrift, Frankfurt
2. Ch'ng LJC, Sandler LM, Kraenzlin ME, Burrin JM, Joplin GF, Bloom SR (1985) Long term treatment of acromegaly with a long acting analogue of somatostatin. Br Med J 290: 284–285
3. Happ J, Gerspach A, Maul FD, Standke R, Böttger B, Althoff P-H, Schöffling K, Hör G (1984) Myocardial Scintigraphy (MS) in Acromegalics. In: Schmidt HAE, Adam WE (eds) Nuklearmedizin. Schattauer, Stuttgart New York, pp 156–157
4. Hopf R, Böhmer D, Kaltenbach M (1977) Röntgenologische Herzvolumenbestimmung. Beschreibung einer neueren Methode mit Durchführung im Sitzen. Fortschr Röntgenstr 127:167–169
5. Lamberts SWJ, Uitterlinden P, Verschoor L, van Dongen KJ, Del Pozo E (1985) Long-Term treatment of acromegaly with the somatostatin analogue SMS 201-995. N Engl J Med 313:1576–1580
6. Musshoff K, Raindell H, Gebhardt W, König K, Roskam H (1967) Die Methode der röntgenologischen Volumenbestimmung des Herzens. Radiologe 7:161–164
7. Schmidt K, Rübesam D, Althoff P-H, Jungmann E, Harris AG, Schöffling K (1989) Organ size reduction in acromegalic patients treated with the somatostatin analog SMS 201-995. Acta Endocrin (Kbh) 120: Suppl 1:80
8. Smallridge RC, Rajfer S, Davia J, Schaaf M (1979) Acromegaly and the heart. An echocardiographic study. Am J Med 66:22–27

The Cardiac Effects of T_3 on Ca Dependent Electrical Activities During β-Adrenoceptor Stimulation and Inhibition

G. Stark, U. Stark, B. Pietsch, K. Hönigl, E. Pilger, H. Bertuch, H. Warnkroß, G. Obermayer, W. Lindner, G. Leb, S. Nagl, and H. A. Tritthart

Department of Internal Medicine and Medical Physics and Biophysics, Karl-Franzens-University of Graz, School of Medicine, Austria

Key-words: Triiodthyronine – Receptors – ECG – Heart rate

Introduction

Hypermetabolism, increased myocardial contractility and tachycardia which are caused by hyperthyroidism resemble the effects of sympathetic hyperactivity. We have tested the acute effects of T3 and of isoproterenol on the electrophysiological properties of isolated spontaneously beating hearts. In addition, the concentrations of the β-receptor-blocking compound (–)propranolol necessary to antagonize the electrophysiological effects of isoproterenol and T3 were also evaluated and compared to the concentration of (–)propranolol which is necessary to block the effects of isoproterenol alone.

Methods

Guinea pigs of either sex, weighing 300–400 g fed ad libitum were injected with 250 IU of heparin one hour before being sacrified by a blow to the neck. The heart was quickly removed and attached to a modified Langendorff type recirculating perfusion system. Tyrode's solution (in mMol/l: NaCl 132.1; KCl 2.7; $CaCl_2$ 2.5; $MgCl_2$ 1.15; $NaHCO_3$ 24.0; NaH_2PO_4 0.42; D-Glucose 5.6) was used as perfusate. Bipolar ECG recordings were taken from the epicardiac surface of the hearts (SST-ECG, Anton Paar KG, Graz, Austria). This bipolar signals contained additionally to the common ECG signals the information about the early atrial and the His bundle activity.

Three different experimental protocols were applied:

1. The effects of 0.01 μM isoproterenol for 10 min on heart rate and on the AV-nodal and His-bundle conduction velocity were studied. Increasing concentrations (from 0.01 μM to 10 μM) of (–)propranolol were then added to the perfusate to test the concentrations needed to antagonize the effects of isoproterenol completely.
2. The effects of 10 μg T_3/100 ml perfusate were studied. The ensuing experimental protocol was the same as described above.
3. The combined influence of 0.1 μM propranolol and of increasing isoproterenol concentrations (0.01–0.03 μM) was studied, to measure the highest catecholamine concentration which could be balanced by 0.1 μM (–)propranolol.

Each drug added to the perfusate was acting for 10 minutes before the experiment was continued. Statistical analysis were done with the paired t-test. All values are expressed as mean ± standard error (SE) of the mean.

Results

T_3, added to the perfusate at a concentration of 10 μM/100 ml, caused no changes of the AH-, HV-interval and of heart rate. Following the administration of 0.01 μM isoproterenol an increase in the spontaneous sinus rate by 24 ± 4% ($p < 0.01$) was detectable. The AH interval was insignificantly prolonged by 16 ± 6% whereas the HV-interval as well as QRS-duration remained within control values. The application of 0.01 μM isoproterenol only, caused an increase of heart rate by 13 ± 4% ($p < 0.01$)

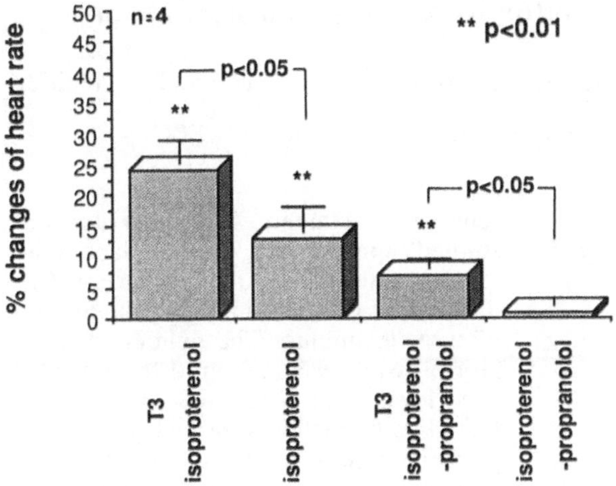

Fig. 1. Changes in heart rate by 0.01 μM isoproterenol alone, T_3 and isoproterenol as well as in the presence of 0.1 μM (−)propranolol

and insignificant changes in AH-, HV- and QRS durations. In hearts perfused with 0.01 μM isoproterenol heart rate completly returned to control values following the application of 0.1 μM of (−)propranolol, whereas the combined effects of T_3 and isoproterenol on the pacemaker activity of the sinus node were not completly antagonized by the same concentration of (−)propranolol (+7 ± 1.4%, $p < 0.05$), sufficient to balance the effects of 0.01 isoproterenol. The concentration of 0.1 μM of (−)propranolol was also able to block the effects of isoproterenol on heart rate up to a concentration of 0.03 μM.

Discussion

The present results show, that T_3 leads to an increased sensitivity of the heart to β-adrenergic stimulation by catecholamines. This is indicated by the significantly higher increase in heart rate following the combined administration of T_3 and isoproterenol than following the administration of isoproterenol alone. These results confirm those found by Levey (1977) and Schwartz (1983). In addition, it could be shown that T_3 needed only the short time span of 10 min to increase the cardiac sensitivity to β-adrenergic stimulation. Therefore it could be speculated, that the mechanism of T_3 on the cardicac electrical activity resembles a "switch on" of the β-receptors in the membrane, either by increasing the density of the receptors and/or the affinity to β-receptor agonists. This fast activation of the β-receptors by T_3 could also explain the reduced effectiveness of 0.1 μM (−)propranolol in T_3 treated hearts by antagonizing the effects of 0.01 μM isoproterenol, whereas in not T_3 treated hearts, the stimulating effects of 0.03 μM isoproterenol could be completely balanced by 0.1 μM (−)propranolol.

References

Kunos G (1977) Thyroid hormone-dependent interconversion of myocardial – and β-adrenoreceptors in the heart. Br J Pharmac 59: 177–189

Levey GS (1971) Catecholamine sensitivity, thyroid hormone and the heart, a reevaluation. Am J Med 50:413–420

Stark G, Huber U, Hofer E, Tritthart HA (1987) Continuous ECG measurements of intracardiac activity from the surface of Langendorff-perfused guinea pig hearts. Basic Res Cardiol 82:437–444

Schwartz HL, Trence D, Oppenheimer JH, Jiang NS, Jump DB (1983) Distribution and metabolism of L- and D-triiodothyronine in the rat: preferential accumulation of L-T3 by hepatic and cardiac nuclei as a probable explanation of the differential biological potency of T3 enantiomers. Endocrinology 113:1236–1243

Williams LT, Lefkowitz RJ, Watanabe AM, Hathaway DR, Besch Jr HR (1977) Thyroid hormone regulation of β-adrenergic receptor number. J Biol Chem 252:2787–2789

Left Ventricular Diastolic Function in Acute Hypothyroidism

S. Wieshammer[1], F. S. Keck[1], J. Waitzinger[2], U. Loos[1], V. Hombach[1], and E. F. Pfeiffer[1]

[1] Zentrum für Innere Medizin und [2] Abteilung Nuklearmedizin, Universität Ulm, FRG

Key-words: Left ventricular function – Diastole – Myocardial relaxation – Hypothyroidism – Radionuclide ventriculography

Introduction

The thyroid state is an important determinant of cardiac performance. This study examines the effects of acute hypothyroidism on left ventricular diastolic function.

Patients and Methods

We studied 9 athyreotic patients (average age 43 ± 3 years) without cardiovascular disease by radionuclide ventriculography with simultaneous right heart catheterization. The patients had had total thyroidectomy and ablative radioiodine treatment for thyroid cancer. To allow for a paired-data analysis, all patients were studied twice once while they were hypothyroid 2 weeks after ceasing triiodothyronine and once while they were euthyroid on thyroxine replacement therapy. The hypothyroid studies were performed prior to a regularly scheduled follow-up total body scan. Pericardial effusion was absent in each patient when hypothyroid as shown by echocardiography. Informed written consent was obtained. The patients were studied supine at rest. A Swan-Ganz catheter was passed to the pulmonary artery. Cardiac output was determined by the thermodilution technique. The pulmonary capillary pressure was measured from a reference level 5 cm below the sternal angle. Gated radionuclide ventriculography was performed in the modified left anterior oblique position after in vivo labeling of red blood cells with 740 mBq of technetium-99m. The variables used to characterize diastolic function were the peak filling rate and the time to peak filling. The latter was defined as the interval from end-systole on the radionuclide time-volume curve to the time of occurrence of peak filling. The peak filling rate was determined in absolute terms from the normalized radionuclide peak filling rate (left ventricular end-diastolic counts/s) and from the end-diastolic volume (thermodilution stroke volume/ejection fraction).

Results

The hemodynamic data are summarized in the Table. Peak filling always occurred during the first half of diastole so that the left atrial contraction did not contribute to the measured peak filling rates. While the time to peak filling was not significantly affected

Table 1. Hemodynamic and radionuclide findings

	Hypothyroid	Euthyroid
Heart rate (beats/min)	70 ± 11	80 ± 14
Systolic blood pressure (mmHg)	124 ± 14	134 ± 22
Pulmonary capillary pressure (mmHg)	6 ± 2	8 ± 2
Endsystolic volume (ml)	32 ± 11	32 ± 7
Enddiastolic volume (ml)	90 ± 19	106 ± 18[a]
Ejection fraction (%)	66 ± 6	70 ± 4
Radionuclide peak filling rate (EDC/s)	3.22 ± 0.91	3.72 ± 0.58
Absolute peak filling rate (ml/s)	287 ± 91	400 ± 118[b]
Time to peak filling (ms)	170 ± 10	159 ± 21

EDC/s, left ventricular enddiastolic counts per second. Values are expressed as the mean ± 1 standard deviation. Differences were analyzed by the Wilcoxon test for paired observations; [a] $p < 0.05$; [b] $p < 0.01$

by the thyroid state, the peak filling rate decreased in all patients when passing from the euthyroid to the hypothyroid state. On average, peak filling rate was by 41 ± 13% lower when the patients were hypothyroid than when they were euthyroid (287 ± 91 ml/s vs 400 ± 118 ml/s, $p < 0.01$).

Discussion

Diastolic filling represents a complex interaction between active myocardial relaxation and the passive viscoelastic properties of the heart. Active relaxation is the major determinant of ventricular filling in early diastole and proceeds rapidly towards completeness so that it does not appreciably contribute to filling beyond the rapid filling phase in the normal heart. It is assumed that the changes in peak filling rate observed in this study reflect hormone-induced changes in active myocardial relaxation because peak filling always occurred early in diastole and the major extrinsic determinants of peak filling rate (i.e. ventricular filling pressure, endsystolic volume, heart rate, and aortic pressure) were not significantly affected by thyroid deficiency. The biochemical mechanism by which thyroid deficiency produces a decrease in relaxation rate may relate to a depressed activity of the sarcoplasmic reticular calcium pump which is under thyroid control [1, 2, 5]. Our data on patients with acute hypothyroidism are consistent with the findings of Strauer and Schulze [4] who found a reduced relaxation velocity in isolated cardiac muscle preparations from cats which had been made hypothyroid 2 months before the experiment day. Our patients had been off triiodothyronine for only 2 weeks and they do not provide a model to study diastolic function in long-standing hypothyroidism. However, an abnormal relaxation was found in chronic hypothyroidism too. Manns et al. [3] demonstrated a prolongation of the isovolumic relaxation period and Vora et al. [6] showed a reduction of the peak thinning rate of the left ventricular posterior wall in patients with long-standing hypothyroidism.

References

1. Dillmann WH, Rohrer D, Popovich A, Barrieux A (1987) Thyroid hormone induced changes in cardiac proteins and mRNAs. In: Loos U, Wartofsky L (eds) Molecular biological approaches to thyroid research. Horm Metabol Res [Suppl 17]:26–29
2. Limas CJ (1978) Calcium transport ATPase of cardiac sarcoplasmic reticulum in experimental hyperthyroidism. Am J Physiol 235: H745–H751
3. Manns JJ, Shepherd AAM, Crooks J, Adamson DG (1976) Measurement of cardiac muscle relaxation in hypothyroidism. Br Med J 1:1366–1368
4. Strauer BE, Schulze W (1976) Experimental hypothyroidism: Depression of myocardial contractile function and hemodynamics and their reversibility by substitution with thyroid hormones. Basic Res Cardiol 71:624–644
5. Suko J (1971) Alterations of Ca^{2+} uptake and Ca^{2+}-activated ATPase of cardiac sarcoplasmic reticulum in hyper- and hypothyroidism. Biochim Biophys Acta 252:324–327
6. Vora J, O'Malley BP, Petersen S, McCullough A, Rosenthal FD, Barnett DB (1985) Reversible abnormalities of myocardial relaxation in hypothyroidism. J Clin Endocrinol Metab 61:269–272

24-Hour ECG-Monitoring in Hyperthyroidism

G. Kahaly, K. von Olshausen, and S. Bischoff

III. Medical Department, University Hospital, Mainz, FRG

Key-words: 24-hour ECG – Hyperthyroidism

The purpose of the study was to follow patients with hyperthyroidism by repeated Holter monitoring during antithyroid therapy in order to answer the following questions:

1. Do hyperthyroid patients exhibit increased supraventricular and ventricular arrhythmias, and if yes, do these arrhythmias decrease during antithyroid therapy?
2. What is the influence of hyperthyroidism on heart rate? Is there a day/night shift or remains heart rate unchanged durin 24 hours?

Patients and Methods

Patients

48 patients (9 male; mean age: 49 ± 11 years) with hyperthyroidism were eligible for the study. The diagnosis of manifest hyperthyroidism was based on elevated peripheral T3 hormone level > 196 ng/ml and a pathological TRH-test (ΔTSH < 0.5 μE/ml). Patients with cardiac or other diseases than hyperthyroidism were excluded from the study: history, clinical examination, electrocardiogram, 2-dimensional echocardiography with doppler and chest x-ray had to be normal. 70% of the patients had Graves' disease, 24% autonomous thyroid function. Goiter was found in 84%, Graves' ophthalmopathy in 54%. All patients were primarily treated by methimazole 5–40 mg per day, 17 patients were later given levothyroxine 25–150 μg per day. Antiarrhythmic or β-blocking therapy was generally not permitted during the study. The mean therapy was 25 ± 17 weeks (range 8–89 weeks).

Methods

All patients were followed by 24 hour Holter monitoring (Reynolds Pathfinder III® system) before and after antithyroid therapy. In 92% a Holter monitoring during therapy (3–9 weeks after initiating therapy, mean 6 ± 2 w) was available. All recordings were analysed twice semiautomatically. Supraventricular premature complexes were roughly classified into rare (< 100/24 h) and frequent (≥100/24 h) complexes. Examples of all types of ventricular premature complexes, all pairs and all ventricular tachycardias were interpreted by a cardiologist. Ventricular arrhythmias were classified according to Lown without class V [4]. For the analysis of heart rate we carefully distinguished between mean heart rate/24 h, heart rate during day and night.

Cardiac arrhythmias and heart rate were compared to those of 50 controls (41 male; mean age 51 ± 8 years, range 30–66 y), who were obviously free of cardiac disease according to examination, stress electrocardiogram, chest x-ray, 2-dimensional echocardiography and left heart catheterization.

Datas were given as mean ± standard deviation. Comparison of 2 samples was performed by the Wilcoxon-test, in case of normal distribution by paired or unpaired t-test. The comparison of 2 or more indices was done by X^2-test (Fisher's exact test) with two-tailed testing. Regression analysis was done by standard linear regression analysis.

Results

The incidence of patients with supraventricular premature complexes remained unchanged during the therapy (88% vs 81%) and was significantly increased compared to controls (38%; $p < 0.001$). The number of patients with >100 supraventricular complexes/24 h decreased during therapy, however, there was still a significant difference compared to controls ($p < 0.001$). The number of patients with supraventricular tachycardias decreased from 11 (25%) to 2 (4%; $p < 0.005$). 4 patients (8%) exhibited atrial fibrillation before therapy, two of whom spontaneously converted to sinus rhythm during therapy.

In general ventricular arrhythmias were rare and remained really unchanged during therapy. Before therapy 15 patients (32%) had complex ventricular arrhythmias (Lown class 3–4), compared to 12 patients (25%) after therapy and 6 patients (12%) in the control group ($p > 0.05$). The median of ventricular premature complexes/24 hours amounted to 2 before therapy and 1 after therapy compared to 1 in the control group. Before therapy 4 patients (11%) had > 100 ventricular premature complexes/24 hours compared to 3 patients (6%) in the control group ($p > 0.05$). The Lown classes showed a weak correlation with age ($r_s = 0.40$; $p < 0.02$) and T4 hormone level ($r_s = 0.37$; $p < 0.05$), but not with T3 hormone level.

In hyperthyroid patients mean heart rate/24 hours as well as mean day and mean night heart rate were significantly elevated as compared to controls (all differences $p < 0.001$). After therapy heart rates were still elevated, but the difference was always ≤10 beats/min compared to normals. Mean heart rate was >100/min in 54% before therapy and in 5% after therapy. The difference between day and night heart rate remained unchanged during therapy and was higher compared to the control group ($p < 0.001$). 5 hyperthyroid patients had a constant heart rate during 24 hours with day/night quotient <1.10. After therapy 4 patients and in the control group 9 patients (18%) had such a constant heart rate profile. Mean heart rate ($r = 0.65$), mean day and mean night heart rate ($r = 0.74$) showed a significant correlation with T3 hormone level.

Discussion

This study demonstrates that ventricular arrhythmias are rare in hyperthyroid patients without cardiac disease. The prevalence of ventricular arrhythmias remains essentially unchanged during antithyroid therapy and is comparable to that of a normal population. The severity of ventricular arrhythmias showed a weak correlation with age thus indicating that age may be one – well known – reason for the occurrence of ventricular arrhythmia in this study group.

However, supraventricular arrhythmias, especially supraventricular tachycardias were found more often in hyperthyroid patients than in normals. Only supraventricular tachycardias were significantly reduced during therapy; the prevalence of supraventricular premature complexes remained essentially unchanged. Since digitalis-toxicity was excluded, hyperthyroidism may have induced supraventricular tachycardias. How much the prevalence of supraventricular premature complexes might decrease down to normal after long lasting therapy can not be answered from this study. Akhtar et al. found supraventricular arrhythmia in only 2 of 60 patients (3%) by means of resting electrocardiogram [1]. The reason for this low prevalence is probably the short recording time. The incidence of atrial fibrillation (8%) was on the lower limit of what was to be expected in hyperthyroid patients [5, 6]. The patients with mitral valve prolapse without regurgitation had no more ventricular arrhythmias than the rest of the study group thus confirming the results of the study of Kraemer et al. [3].

The general clinical "experience" that hyperthyroid patients have elevated heart rates was confirmed by this study [2, 7]. Mean day heart rate amounted to 100 ± 13/min. However, this increased heart rate is not kept constant during 24 hours, but an even more pronounced day/night shift than the control group and is hardly influenced by short-term antithyroid therapy. The hyperthyroid state induces a parallel movement of the heart rate curve which is similar to normal after therapy. The closest correlation between T3 hormone level and human heart rate was found for night heart rate which is least influenced by sympathetic tone. The cardiac strong feelings and palpitations are mainly caused by sinus tachycardia and/or supraventricular arrhythmias. Ventricular arrhythmias were too rare in this study to be responsible for the symptoms of the majority of patients. Antiarrhythmic therapy is definitely not necessary in these patients.

References

1. Akhtar M, Singh SJ, Krishnamurti S (1987) Cardiovascular manifestation in thyroid disorders. Indian Heart J 203–207
2. Forfar JC, Caldwell GC (1985) Hyperthyroid heart disease. Clin Endocrinol Metab 14: 491–508
3. Kraemer HM, Kligfield P, Devereux RB, Savage DD, Kraemer-Fox R (1984) Arrhythmias in mitral valve prolapse: effect of selection bias. Arch Intern Med 144:2360–2364
4. Ryan M, Lown B, Horn H (1975) Comparison of ventricular ectopic activity during 24-hour monitoring and exercise testing in patients with coronary heart disease. N Engl J Med 292:224–229
5. Sandler G, Wilson GM (1959) The nature and prognosis of heart disease in thyrotoxicosis. Q J Med 28:347–369
6. Staffurth JS, Gibbered MC, Tangfui SNG (1977) Arterial embolism in thyrotoxicosis with atrial fibrillation. Br Med J 2:688–690
7. Symons C (1979) Thyroid heart disease. Br Heart J 41:257–262

Effects of Propranolol Isomers in Hyperthyroid and Euthyroid Patients

B. Pietsch, H. Warnkroß, G. Obermayer, G. Stark, S. Sager, W. Lindner, W. Klein, and G. Leb

Department of Internal Medicine and Institute of Pharmaceutical Chemistry, University of Graz, Austria

Key words: Hyperthyroidism – Propranolol isomers – Deiodeination

Introduction

The effects of Propranolol (prop.) as a racemate have been described extensively. In peripheral thyroid hormone metabolism, prop. inhibits the T3/T4 conversion with a simultaneous increase in rT3.

Until now in hyperthyroidism the drug has been used symptomatically like other beta-blocking agents because of an increased number of beta-adrenoceptors.

The present study evaluated the activity of the isomers used separately in hyperthyroid patients compared to normal controls. We also looked at whether the activity can be ascribed to beta-receptor antagonism [1].

Patients and Methods

Ten patients with untreated hyperthyroidism of recent onset and nine healthy euthyroid controls (age 37 ± 10 years, range from 21 to 64) of comparable body mass index were studied. After informed consent, all probands randomly received R- or S-prop. (40 mg t.i.d.) for 5 days separated by a placebo pause.

We measured cardiac parameters (blood pressure, heart rate, ECG) and on day 1, 3 and 5 all peripheral thyroid parameters, pituitary hormones, parameters of glucose and lipid metabolism and plasma levels of prop. isomers using high-pressure liquid chromatography [2]. For phenotypical classification of prop. metabolism (poor or extensive metabolizer) we compared urine samples for spartein metabolic rate.

Statistical Analysis

Significances of the differences were evaluated by the two-tailed unpaired t-test. Values were considered to be significant at $p < 0.05$. In cases of wide interindividual variance without mathematical significance, percentual values are shown.

Results

As expected, plasma levels of prop. varied widely among the individuals. On average, S-prop. concentrations were higher than R-prop. levels and both were higher in the euthyroid than in the hyperthyroid group. In the euthyroid group, we found two "poor metabolizers" with high prop. levels. There was no inversion from R-prop. to S-prop. or vice versa.

In peripheral thyroid hormone metabolism, only R-prop. was active. In the euthyroid group T3 decreased significantly after 5 days ($p < 0.01$) as did fT3 and the T3/T4-ratio. T3, fT3 and the T3/T4-ratio in hyperthyroid patients were similar. In contrast, rT3 increased in both groups within 5 days (+50%, $p < 0.01$). The T4 levels remained unchanged in both groups, in euthyroid probands fT4 increased (+30%, $p < 0.05$).

Cholesterol and LDL decreased slightly in the controls receiving S-prop. There was no change in blood sugar or insulin metabolism. Blood pressure and heart rate fell significantly ($p < 0.01$) in all S-prop. treated probands.

Discussion

Since the effect of R-prop. seems independent of its beta-blocking action, several concepts have been proposed. There is scant evidence for a membrane-stabilizing, quinidine-like effect in vivo at the dosage used. Structural similarity to tyrosine also does not solve the problem. A stereospecific decrease in liver ATP-content and T4 uptake could be possible [3].

We concluded that prop. stereo-specifically inhibits the 5′-deiodeinase with accumulation of rT3 and decrease of T3.

Conclusion

Because of the absence of cardiac effects, R-prop. could be used as an auxiliary medication in hyperthyroid patients with relative or absolute contraindications to beta-blockers, i.e. obstructive airway disease, congestive heart failure, peripheral arterial disease, diabetes mellitus or pregnancy.

References

1. Barrett AM, Cullum AC (1968) The biological properties of the optical isomers of propranolol and their effects on cardiac arrhythmias. Br J Pharmacol 34:43–55
2. Lindner W, Leitner CH, Uray G (1984) Liquid chromatographic separation of enantiomeric alkanolamines via diastereomeric tartaric acid monoesters. J Chromatogr 316:605–616
3. Krenning EP, Docter R, Bernard HF, Visser RJ, Hennemann G (1982) Decreased transport of thyroxine (T4), 3,3′,5-triiodothyronine (T3) and 3,3′,5′-triiodothyronine (rT3) into rat hepatocytes in primary culture due to a decrease of cellular ATP content and various drugs. FEBS Lett 140:229

The Effect of Treatment with Propranolol, Verapamil and Dantrolene on the in vitro Performance of the Hyperthyroid Rat Heart

N. Butkow, J. Musiker, J. Grote, A. M. Wheatley, and C. Rosendorff

Department of Medical Physiology and the MRC/University Circulation Research Unit, University of the Witwatersrand, Johannesburg, South Africa

Key words: Hyperthyroidism – Verapamil – Propranolol – Myocardial contractility – Heart rate

Introduction

The hyperthyroid myocardium exhibits a number of alterations, including tachycardia, cardiac hypertrophy, enhanced calcium fluxes across the sarcolemma and the sarcoplasmic reticulum, and an increase in the number of myocardial beta-receptors (Morkin et al. 1983). To define the role that these processes might play in the pathogenesis of hyperthyroidism, we investigated the effect of treatment of hyperthyroid rats with three drugs that interfere with some of these mechanisms in isolated perfused hearts.

Methods

Hyperthyroidism was induced in rats by daily injection of L-thyroxine (1 mg · kg^{-1} · day^{-1}) for 7 days and then, together with a maintenance dose of thyroxine (0.25 mg · kg^{-1} · day^{-1}), were treated for 14 days with one of the following: Propranolol (10 mg · kg^{-1} · day^{-1}) a beta-adrenergic blocker, verapamil (10 mg · kg^{-1} · day^{-1}), a calcium channel blocker and dantrolene (5 mg · kg^{-1} · day^{-1}), a sarcoplasmic reticulum calcium blocker. 24 hours after the final dose, the rats were killed, the hearts removed and perfused with Krebs-Henseleit buffer in the non-working mode (Marcus et al. 1987). Cardiac function (heart rate, coronary flow and dP/dt_{max}) were measured *in vitro* (Marcus et al. 1987) at spontaneous heart rate and at paced rates. Dry heart mass to body-mass ratios were also obtained. Statistical analysis was carried out using a ANOVA procedure with Tukey's correction for unequal cell sizes.

Results

Verapamil treatment reversed the thyroxine-induced tachycardia 267 ± 8.8 beats · min^{-1}, which was not dissimilar to heart rates obtained in the control group (Table 1). Neither propranolol or dantrolene altered hyperthyroid heart rate. Propranolol reduced the enhanced contractile response, however, unlike the action of verapamil, this effect was maintained at paced heart rates (Table 1), implying a direct negative inotropic action. Both propranolol and verapamil partially reversed the development of the hypertrophy of hyperthyroidism (Table 1). Values for the drug treated groups were still significantly higher than that seen in the euthyroid saline treated group (0.53 ± 0.01 mg · g^{-1}, $p < 0.01$). None of the drug treatments affected coronary flow.

Discussion

The only drug treatment that significantly altered heart rate was verapamil. It is known to possess negative chronotropic activity both *in vivo* and *in vitro* (Singh et al. 1982), although its effect has never been demonstrated before in the hyperthyroid state. It was surprising that propranolol was ineffective on thyroxine-induced tachycardia, as it is widely used in clinical situations (Feely and Peden 1984). In animals, however, propranolol has been found to reduce heart rate to the same extent in hyperthyroid and euthyroid (Strauer and Scherpe 1975; Gross and Lues 1985).

Propranolol treatment effectively reduced contractility. It has been found to cause a greater depression of contractility in the hyperthyroid, than in the euthyroid heart (Strauer and Scherpe 1975; Rutherford et al. 1979). Although verapamil did reduce contractility, this was probably associated with its negative chronotropic action (Singh et al. 1982). Propranolol and verapamil were equally effective in reducing the hypertrophy of hyperthyroidism, but not to control levels. Although verapamil has never been investigated in this regard, propranolol has been found to reduce but not reverse this hypertrophy (Gross and Lues 1985).

Table 1. Heart rate and dP/dt_{max} (measured *in vitro*) and dry heart mass to body mass ratios of hearts following various treatment schedules

	Spontaneous heart rate (beats · min^{-1})	dP/dt_{max} (unpaced) (mmHg · sec^{-1})	dP/dt_{max} (paced) (mmHg · sec^{-1})	Dry heart mass: body mass ratio (mg · g^{-1})
Thyroxine	331 ± 5.6	4121 ± 57	4271 ± 71	0.92 ± 0.02
Thyroxine and propranolol	312 ± 5.3	3782 ± 72[a]	3854 ± 85[a]	0.70 ± 0.01[b]
Thyroxine and verapamil	267 ± 8.8[b]	3777 ± 54[a]	4153 ± 53	0.74 ± 0.02[b]
Thyroxine and dantrolene	307 ± 9.2	3880 ± 101	3955 ± 66	0.99 ± 0.04
Thyroxine and Saline	272 ± 7.7[b]	3485 ± 65[b]	3879 ± 65[a]	0.69 ± 0.02[b]
Saline	244 ± 5.9[b]	3065 ± 61[b]	3604 ± 113[b]	0.52 ± 0.01[b]

[a] $p < 0.01$ vs thyroxine; [b] $p < 0.001$ vs thyroxine

In conclusion it appears that verapamil primarily effects sinoatrial frequency, while propranolol exerts a negative inotropic action on the hyperthyroid myocardium. The inability of dantrolene to exert an action may reflect the insensitivity of myocardium to dantrolene. Both calcium and adrenergic mechanisms appear to play a role in the genesis of hypertrophy in hyperthyroidism.

References

Feeley J, Peden N (1984) Use of beta-adrenoreceptor blocking drugs in hyperthyroidism. Drugs 27:425–446

Gross G, Lues I (1985) Thyroid-dependent alterations of myocardial adrenoreceptors and adrenoreceptor mediated responses in the rat. Naunyn-Schmiedebergs Arch Pharmacol 329: 427–439

Marcus RH, Butkow N, Wheatley AM, Lippe I, Norton G, Rosendorff C (1987) Independent mechanisms for the chronotropic and inotropic responses in hyperthyroidism. Basic Res Cardiol 82:261–270

Morkin E, Flink IL, Goldman S (1983) Biochemical and physiological effects of thyroid hormone on cardiac performance. Prog Cardiovasc Dis 25:435–465

Rutherford JD, Vatner SF, Braunwald E (1979) Adrenergic control of myocardial contractility in conscious hyperthyroid dogs. Am J Physiol 237:H590–H596

Singh BN, Hecht HS, Nadamanee K, Chew CYC (1982) Electrophysiologic and hemodynamic effects of slow-channel blocking drugs. Prog Cardiovasc Dis 25:103–132

Strauer BE, Scherpe A (1975) Experimental hyperthyroidism III: Contractile response to propranolol of the intact heart and of the isolated myocardium. Basic Res Cardiol 70: 237–245

Radioimmunoassay of Plasma and Urinary Norepinephrine

B. Manz[1], M. Lorey[1], K. Pollow[1], U. Krause[2], and J. Beyer[2]

[1] Department of Experimental Endocrinology and [2] Department of Internal Medicine, Endocrinology and Metabolism; Joh. Gutenberg-Universität Mainz, FRG

Key words: Radioimmunoassay – Plasma – Urinary norepinephrine

Introduction

Various analytical methods, such as fluorimetry, radioenzymic assay and in particular liquid chromatography are used for the analysis of norepinephrine (NA) in body fluids and tissue homogenates. These procedures, however, often lack sensitivity, are expensive and/or time consuming. Basing on our previous reports on the radioimmunoassay of chemically modified serotonin[1], 5-hydroxy-3-indole acetic acid[2] and normetanephrine (NMN)[3], a sensitive radioimmunoassay of the N-acetyl,3-methoxy analogue of urinary and plasma norepinephrine was developed.

Methods

Radioimmunoassay

The antiserum was raised in a rabbit against a conjugate of bovine serum albumin with normetanephrine hemisuccinamide[3]. Polyethylene glycol 4000 (Merck, Darmstadt, FRG) in combination with goat anti-rabbit IgG was used to separate bound and unbound ^{125}I-Bolton-Hunter reagent-NMN conjugate. A specific one tube sample preparation was established. After solid phase extraction of NA using immobilized m-aminoboronic acid, NA was converted enzymatically to NMN using rat liver catechol-O-methyltransferase and S-adenosyl-L-methionine p-toluenesulfonate as coenzyme. The enzymatic reaction was terminated by the N-acetylation of NMN with acetic anhydride. The resulting stabile N-acetylnormetanephrine was then determined. This sample preparation allows the processing of large series within one working day.

High Performance Liquid Chromatography (HPLC)

Urines were stabilized with 1 ml glycin/sulfuric acid buffer per 100 ml urine (100 mg glycin dissolved in 1 ml 5 N sulfuric acid). 1 ml aliquots were adjusted to pH 8.55 with TRIS-phosphate buffer (TRIS 121.14 g/l, Na_2HPO_4 5.0 g/l, EDTA-Na_2, 50 g/l) and absorbed to Al_2O_3. After two rinses with distilled water and one rinse with phosphate buffer (Na_2HPO_4, 5 g/l, pH 8.4), catecholamines were desorbet with 0.1 molar perchloric acid. These extracts were subjected to HPLC with postcolumn derivatization and fluorescence detection[4].

Results and Discussion

The minimal detectable concentration of NA was 0.2 nmol/l (20 pg/ml) plasma or 1 pg/tube. Recovery (including extraction, enzymatic methylation and acetylation) was 90 ± 3%, the intra-assay precision (CV) for urine samples was 7% ($n = 10$) at a level of 0.9 μmol/l, and 15% ($n = 10$) at a level of 0.22 μmol/l. The inter-assay CV was 9% at a level of 0.9 μmol/l. The only substances which significantly cross-reacted with the antibody were N-acyl derivatives of normetanephrine which were not detectable in the m-aminoboronic acid extract of plasma or urine when the acetylation step was omitted. To validate the clinical usefulness of this assay, a comparison with HPLC was performed. Both, radioimmunoassay and HPLC accurately identified two patients with known pheochromocytoma. A correlation of $r = 0.91$ was demonstrated be-

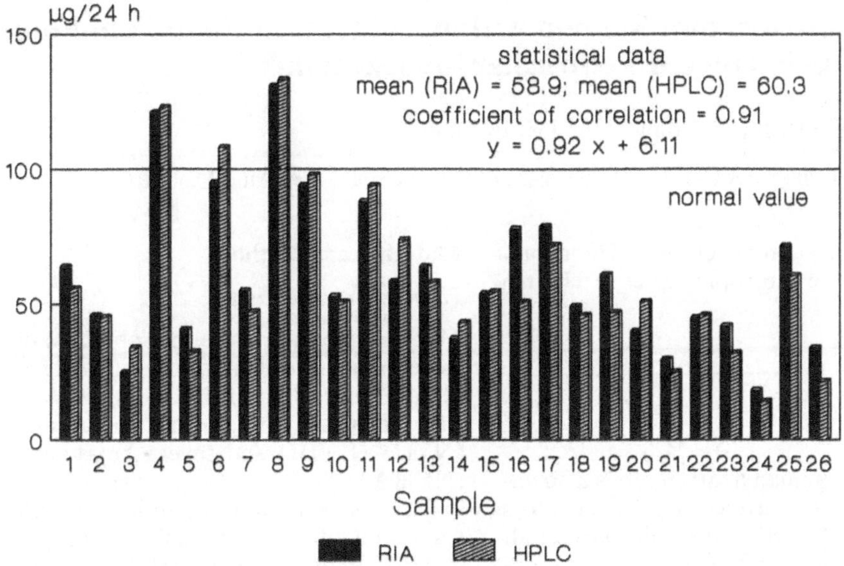

Fig. 1. Determination of norepinephrine in urine. Comparison of HPLC and RIA data

tween the two assays in a comparison of normal and pathological urines (Fig. 1). A simultanous determination of NA and its metabolits NMN in normal and pathological sera showed that both parameters were raised in case of pheochromocytoma.

References

Manz B, Kosfeld H, Belovsky O, Grill HJ, Pollow K (1986) Direkte radioimmunologische Bestimmung des Serotonins in normalen und pathologischen Seren. Arztl Lab 32:135–140

Manz B, Grill HJ, Belovsky O, Kleinböhl I, Heubner A, Pollow K (1987) Radioimmunoassay of 5-hydroxy-3-indole acetic acid. J Clin Chem Clin Biochem 25:101–106

Manz B, Bartolic M, Heyn S, Pollow K (1988) Screening for pheochromocytoma by direct radioimmunoassay of urinary normetanephrine. Acta Endocronol [Suppl] 287:245

Kringe KP, Neidhart B, Lippmann Ch (1982) Practical aspects of the routine determination by HPLC of free noradrenaline and adrenaline in urine and plasma. In: Molnar (ed) Practical aspects of modern HPLC. Walter de Gruyter, Berlin New York, pp 241–273

The β_2-Adrenoceptor Subpopulation and Its Contribution to Force Generation in Human Ventricular Myocardium*

M. Böhm, B. Pieske, P. Schnabel, and E. Erdmann

Medizinische Klinik I der Universität München. Klinikum Großhadern, München, FRG

Key words: β_2-adrenoceptor – Heart failure – Positive inotropic effect – Human myocardium

Introduction

In the failing human heart, there is a downregulation of cardiac β-adrenoceptors (Bristow et al. 1982, 1984; Ginsburg et al. 1983; Böhm et al. 1988a). As a consequence, the positive inotropic effect of β-adrenoceptor agonist is reduced under experimental (Bristow et al. 1982; Fowler et al. 1986; Böhm et al. 1988a, b) and clinical conditions (Colucci et al. 1988). Increased levels of noradrenaline, imposing a permanent β-adrenergic stimulus on the heart of patients with heart failure (Chidsey et al. 1962, Cohn et al. 1984), are regarded to initiate β-adrenoceptor downregulation. Since noradrenaline primarily stimulates β_1-adrenoceptors (Gille et al. 1985) one would expect that β_1-adrenoceptors are more affected by downregulation than the β_2-adrenoceptor subpopulation. If this is true, the stimulation of β_2-adrenoceptors which have been identified in the human myocardium by radioligand- and functional studies (Brodde et al. 1983, 1984, 1986) could be a usefull pathway to increase force of contraction in heart failure. Therefore, cardiac β-adrenoceptors and the β_1- and β_2-adrenoceptor subpopulation were studied with radioligand binding experiments. Moreover, the effect of the β_2-adrenoceptor agonist dopexamine (Brown et al. 1985; Smith et al. 1987) on force of contraction and adenylate cyclase activity was studied in isolated myocardium from failing hearts.

* Experimental work was supported by the Deutsche Forschungsgemeinschaft and Friedrich-Baur-Stiftung, Munich (FRG)

Materials and Methods

Human Cardiac Tissue

Myocardial tissue was either obtained during cardiac transplantations or mitral valve replacement operations. Patients were classified in groups with moderate heart failure (NYHA II–III) and severe heart failure (NYHA IV).

Patients received diuretics, nitrates, Ca^{2+}-antagonists and enalapril in some cases. Patients receiving catecholamines or β-blockers were withdrawn from the study.

Radioligand binding Experiments

The nonselective, hydrophilic ligand ^{3}H-CGP 12.177 was used. Competition experiments were performed with the selective β_1-adrenoceptor antagonists CGP 207.12 A and the β_2-selective antagonist ICI 118.551. Competition curves were analysed with the non-linear curve fitting program SCTFIT according to De Lean et al. (1982). Further experimental details are published elsewhere (Böhm et al. 1988a, b, 1989).

Contraction Experiments

Cardiac force of contraction was recorded in isolated, electrically driven (1 Hz) papillary muscle strips from patients with NYHA II–III or NYHA IV. For further details see Böhm et al. (1988a, b).

Adenylate Cyclase Assay

Adenylate cyclase activity was measured in broken cell preparations according to Kruse and Scholz (1978). Cyclic AMP was determined with a protein binding assay (Gilman 1970).

Abbreviations: ms = millisecond; mN = milli Newton; cAMP = cyclic adenosine-3′-5′monophosphate

Results

Cardiac β-Adrenoceptors

In the failing myocardium, there was a reduction in the number of β-adrenoceptors from 87.9 or 97 fmol/mg protein in two nonfailing hearts to 57.8 ± 4.6 fmol/mg protein ($n = 6$) in failing hearts. The reduction in the total amount of β-adrenoceptors was accompanied by a reduction of the β_1-subpopulation, whereas the number of β_2-adrenoceptors was not detectably changed. This leads to an increased β_2- to β_1-adrenoceptor ratio in the failing myocardium of 38.6/61.4 compared to 21/79 in the normal myocardium.

Radioligand binding data are summarized in Table 1.

Force Contraction and Adenylate Cyclase Activity

Fig. 1A shows typical force recordings in papillary muscle strips from a patient with moderate heart failure (NYHA II–III) due to mitral valve disease. Dopexamine alone failed to increase force of contraction but produced a positive inotropic effect in the presence of milrinone. Cumulative concentration-response curves (Fig. 1B) demonstrate the positive inotropic effects of dopexamine alone, dopexamine in the presence of milrinone, isoprenaline and Ca^{2+}. Dopexamine alone did not increase force of contraction but exerted contraction-dependent positive inotropic effects after preincubation with milrinone.

However, the positive inotropic effect of isoprenaline was more potent and efficacious than the effect of dopexamine plus milrinone. Ca^{2+} was studied in order to meassure the maximal possible effect in each individual preparation. In NYHA II–III, the positive inotropic effect of isoprenaline amounted to about 70% of the maximal positive inotropic effect of Ca^{2+}. The concentration-response curve fordopexamine in the presence of milrinone was shifted to the right by ICI 118.551 but was unaffected by CGP 207.12 A.

Dopexamine concentration-dependently stimulated adenylate cyclase activity to 236.3 ± 25.4% ($n = 6$) of basal activity at 100 µmol/l in NYHA IV. Like in the experiments on force of contraction ICI 118.551 produced a rightward shift of the concentration response curve whereas CGP 207.12 A hade no effect. The pD_2-valves are summarized in Table 2.

Discussion

The major findings of the present study are that cardiac β-adrenoceptors are reduced in failing myocardium. This downregulation affects primarily the β_1-adrenoceptor subpopulation, leaving the β_2-adrenoceptor population unchanged. However, dopexamine alone failed to increase force of contraction. In the presence of milrinone, a positive inotropic response was observed. Both, the increase of force of contraction and stimulation of adenylate cyclase activity was mediated by β_2- but not β_1-adrenoceptors.

In patients with heart failure, a permanent β-adrenergic stimulus is imposed on the heart by a compensatory activation of the sympathetic nervous system (Packer 1988). As a consequence, increased noradrenaline levels can be measured in the blood of these patients (Chidsey et al. 1960; Cohn et al.

Table 1. Identification of β_1- and β_2-adrenoceptor subtypes in nonfailing (NF) and failing (NYHA IV) human myocardium determined by competition of CGP 207.12 A and ICI 118.551 to ^{3}H-CGP 12.177 binding

		CGP 207.12 A					ICI 118.551				
	B_{max} (fmol/mg protein)	β_1 (%)	β_2 (%)	K_H nmol/l	K_L nmol/l	β_1 selectivity	β_1 (%)	β_2 (%)	K_H nmol/l	K_A nmol/l	β_2-selectivity
NF	87.9	80	20	7.0	3177	454	80	20	5.8	1236	213
n = 2	96.0	78	22	7.0	4628	661	76	24	4.3	819	191
NYHA IV	57.8	61.4	38.6	7.8	5370	714	64.8	35.4	4.6	968	224
n = 5	±4.6	±3.0	±3.0		(3157–	±90	±3.5	±3.6		(752–	±21
				(6.1–9.9)	9132)				(3.3–6.3)	1245)	

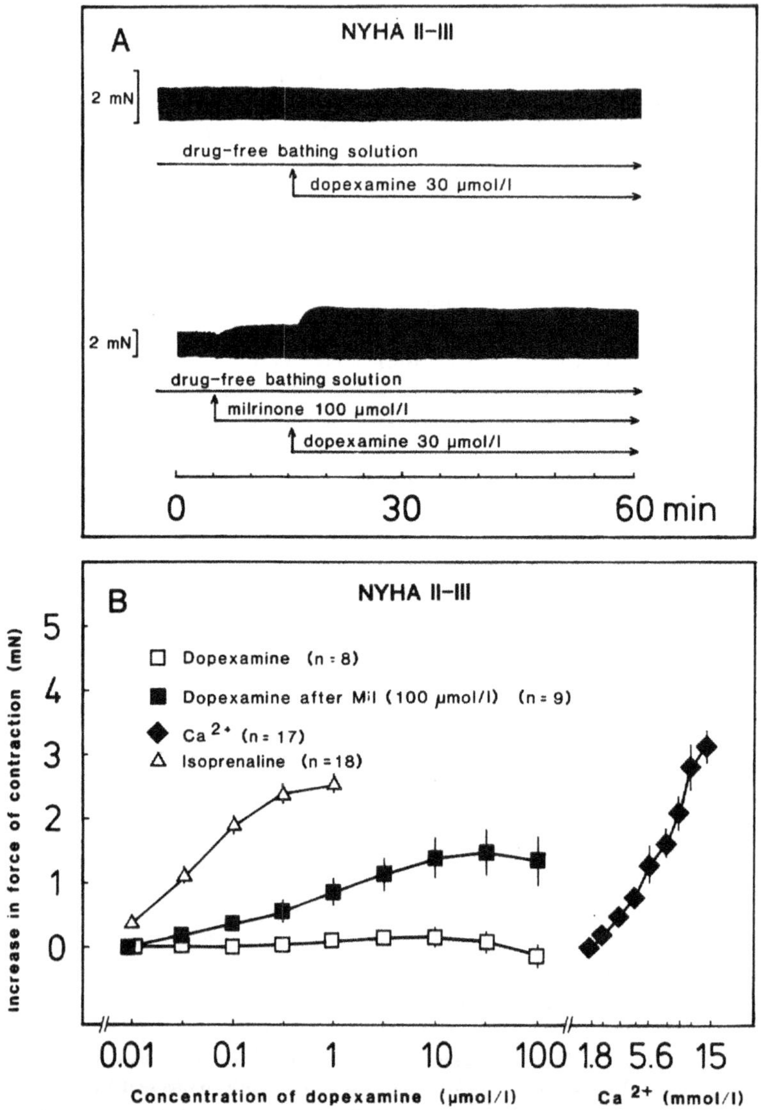

Fig. 1 Orginal tracing **(A)** illustrating force generation after dopexamine alone (30 µmol/l, upper panel) and dopexamine in the presence of milrinone (lower panel) and cumulative concentration-response curves for isoprenaline, dopexamine, dopexamine after milrinone and Ca^{2+} in isolated, electrically driven papillary muscle strips from patients with moderate heart failure (NYHA II–III). Basal force of contraction was 1.8 ± 0.2 mN (n = 52). Modified from Böhm et al. (1989)

Table 2. pD_2 values of the effect of dopexamine (Dopex) on adenylate cyclase activity and force of contraction

	Dopex	Dopex + CGP 207.12 A	Dopex + ICI 118.551
Adenylate cyclase activity	5.48 ± 0.24[a]	5.19 ± 0.17[a]	4.66 ± 0.1
Force of contraction	5.78 ± 0.77[a]	6.32 ± 0.41[a]	4.42 ± 0.48

[a] $p < 0.05$ vs Dopex + ICI 118.551
Experiments on force of contraction were performed in the presence of 100 µmol/l milrinone.
Modified from Böhm et al. (1989).

1984). Prolonged agonist stimulation produces downregulation of their receptors with consequently reduced agonist-stimulated adenylate cyclase activity (Sibley and Lefkowitz 1984). The agonist-induced downregulation is the most likely explanation for the reduced number of β-adrenoceptors in the failing myocardium observed in this and previous studies (Bristow et al. 1982, 1984; Böhm et al. 1988a, b). The number of β_1- but not the number of β_2-adrenoceptors was reduced in NYHA IV. This finding provides evidence that noradrenaline-induced downregulation specifically affects β_1-adrenoceptors. This is supported by the findings that noradrenaline induced stimulation of adenylate cyclase is mainly mediated by β_1-adrenoceptors (Gille et al. 1985). Moreover, there is no good evidence that in heart failure adrenaline, which stimulates β_1- and β_2-adrenoceptors, is excessively increased (Cohn et al. 1984).

Dopexamine stimulates selectively cardiac β_2-adrenoceptors (Brown et al. 1985, Smith et al. 1987) and produces haemodynamic improvement in patients with congestive heart failure (Tan et al. 1987). The increase in force of contraction by dopexamine in the presence of milrinone and stimulation of adenylate cyclase was mediated by β_2-adrenoceptors. These findings demonstrates that β_2-adrenoreceptors are capable of coupling to myocardial adenylate cyclase thereby increasing force of contraction. Notwithstanding the preserved β_2-adrenoceptors population, stimulation of β_2-adrenoceptors by dopexamine failed to reliably increase force of contraction. Although partial agonist properties of dopexamine could contribute to this lack of effect, stimulation of cardiac β_2-adrenoceptors might not be sufficient to maintain cardiac force of contraction in heart failure. The beneficial haemodynamic effects of dopexamine in patients with heart failure might, therefore, be due to effects on peripheral circulation such as after- or preload reduction.

References

Böhm M, Beuckelmann D, Brown L, Feiler G, Lorenz B, Näbauer M, Kemkes B, Erdmann E (1988) Reduction of beta-adrenoceptor density and evaluation of positive inotropic responses in isolated, diseased human myocardium. Eur Heart J 9:844–852

Böhm M, Diet F, Feiler G, Kemkes B, Kreuzer E, Weinhold C, Erdmann E (1988) Subsensitivity of the failing human heart to isoprenaline and milrinone is related to beta-adrenoceptor downregulation. J Cardiovasc Pharmacol 12: 726–732

Böhm M, Pieske B, Schnabel P, Schwinger R, Kemkes B, Klövekorn, Erdman E (1989) Reduced effects of dopexamine on force of contraction in the failing human heart despite preserved β_2-adrenoceptor subpopulation. J Cardiovasc Pharmacol, in press

Bristow MR, Ginsburg R, Minobe W, Cubiciotti RS, Sageman WS, Lurie K, Billingham ME, Harrison DC, Stinson EB (1982) Decreased catecholamine sensitivity and beta-adrenergic-receptor density in failing human hearts. N Engl J Med 307:205–211

Bristow MR, Kantrowitz NE, Ginsburg R, Fowler MR (1985) Betaadrenergic function in heart muscle disease and heart failure. J Mol Cell Cardiol 17 [Suppl 2]:41–52

Bristow MR, Ginsburg R, Umans V, Fowler M, Minobe W, Rasmussen R, Zera P, Menlove R, Shah P, Jamieson S, Stinson EB (1986) β_1- and β_2-Adrenergic receptor subpopulatons in nonfailing and failing human ventricular myocardium: coupling of both receptor subtypes to muscle contraction and selective β_1-receptor down-regulation in heart failure. Circ Res 59:297–309

Brodde OE, Karad K, Zerkowski HR, Rohm N, Reidemeister JCh (1983) Coexistence of β_1- and β_2-adrenoceptors in human right atrium. Direct indentificaton by (I)-125iodocyanopindolol binding. Circ Res 53:752–758

Brodde OE, O'Hara N, Zerkowski HR, Rohm N (1984) Human cardiac β-adrenoceptors: both β_1- and β_2-adrenoceptors are functionally coupled to the adenylate cyclase in the right atrium. J Cardiovasc Pharmacol 6:1184–1191

Brodde OE, Schüler S, Kretsch R, Brinkmann M, Borst HG, Hetzer R, Reidemeister JCh, Warnecke H, Zerkowski HR (1986) Regional distribution of β-adrenoceptors in the human heart: coexistence of functional β1- and β2-adrenoceptors in both atria and ventricles in severe congestive cardiomyopathy. J Cardiovasc Pharmacol 8:1235–1242

Brown RA, Dixon J, Farmer JB, Hal JC, Humphries RG, Ince F, O'Connor SE, Simpson WT, Smith GW (1985) Dopexamine: a novel agonist at peripheral dopamine receptors and β_2-adrenoceptors. Br J Pharmacol 85:599–608

Chidsey CA, Harrison DC, Braunwald E (1962) Augmentation of the plasma noradrenaline response to exercise in patients with congestive heart failure. N Engl J Med 267:650–654

Cohn JN, Levine TB, Olivari MT, Garberg V, Lura D, Francis GS, Simon AB, Rector T (1984) Plasma noradrenaline as a guide to prognosis in patients with chronic congestive heart failure. N Engl J Med 311:819–823

Colucci WS, Leatherman GF, Ludmer PL, Gauthier DF (1987) β-adrenergic inotropic responsiveness of patients with heart failure: studies with intracoronary dobutamine infusion. Circ Res 61 [Suppl I]:82–86

De Lean A, Hancock AA, Lefkowitz RJ (1982) Validation and statistical analysis of a computer modeling method for quantitative analysis of radioligand binding data for mixtures of pharmacological receptor subtypes. Mol Pharmacol 21:5–16

Gille E, Lemoine H, Ehle B, Kaumann AJ (1985) The affinity of (−)-propranolol for β_1- and β_2-adrenoceptors of human heart. Differential antagonism of the positive inotropic effects and adenylate cyclase stimulation by (−)-noradrenaline and (−)-adrenaline. Naunyn-Schmiedebergs Arch Pharmacol 331:60–70

Gilman AG (1970) A protein binding assay for adenosine 3′,5′-cyclic monophosphate. Proc Natl Acad Sci USA 67:305–312

Ginsburg R, Bristow MR, Billingham ME, Stinson EB, Schroeder JS, Harrison DC (1983) Study of the normal and failing isolated human heart: decreased response of failing heart to isoproterenol. Am Heart J 106:535–540

Kruse E, Scholz H (1987) Effect of theophylline on myocardial adenylate cyclase activity. Experientia 34:504–505

Packer M (1988) Neurohormonal interactions and adaptations in congestive heart failure. Circulation 77:721–730

Sibley DR; Lefkowitz RJ (1985) Molecular mechanisms of receptor desensitization using the beta-adrenergic receptor-coupled adenylate cyclase system as a model. Nature 317: 124–129

Smith GW, Hall JC, Farmer JB, Simpson WT (1987) The cardiovascular actions of dopexamine hydrochloride, an agonist at dopexamine receptors and β_2-adrenoceptors in the dog. J Pharm Pharmacol 39:636–641

Tan LB, Litter WA, Murray RG (1987) Beneficial haemodynamic effects of intravenous dopexamine in patients with low-output heart failure. J Cardiovasc Pharmacol 10:280–286

Efficacy of Alpha-Methyldopa in Ventricular Arrhythmias by Decrease of Sympathetic Activity

P. Brugger

Pensionsversicherungsanstalt der Arbeiter, Landesstelle Salzburg, Austria

Key words: Alpha-methyldopa – Ventricular arrhythmias – Sympathetic activity

Introduction

Identifying patients at increased risk of sudden death continues to be a key problem in contemporary cardiology. It has been recognized that certain types of ventricular premature beats (specifically, repetitive forms or runs of ventricular tachycardia) enhances the risk for sudden cardiac death [4, 27, 29] and that patients with coronary artery disease (CAD) and symptomatic ventricular tachycardia or ventricular fibrillation in their history, are especially prone to sudden death.

Moreover, their suppression with antiarrhythmic drugs prevents a recurrence of arrhythmia and improves survival [7]. But treatment of these arrhythmias is difficult and often frustrating because of frequent failure of antiarrhythmic agents, and a high incidence of side-effects associated with currently available drugs. Therefore, there is a undimineshed need of a well tolerated antiarrhythmic agent.

Alpha-methyldopa, a centrally acting antihypertensive, was investigated for its effect on the heart in patients with coronary artery disease for antiarrhythmic properties. Direct effects of alpha-methyldopa on ventricular arrhythmias were not yet investigated but may be of interest because alpha-methyldopa inhibits the central sympathetic activity.

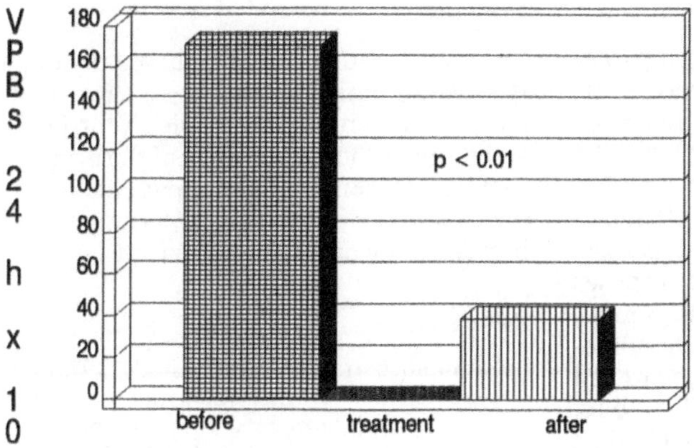

Fig. 1. Effects of alpha-methyldopa on ventricular arrythmias

Patients and Methods

The study was conducted in 14 patients (12 men, 2 women), aged 60 ± 9 (range 47–71) years with at least Lown grade IVa per 24 hrs. Cardiac diagnosis was coronary artery disease in all patients.

All patients were treated with alpha-methyldopa 250 mg twice a day. This treatment was continued during a two weeks period. Arrhythmia monitoring was performed before and after the treatment by 24 hr Holter recordings using the Reynolds Pathfinder II system.

For the maximal grading of ectopic activity we used a modified Lown's classification of ventricular arrhythmias [3, 20].

Results

For all coronary patients a daily dose of alpha-methyldopa dose of 500 mg caused a significant reduction of VPCs by 78% ($p < 0.01$) whereat this ventricular extrasystoles decreased significantly from 1712 ± 2091 to 387 ± 295 (fig. 1). A similar result was also found for couplets, which showed a significant reduction of 95% ($p < 0.0001$) with a decrease from 27 ± 48 to 1.1 ± 1.7 after treatment with alpha-methyldopa (fig. 2). Ventricular tachycardia, present in 5 of 14 patients, were prevented in all cases by alpha-methyldopa. The maximal grade of arrhythmias according to Lown's classification showed a significant improvements in the Lown grades from 4.4 to 3.3 in all patients ($p < 0.001$). No adverse reactions were noted under the drugs therapy.

Statistics

An applied test includes matched-pairs Wilcoxon signed-ranks test. A p value of less than 0.05 has been accepted as the limit of significance.

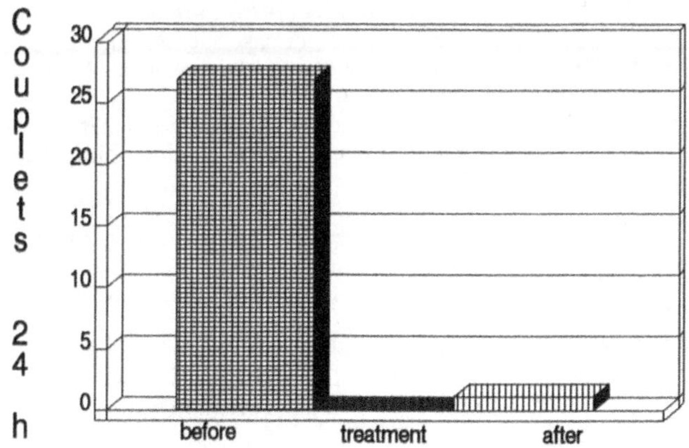

Fig. 2. Antiarrhythmic efficacy of alpha-methyldopa on Couplets; $p < 0.0001$

Discussion

It has long been recognized that sympathetic neural activity predisposes to cardiac arrhythmias and increases cardiac vulnerability to ventricular fibrillation [6, 13, 19, 21, 25, 32]. Enhanced sympathetic activity, whether elicited by electrical stimulation of hypothalamic centers or of stellate ganglia increases sympathetic tone and predisposes to various arrhythmias [9, 17, 32]. Similar effects can be induced with sympathomimetic drugs [11, 28]. Conversely, the heart can be protected against arrhythmias by reduction of sympathetic neural traffic achieved either surgically [5, 10, 16, 18, 22, 24, 31] or pharmacologically [1, 2, 8, 11, 12, 14, 15, 28]. Because it has been documented that the presence of complex forms of ventricular premature beats is associated with a threefold increased incidence of sudden cardiac death in the 5 year period after acute myocardial infarction [29, 30], there is a great importance of treatment of these ventricular arrhythmias.

The main problem in antiarrhythmic therapy occurs in the fact that available drugs are not able to reduce ventricular arrhythmias in all of the treated cases.

Therefore there is a need of new antiarrhythmic drugs. In this connection our experiences with alpha-methyldopa are of great interest, since they demonstrate for the first time that under this treatment there could be verified a significant decrease of couplets from 27 ± 48 to 1.1 ± 1.7. A similar result was also found for ventricular premature beats, which revealed a significant decrease from 1712 ± 2091 to 387 ± 295. Moreover ventricular tachycardia, present in 5 of 14 patients, were prevented by alpha-methyldopa.

The efficacy of alpha-methyldopa in ventricular arrhythmias is caused by inhibition of noradrenaline synthesis and reduced sympathetic tone.

In addition to that investigations of Philippu and Schümann [26] are worth mentioning since they showed a loss of noradrenaline from guinea-pig hearts after alpha-methyldopa treatment. Moreover Muscholl and Rahn [23] found in patients treated with alpha-methyldopa a diminished urinary excretion of noradrenaline.

Conclusion

Our results indicate that alpha-methyldopa is a useful antiarrhythmic agent for treatment of patients with complex ventricular arrhythmias. The properties of the drug are such that under its influence patients suffering from ventricular tachycardia may expect protection against tachycardia episodes.

References

1. A multicentre international study (1975) Improvement of prognosis of myocardial infarction by long-term beta-adrenoceptor blockade using practolol. Br J Med 3:735–740
2. Ahlmark G, Saetre H (1976) Long-term treatment with beta-blockers after myocardial infarction. Eur J Clin Pharmacol 10: 77–83
3. Bethge KP, Klein H, Lichtlen PR (1970) Koronare Herzerkrankung, Rhythmusstörungen und plötzlicher Herztod. Internist Welt 2:107–117
4. Bigger JT, Weld FM, Rolnitzky LM (1981) Prevalence, characteristics and significance of ventricular tachycardia (three or more complexes) detected with ambulatory monitoring in the late hospital phase of acute myocardial infarction. Am J Cardiol 48: 815–823
5. Cox WV, Robertson HF (1936) The effect of stellate ganglionectomy on the cardiac function of intact dogs and its effect on the extent of myocardial infarction and on cardiac function following coronary artery occlusion. Am Heart J 12:285–300
6. Erlij D, Mendez R (1964) The modification of digitalis intoxication by excluding adrenergic influences on the heart. J Pharmacol Exp Ther 144:97–193
7. Garrey WE (1908) Some effects of cardiac nerves upon ventricular fibrillation. Am J Physiol 21:282–300
8. Grossmann MA (1976) Cardiac arrhythmias in acute CNS disease-successfull management with stellate ganglion block. Arch Intern Med 136:203–207
9. Han J, Garcia de Jalon P, Moe G (1964) Adrenergic effects on cardiac vulnerability. Circ Res 14:516
10. Harris AS, Estandia A, Tillotson RF (1951) Ventricular ectopic rhythms and ventricular fibrillation following cardiac sympathectomie and coronary occlusion. Am J Physiol 165:505–512
11. Hoff HE, Nahum LH (1934) The role of adrenaline in the production of ventricular rhythms and their supression by acetyl-beta-

methyl-choline chloride. J Pharmacol Exp Ther 52:235–245
12. Hoff HE, Nahum LH (1935) The nature of ventricular fibrillation following electric schock and its prevention by acetyl-beta-methyl-choline chloride. Am J Physiol 110: 680
13. Hunt R (1899) Direct and reflex acceleration of the mammalian heart with some observations on the relations of the inhibitory and accelerator nerves. Am J Physiol 2:395–470
14. Kelliher G, Roberts J (1974) A study of the antiarrhythmic action of certain beta-blocking agents. Am Heart J 87:458–467
15. Khan MI, Hamilton JT, Manning GW (1972) Protective effects of beta-adrenoceptor blockade in experimental coronary occlusion in conscious dogs. Am J Cardiol 30:832–837
16. Kliks BR, Burgess M, Abildskov JA (1975) Influence of sympathetic tone on ventricular fibrillation threshold during experimental coronary occlusion. Am J Cardiol 36:45–49
17. Korteweg GCJ, Boeles TF, Tencate J (1975) Influence of stimulation of some subcortical areas on electrocardiogram. J Neurophysiol 20:100
18. LeRoy GV, Snider SS (1941) The sudden death of patients with few symptoms of heart disease. JAMA 117:2019–2024
19. Levy AG (1913) The exciting causes of ventricular fibrillation in animals under chloroform anesthesia. Heart 4:319–378
20. Lown B, Wolf M (1971) Approaches to sudden death from coronary heart disease. Circulation 44:130
21. Lown B, Verrier RL, Rabinowitz SH (1977) Neural and psychologic mechanisms and the problem of sudden cardiac death. Am J Cardiol 39:890–902
22. McEachern G, Manning GW, Hall GE (1940) Sudden occlusion of coronary arteries following removal of cardiosensory pathways. Arch Intern Med 65:661–670
23. Muscholl E, Rahn KH (1966) Nachweis von alpha-Methylnoradrenalin im Harn von Hypertonikern während einer Behandlung mit alpha-Methyldopa. Klin Wochenschr 44:1412–1413
24. Otto HL (1927) Über die Beziehungen der Accelerantes zu den Folgen der Unterbindung von Coronargefäßen. Arch Ges Physiol 217:528–530
25. Pearle DL, Gillis RA (1974) Effect of digitalis on response of the ventricular pacemaker to sympathetic neural stimulation and to isoproterenol. Am J Cardiol 34: 704–710
26. Philippu A, Schuemann HJ (1965) Effect of alpha-methyldopa, alpha-methyldopamine, and alphamethylnorepinephrine on the norepinephrine content of the isolated heart. Life Sci 4:2039–2046
27. Podrid JP (1985) Treatment of ventricular arrhythmia. Applications and limitations of noninvasive vs invasive approach. Chest 88:121–128
28. Rabinowitz SH, Verrier RL, Lown B (1976) Muscarinic effects of vagosympathetic trunk stimulation on the repetive extrasystole (RE) threshold. Circulation 53:622–627
29. Ruberman W, Weinblatt E, Goldberg JD, Frank CW, Shapiro S (1977): Ventricular premature beats and mortality after myocardial infarction. N Engl J Med 279:750–757
30. Ruberman W, Weinblatt E, Goldberg J, Frank CW (1980): Sudden death of myocardial infarction: runs of ventricular premature beats and R-on-T as high risk factors (abstr). Am J Cardiol 45:444
31. Shumaker HB, Riberl A, Boone RD, et al. (1954) Ventricular fibrillation in the hypothermic state. IV. The role of extrinsic cardiac innervation. Ann Surg 143:223–229
32. Verrier RL, Calvert A, Lown B (1975) Effect of posterior hypothalamic stimulation on the ventricular fibrillation threshold. Am J Physiol 228:923

Hemodynamic Effects of Amrinone and Changes in Norepinephrine (NE) Plasma Concentration

D. Jäger[1], A. Machraoui[1], W. Reier[1], J. Gude[1], G. Johannsen[2], and J. Barmeyer[1]

[1] Department of Cardiology and [2] Institute of Clinical Chemistry and Laboratory of Medicine, University Medical School "Bergmannsheil" Bochum, FRG

Key words: Amrinone – Norephrine – Hemodynamic effects

Introduction

Plasma NE concentration of patients with severe heart failure (NYHA class (III-)IV) was found to be about three times higher than it was evaluated in those patients with normal hemodynamic function or mild heart failure (NYHA class I and II) [1, 2], and there is a negative correlation between circulating catecholamines and myocardial beta-receptor density [2, 3, 4]; treatment of severe heart failure with catecholamines will be rather ineffectiv.

Amrinone, a nonglycoside and noncatecholamine cardiotonic agent with combined positiv inotropic and vasodilating properties improves hemodynamic function in most of the cases of "refractory" heart failure without stimulating down regulated beta receptors [5].

Methods

12 patients, aged 35 to 63 years, with heart failure class III (n = 3) or IV (n = 9) caused by advanced coronary artery disease and/or hypertension were included in the study. Hemodynamic testing was performed at baseline and 20 minutes after the intravenous administration of amrinone (bolus injection, 1.5 mg/kg). NE plasma concentration also had been estimated at baseline and 20 minutes after administration of amrinone. All patients received optimal doses of digitalis, diuretics and vasodilators.

Results

Bolus injection of amrinone caused increase in cardiac output and stroke volume index significantly by 33% and 27% respectivly. Pulmonary capillary wedge pressure was not decreased significantly: 11%; but amrinone decreased mean right atrial pressure significantly by 22%. Heart rate and arterial blood pressure both remained unaltered. Futhermore we evaluated decrease in NE plasma level also significantly by 26%. In mild heart failure (NYHA I and II) NE plasma concentration was 390 (±100) pg/ml (normally <500 pg/ml), in our study group NE plasma level ranged at 1160 (±345) pg/ml).

Table 1. Hemodynamic Changes After Intravenous Amrinone Bolus Injection (12 Patients; NYHA III: n = 3; NYHA IV: n = 9)

	Control	Amrinone (1.5 mg/kg)
CI (l/min/m^2)	1.77 ± 0.50	2.36 ± 0.55[a]
SVI (ml/m^2)	19.5 ± 6.8	24.8 ± 7.4[a]
HR (beats/min)	93 ± 19	98 ± 22[b]
SAP (mmHg)	111 ± 6	118 ± 15[b]
DAP (mmHg)	75 ± 5	76 ± 6[b]
PCWP (mmHg)	29.7 ± 7.0	26.3 ± 7.6[b]
RAP (mmHg)	13.6 ± 4.7	10.6 ± 3.6[a]
SO2PA (%)	50.3 ± 10.5	61.4 ± 9.8[a]
NE (pg/ml)	1160 ± 345	859 ± 246[a]

[a] $p < 0.05$; [b] p not significant
CI = cardiac index; DAP = diastolic arterial pressure; HR = heart rate; NE = plasma norepinephrine concentration; PCWP = mean pulmonary capillary wedge pressure; RAP = mean right atrial pressure; SAP = systolic arterial pressure; SO2PA = central venous O2 saturation; SVI = stroke volume index

Discussion

Most hemodynamic parameters improved significantly when amrinone was administered by bolus injection in 12 patients with severe heart failure which were chronicly treated with digitalis, diuretics and vasodilators. Hemodynamic improvement was found contrarily to decrease in NE plasma concentration, this finally will lead to increase density of beta receptors (μp regulation) in the sarcolemmal membrane.

References

1. Chatterjee K (1984) Angiotensin-Conversions-Enzym-Hemmer (ACE-Hemmer) bei Herzinsuffizienz. In: Sobel B, Julien D, Hugenholtz P (eds) Perspectives in Cardiology. Current Medical Literature Ltd., London, pp 178–180
2. Lehmann M, Rühle K, Schmid P, Klein H (1983) Hämodynamik, Plasmakatecholaminverhalten und Beta-Rezeptoren-Dichte bei Trainierten, Untrainierten und Herz-Insuffizienten. Z Kardiol 72:529–536
3. Baumann G, Riess G (1982) Verhalten kardialer Beta-Rezeptoren bei akutem Myokardinfarkt und chronischem Herzversagen. Mögliche Rolle von H2-Rezeptor-Agonisten im katecholamin-refraktären Myokard. Herz/Kreisl 14:169–178
4. Drici MD, Sbirrazzuoli V, Gibelin P, Kreitmann P, Candito P, Baudouy M, Lapolus P, Morand P (1988) Human myokardium beta adrenoreceptor regulation: relationship between density and norepinephrine Plasma Levels. Eur Heart J 9, [Suppl]:115
5. Honerjäger P , Schäfer-Korting M, Reiter M (1981) Involvement of cyclic AMP in the direct inotropic action of amrinone. Naunyn Schmiedebergs Arch Pharmacol 318:112–120

Catecholamine-Induced Cardiomyopathy Caused by Abuse of Ephedrine

D. Meyer, R. Winterhoff, U. Stierle, K. Sack, and A. Sheikhzadeh

Clinic of Cardiology and Clinic of Internal Medicine, University of Lübeck, FRG

Key words: Catecholamine – Ephedrine – Cardiomyopathy

It is well-known that pheochromocytoma, a catecholamine-releasing tumor, may produce cardiomyopathy with symptoms like cardiac enlargement, congestive heart failure and tachycardia. In most cases this condition is reversible after treatment. We want to report a case of reversible severe cardiomyopathy due to catecholamine (ephedrine) abuse.

Case Report

A 41 year-old female was admitted to our hospital because of biventricular heart failure which has lasted for at least 6 months. History reported abuse of a drug containing ephedrine and theophylline for more than ten years because of bronchial asthma. Physical examination revealed a patient in a marked reduced state. Striking were the marked edema in the lower extremities combined with distended neck veins. Edematous infiltrations of the eyelids as well as pronounced anasarca were also present. Auscultation revealed a soft S_1 with a pronounced P_2 and a gallop rhythm. A 2/6 apical systolic murmur and a 1–2/6 systolic murmur at the lower right sternal border with positive Carvallo sign were noticed. Dyspnoe and pulmonary rales as sign of pulmonary congestion were not present. The liver was enlarged. The heart rate was 112 bpm and arterial blood pressure 180/80 mmHg. ECG demonstrated regular sinus rhythm with unspecific ST-T changes. Chest X-ray revealed cardiomegaly with signs of pulmonary hypertension and pulmonary congestion. Echocardiography yielded the following results: LVEDD 53 mm, LVESD 44 mm, fractional shortening 17%, ES-distance 18 mm, DE-amplitude 15 mm; Interventricular septum: enddiastolic 15 mm, endsystolic 15 mm; posterior wall: endsystolic 10 mm, enddiastolic 14 mm; RV enddiastolic 27 mm. Catheterization showed a dilated LV with increased LVEDV and LVESV, ejection fraction was 22%. Mitral and tricuspid regurgitation were present.

Hemodynamic parameters: LVEDP 40 mmHg, PAP 70/40 (50) mmHg. A diastolic plateau in all cardiac chembers was recorded. The overshoot in the Valsalva maneuver was absent.

The laboratory findings were normal except the following: potassium 3.12 mval/l, creatinine 172 μmol/l, creatine kinase 114 U/l, HBDH 270 U/l, LDH 494 U/l, elevated α2-globuline fraction, aldosterone 845 μg/l, theophylline blood level 26 μg/ml.

Blood gas analysis revealed a reduced arterial oxygen saturation of 64%. In the 24-hour collected urine vanillylmandelic acid was 8.4 mg/24 h (normal < 6 mg/24 h) and catecholamine 147 μg/day (normal < 100 μg/day). An infection including a viral cause as well as a systemic disease could be excluded by several laboratory investigations.

One year after termination of the ephedrine abuse all clinical, electrocardiographic and echocardiographic findings returned to normal. The patient is now pregnant in the 24th week.

Comment

This report demonstrates a severe dilated and restricted cardiomyopathy caused by ephedrine which has been reported to our knowledge only once in literature [1]. Van Mieghem et al. had nearly similar findings in their patient who had complete recovery from his symptoms of cardiac failure within two years. Fundamentally for the development of an ephedrine-induced cardiomyopathy is a longstanding regular intake of this drug in a dosage which is much higher than the therapeutic one. The regular dose is 15–30 mg/day for the treatment of asthmatic complaints [2]. Our patient had a daily ingestion of 150 mg ephedrine for more than ten years which was responsible for her cardiomyopathy. This pathologic reaction was aggravated by the fact that the same drug

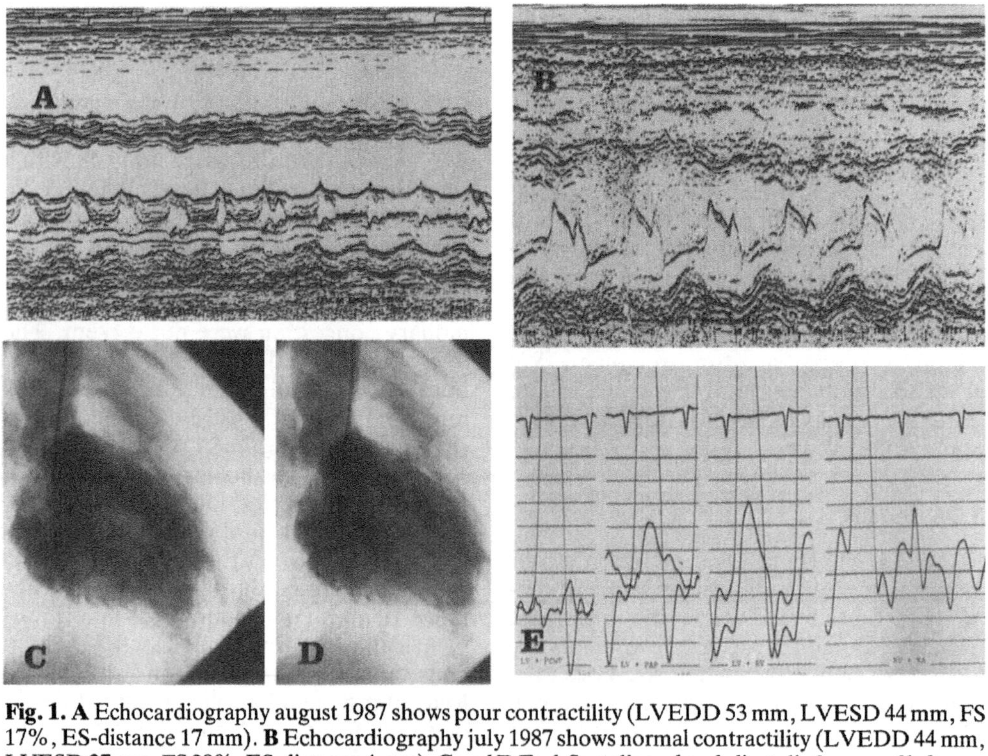

Fig. 1. A Echocardiography august 1987 shows pour contractility (LVEDD 53 mm, LVESD 44 mm, FS 17%, ES-distance 17 mm). **B** Echocardiography july 1987 shows normal contractility (LVEDD 44 mm, LVESD 27 mm, FS 39%, ES-distance 4 mm). **C** and **D** End-Systolic and end-diastolic frames of left ventricular angiography: EF 22%. **E** Hemodynamic parameter shows extremely elevated right ventricular and left ventricular end-diastolic pressures

combination also contained theophylline which is well-known for its cardiotoxic enhancement of the ephedrine toxicity. The total amount of daily intake of theophylline was in the normal range (750 md/day). The patient of van Mieghem et al. had taken ephedrine for more than 15 years with progressive increase of dosage to about 400 mg/day which is much more than our patient has ingested.

From these both reports we can draw the conclusion that continuous intake of toxic ephedrine doses may lead to severe cardiomyopathy which is completely reversible after withdrawal of the drug.

The mechanism which causes this type of cardiomyopathy seems to be an excessive stimulation of the noradrenergic system. A similar clinical picture can be seen in patients with pheochromocytoma [3, 4].

The pronounced sympathetic stimulation has been documented in our patient by the elevated blood level catecholamines in the collected 24-hour urine sample. The exact pathologic mechanism and its clinical implications have been reported elsewhere [1].

References

1. Van Mieghem W, Stevens E, Cosemans J (1978) Ephedrine-induced cardiomyopathy. Br Med J I:816
2. Weiner N (1985) Norepinephrine, epinephrine and the sympathetic amines. In: Goodman and Gilman (eds) The pharmaceutical basis of therapeutics. MacMillan, New York, Toronto and London, p 169
3. Szczeklik A, Nigankowski R, Uruk J (1977) Myocardial infarction in status asthmaticus. Lancet I:658–659
4. Sheikhzadeh A, Fatourechi V, Paydar D, Nazarian I (1983) Unusual cardiovascular manifestations in a case of pheochromocytoma. Clin Cardiol 6:136–142

The Heart in Various Endocrine Systems

Cardiac Function in Adrenal Insufficiency – An Echocardiographic Study

R. Griebenow, L. Krämer, U. Frangenberg, B. Allolio, D. Kaulen, W. Winkelmann, and W. Kaufmann

Medizinische Universitätsklinik II, Köln, FRG

Key words: Adrenal insufficiency – Cardiac function – Echocardiography

Though it is not known that physiological concentrations of cortisol directly influence cardiac function corticosteroids may by their multiple interactions with other hormones important for the cardiovascular system have an indirect effect on cardiac performance (Kunos et al. 1980; Bakiri et al. 1983; Whitworth et al. 1985). It was the aim of this study to investigate systolic and diastolic left ventricular function noninvasively by echocardiography in patients with adrenal insufficiency.

Patients and Methods

Six patients (5 female, 1 male, mean age: 34.5 years) with adrenal insufficiency (M. Addsion: 5, after operative removal of a crainiopharyngeoma: 1) have been studied by two-dimensional echocardiography. Echocardiograms have been taken in the left lateral position at rest and were registered as double-M-mode echocardiograms at the level of the aorta and the left ventricle (100 mm/s). Computer-aided evaluation of the echocardiograms was performed according to the methods described by Traill and Gibson (1979). Cortisol was determined by RIA (NEN). All patients were not in overt Addsion crisis but had deteriorated because of inadequate substitution therapy and showed circadian variations of cortisol concentrations which did not exceed 1 μ/100 ml (normal: 12.8 ± 6.4 μg/100 ml). For comparison a group of 24 healthy volunteers has been studied (22 male, 2 female, mean age: 23 years).

Results

	Adrenal insufficiency	Normals		p
HR	75 ± 17	66 ± 10	min^{-1}	ns
RR_s	110 ± 18	124 ± 10	mmHg	0.005
RR_d	71 ± 10	73 ± 8	mmHg	ns
PEP	90 ± 14	85 ± 14	ms	ns
LVET	276 ± 49	303 ± 17	ms	ns
EDD	49 ± 7	50 ± 4	mm	ns
ESD	33 ± 4	32 ± 3	mm	ns
dD/dt_s	10.0 ± 0.8	10.6 ± 1.6	cm/s	ns
FS	32 ± 5	37 ± 5	%	ns
IVR	74 ± 21	61 ± 13	ms	ns
FP	394 ± 120	479 ± 117	ms	0.05
RFP	94 ± 17	102 ± 30	ms	ns
dD/dt_d	18.4 ± 3.6	17.8 ± 4.1	cm/s	ns

(x ± sd)
dD/dt: maximal velocity of systolic (s) and diastolic (d) change in LV-diameter
(RFP: (rapid) filling period)

Discussion

Arterial hypotension is a frequent clinical finding in patients with adrenal insufficiency (Nerup 1974). In our group systolic blood pressure was significantly lower than in the normal controls but was well above those values found in Addison's crisis. This finding and the normal values for enddiastolic left ventricular dimension indicate that hormone substitution (cortisone and mineralocorticoids) has already had a substantial effect leading to normalization of intravascular volume (Falkheden ans Sjögren 1964), though the clinical status had not completely returned to normal. As might be expected form these data indicating normal preload and reduced afterload we were not able to demonstrate any sign of systolic functional impairment in our patients with adrenal insufficiency. This is in accordance with the results of Knowlton and Baer (1983) who have shown that in patients with Addison's disease the occurrence of cardiac failure cannot be related to the hormonal disorder. Up to now there are no data on diastolic left ventricular filling in adrenal insufficiency. In our group of patients we were not able to demonstrate any abnormality of diastolic left ventricular filling as studied by echocardiography.

References

1. Bakiri F, Benmiloud M, Vallotton MB (1983) The renin-angiotensin system in panhypopituitarism dynamic studies and therapeutic effects in Sheehan's syndrome. J Clin Endocrinol Soc 56:1042–1047
2. Falkheden Th, Sjögren B (1964) Extracellular fluid volume and renal function in pituitary insufficiency and acromegaly. Acta Endocrinol 46:80–88
3. Knowlton AI, Baer L (1983) Cardiac failure in Addision's disease. Am J Med 74:829–836
4. Kunos G, Mucci L, O'Regan (1980) The influence of hormonal and neuronal factors on rat heart adrenoceptors. Br J Pharmacol 71: 371–386
5. Nerup J (1974) Addison's Disease – clinical studies – A report of 108 cases. Acta Endocrinol 76:127–1411
6. Traill TA, Gibson DG (1979) Left ventricular relaxation and filling: study by echocardiography. In: Yu PN, Goodwin JF (eds) Progress in cardiology, vol 8. Lea & Febiger, Philadelphia, pp 39–71
7. Whitworth JA, Butty J, Saines D, Scoggins B, Thatcher R (1985) The effects of ACTH on the renin-aldosterone system in normotensive man. Clin Exp Hypertension 7:1361–1376

Atrial Natriuretic Peptide (ANP) in Syndrome of Inappropriate Antidiuretic Hormone Secretion (SIADH)*

P. Gross[1], M. Ketteler[1], C. Hausmann[1], A. Schömig[1], and R. Lang[2]

[1] Departments of Medicine and [2] Pharmacology[1], University of Heidelberg, Heidelberg, FRG

Key words: Atrial natriuretic peptide – Hyponatremia – Syndrome of inappropriate ADH secretion

Introduction

The syndrome of inappropriate antidiuretic hormone secretion (SIADH) is a state of disturbed body fluid volume homeostasis and altered sodium balance [1]. The potential role of atrial natriuretic peptide (ANP) as an indicator of the alterations of body fluid volume in SIADH or as a mediator of the associated negative sodium balance has not been evaluated systematically.

Methods

We therefore studied 15 patients with SIADH of different etiologies. Our evaluation included the following:

* Part of this data has been reported in a manuscript which is currently in press by the European Journal of Clinical Investigation.

Table 1. General observations in 15 patients with SIADH

	Plasma sodium concentration (mM/l)	Plasma osmolality (mosm/kg H_2O)	Plasma urea concentration (mg/dl)	Plasma creatinine concentration (mg/dl)	Plasma urate concentration (mg/dl)	Urinary sodium concentration (mM/l)
SIADH (n = 15)	126.5 ± 0.8	264 ± 2	19.1 ± 1.6	0.76 ± 0.06	3.0 ± 0.3	82 ± 8.5

1. a history and a complete physical examination;
2. an evaluation of the patient's medical record;
3. a standardized blood sample obtained at approximately 8.30 a.m. after a 40 min. period of supervised rest in the supine position;
4. a 24 h-urinary collection.

Criteria to Diagnose SIADH

In accordance with established literature [6] we used the following criteria:

a) presence of hyponatremia together with hypoosmolality;
b) urine less than maximally dilute (maximal dilution: approximately 50 mosm/kg H_2O);
c) urinary sodium concentration >30 mM/l;
d) no treatment by diuretics;
e) no evidence of cardiac failure, cirrhosis of the liver, volume contraction or drug induced hyponatremia;
f) presence of an underlying illness compatible with SIADH;
g) presence of a normal plasma creatinine concentration (0.5–1.1 mg/dl and a low or normal plasma urate concentration (<4 mg/dl).

Specific Measurements

Plasma renin activity (PRA; normal range of values in our laboratory: 0.2–2 ng AI/ml × h), plasma aldosterone concentrations (PA; normal range: 2–10 ng/dl) and plasma concentrations of arginine vasopressin (AVP, normal range 3–7 pg/ml at a normal plasma osmolality) were all determined by sensitive radioimmunoassays as described previously [4]. Plasma concentrations of norepinephrine (NE; normal range: 0.5–2 nM/l) were determined radioenzymatically as described [4]. Plasma ANP was measured by RIA as described [4, 7]. In 48 healthy medical students ANP was 13.4 ± (SEM) 1.2 fM/ml by this RIA. In 14 patients with advanced hyponatremic heart failure (NYHA: stages III and IV) ANP was 35.2 ± 6 fM/ml by this RIA.

Results

The underlying illnesses of the 15 patients with SIADH were the following: CNS disease (n = 5); pulmonary disease (n = 5); oropharyngeal carcinoma (n = 4); other (n = 1).

Mean age was 58 ± 1 years (ratio females/males: 6/9). At the time of study patients had been in the hospital for a mean of 13 days. During this time, the degree of hyponatremia and patients' body weight had both remained stable. Measured oral fluid intake was 2.25 ± 0.21/24 h in patients with SIADH.

Results of laboratory measurements are in Tables 1 and 2.

Table 2. Specific observations in 15 patients with SIADH

	PRA (ng AI/ml × h)	Plasma aldosterone concentration (ng/dl)	Plasma norepinephrine concentration (nM/l)	Plasma AVP concentration (pg/ml)	Plasma ANP concentration (fM/ml)
SIADH (n = 15)	1.1 ± 0.2	7.7 ± 0.5	2.02 ± 0.2	7.9 ± 2	18.5 ± 2.4

Discussion

In the 15 patients of our study the criteria of SIADH quoted above were fully met. AVP was 7.9 ± pg/ml in the presence of hypo-osmolality, a value that is compatible with SIADH. Therefore our study provided an adequate data base to examine plasma ANP in SIADH.

Individual case reports in the literature have indicated elevated ANP in SIADH [2]. In fact, such would be an attractive concept with respect to the alterations of body fluid volume and negative sodium balance of SIADH. Furthermore a direct stimulation of ANP by AVP in the heart [5] and an antagonism between AVP and ANP in the collecting duct of the kidney [3] have been shown; this may be considered as further suggestive evidence of a significant relationship between both hormones.

However, we found ANP of this SIADH to be no different from normal control. We have no proven explanation for the discrepancy between findings. Clearly, our assay was able to detect elevated ANP, as demonstrated in hyponatremic heart failure. A potential explanation may be related to the duration and stability of the observed SIADH.

In our study, the observed patients had suffered SIADH for a period of at least 13 days and possibly much longer. The observed stability of their hyponatremia may be an indication of a relatively stable new balance of water metabolism achieved and maintained chronically in this SIADH. It is therefore possible that the chronicity of this SIADH is associated with a degree of ANP stimulation which is different from that of acute SIADH, i.e. before the achievement of stable water balance.Thus, elevated ANP was mainly described in response to acute volume changes [2].

Therefore, studies of ANP in response to acute volume load in chronic stable SIADH should also be undertaken to broaden the scope of the unexpected findings presented above.

Acknowledgements: We are indebted to Prof. W. Fiehn for his laboratory support of the study, to Prof. E. Hackenthal for his measurements of PRA, to Prof. P. Vecsei for measuring aldosterone and to Prof. W. Rascher, Essen, FRG, for measuring AVP.

References

1. Bartter FC, Schwartz WB (1967) The syndrome of inappropriate secretion of antidiuretic hormone. Am J Med 42:790–806
2. Cogan E, DeBieve MF, Pepersack T, Abramow M (1986) High plasma levels of atrial natriuretic factor in SIADH. N Engl J Med 314:1258–1259
3. Dillingham MA, Anderson RJ (1986) Inhibition of vasopressin by atrial natriuretic factor. Science 231:1572–1573
4. Gross P, Ketteler M, Hausmann C, Reinhard C, Schömig A, Hackenthal E, Ritz E, Rascher W (1988) Role of diuretics, hormonal derangements, and clinical setting of hyponatremia in medical patients. Klin Wochenschr 66:662–669
5. Manning PT, Schwartz D, Katsube NC, Holmberg SW (1985) Vasopressin stimulated release of atriopeptide: endocrine antagonists in fluid homeostasis. Science 229:395–397
6. Martinez-Maldonado M (1980) Inappropriate antidiuretic hormone secretion of unknown origin. Kidney Int 17:554–567
7. Rascher W, Tulassay T, Lang RE (1985) Atrial natriuretic peptide in plasma of volume-overloaded children with chronic renal failure. Lancet II:303–305

Effects of Vasopressin on the Canine Coronary Circulation: Evidence for a Small Vessel Constrictor Action and Modulation of Vascular Control

D. Franzen, M. Zhao, R. Forman, and C. Eng

Medizinische Klinik III, University of Cologne, FRG and Department of Cardiology, Albert Einstein College, New York, USA

Key words: Vasopressin – Autoregulation – Coronary flow

The effects of vasopressin on cardiovascular dynamics and myocardial oxygen metabolism have been extensively studied by Nakano (1967). Decreased coronary flow and myocardial contractile force following vasopressin infusion were shown to be due to its vasoconstrictor effect. A specific and selective vasoconstrictor action on small coronary vessels was suggested by Altura using direct in vivo microscopy (1973).

In the following study the implications of a (predominant) small vessel vasoconstrictor action of vasopressin were tested on transmural blood flow distribution, coronary reserve and coronary autoregulation.

Intracoronary infusion of vasopressin in open-chest dogs resulted in a uniform reduction of basal coronary blood flow in the subepicardial-, the mid- and the subendocardial layer using the microsphere method. Systemic hemodynamics were not affected. This unique feature of a uniform transmural flow reduction by vasopressin is in marked contrast to the transmural flow gradient created by a decrease in flow due to a stenosis of an epicardial coronary vessel or a large vessel constrictor. The findings suggest that the small vessel vasoconstrictor action of vasopressin resulted in a uniform transmural flow reduction.

The decrease in flow following infusion of vasopressin resulted in ischemia as shown by decrease in myocardial contractile force and by lactate production in the local vein blood and myocardial tissue. Despite ischemia, the coronary bed demonstrated a reactive hyperemic response to a 15 second coronary occlusion. Thus, the coronary system exhibited significant reserve at a time when both flow and contractility were decreased (ischemia). However, when coronary flow was decreased to a comparable level by a stenosis (screw clamp) or constriction (phenylephrine) of a large coronary artery, the reactive hyperemic response was completely abolished.

The autoregulatory response during vasopressin infusion was studied constructing pressure-flow relationships by varying the coronary inflow pressure. Despite ischemia, the coronary bed retained its ability to regulate coronary blood flow or to defend a given level of coronary flow over a range of coronary perfusion pressures. This is in contrast to the metabolic theory of autoregulation (e.g. the adenosine hypothesis) and suggests a role for a myogenic mechanism.

The observation that vasopressin exerts a special effect on the actual site of vascular control (autoregulation) is extended by our findings on the effect of vasopressin on a maximally vasodilated bed produced by i.v. carbochromen or i.c. adenosine. Vasopressin infusion in a previous passive, e.g. non-regulating vascular bed resulted in restoration of autoregulation. Phenylephrine infusion in a maximal vasodilated bed decreased coronary flow, however it did not restore autoregulation.

The presented findings suggest that vasopressin is a small vessel constrictor. In addition, it obtains a unique property to modulate the actual site of vascular control in the coronary circulation by maintaining autoregulation during ischemia and by restoring autoregulation in a previous non-regulating coronary bed.

References

Altura BM (1973) Selective microvascular constrictor actions of some neurohypophyseal peptides. Eur J Pharm 24:49–60

Nakano J (1967) Studies on the cardiovascular effects of synthetic vasopressin. J Pharmacol Exp Ther 157/1:19–31

Angiotensin I Forming Angiotensinogenases (Renin-Like Enzymes) in the Heart – Evidence for Their Location in the Coronaries*

H. Dahlheim, M. Thurnreiter, M. Plaschke, W. Reiter, I. Durasin, and J. Rosenthal

Department of Physiology, University of Munich and Ulm University Medical Center, FRG

Key words: Renin-angiotensin system – Heart – Fast protein liquid chromatography

Introduction

Previous investigations demonstrated the presence of renin or renin-like enzymes (angiotensin I forming angiotensinogenases = AIFAs) in the heart. Other studies indicated the existence of similar enzymes in extracardiac (extrarenal) vascular walls (for a comprehensive survey see [1]). – The question thus arises whether the AIFAs demonstrated in the heart are contained in the coronaries. The present study was designed to identify and biochemically characterize AIFAs in cardiac tissues of the rat and to compare them with the enzymes in extracardiac (extrarenal) vascular walls. For this purpose, Fast Protein Liquid Chromatography (FPLC) of cardiac AIFAs and extracardiac (extrarenal) vascular wall AIFAs was applied and the pH optima of the separated enzymes measured.

Methods

Sprague-Dawley rats (230–330 g body weight) of either sex were used. Preparation of tissue extracts and measurements of enzyme activities have been previously described [3, 4]. AIFA activities were determined by the angiotensin I radioimmunoassay using purified rat angiotensinogen as substrate. FPLC techniques (Pharmacia, Uppsala, Sweden) were used for separation and characterization of the enzymes. (Anion exchanger: Q-Sepharose fast flow; column: HR 10/10; buffer system: 0.02 M TRIS/0.02 M TRIS + 1 M NaCl, pH 7.4; Isochromatofocusing: Mono P; column: HR 5/20; start buffer: 0.025 M BISTRIS, pH 7.1; elution buffer: Polybuffer 74 (Pharmacia), pH 4.05).

Results

Three pH optima (5.6; 5.1; 4.0) were found for cardiac AIFAs. Separation of these enzymes was achieved subsequently by FPLC anion exchange chromatography (elution volume: 21.0 ml (pH optimum 5.6), 13.0 ml (pH optimum 5.1), 24.3 ml (pH optimum 4.0). AIFA-5.6 (pH optimum at 5.6) was contained mainly in ventricles, AIFA-5.1 predominantly in atria and in the remaining tissues of the heart. AIFA-4.0 was located in atria, but to a lesser extent than AIFA-5.1, and was also present in plasma. Highest cardiac AIFA activity (in ng AI/g · h) was found in septum 266 ± 148, n = 7; left ventricle 224 ± 55, n = 8; right ventricle 189 ± 24, n = 8; atria/auricles 227 ± 65, n = 6. Significantly lower values were obtained for SHR: left ventricle 136 ± 27, n = 8, $p < 0.01$; right ventricle 120 ± 6.5, n = 8, $p < 0.01$. For atrial AIFAs seven isoelectric points (6.5; 6.2; 5.9; 5.7; 5.2; 4.95; 4.8) were measured.

Discussion

The data obtained demonstrate the existence of several AIFAs in cardiac tissues of the rat. Since the pH optima and FPLC elution volumes of cardiac tissue and extracardiac (extrarenal) vascular wall enzymes were found to be identical, we assume that the cardiac enzymes are located in the coronaries. In view of the pH optima and FPLC elution volumes, (ventricular) AIFA-5.6 is identical with the enzyme present in extracardiac arteries and (atrial)

* Supported by the "Deutsche Forschungsgemeinschaft"

AIFA-5.1 with that enzyme contained in veins of normotensive rats. AIFA-5.1 was also observed in isolated aortic smooth muscle cells of the rat and its activity is distinctly elevated in arterial walls of SHR [3, 4]. The number of isoelectric points found indicate that there are more than 3 cardiac AIFAs. Five of these isoelectric points were also obtained by Kim et al. [2] for AIFAs present in plasma and kidney of the rat. The authors further demonstrated that the enzymes affect renal function when intravenously administered. We assume that there is an intrinsic RAS in the heart which is located in coronaries and which participates in control of coronary blood flow. The therapeutic effects of ACE-inhibitors on cardiac function may be mediated by these enzymes. The presence of AIFAs in extravascular cardiac structures cannot be excluded by the present study.

References

1. Dahlheim H, Jacob ICM, Pschorr J, Rosenthal J (1983) The renin-angiotensin system in the extrarenal vascular walls: an approach to studies in humans. In: Fotherby K, Pal SB (eds) Hormones in normal and abnormal tissues, vol III. Walter de Gruyter, Berlin, pp 251–284
2. Kim SH, Lloyd MC, Sessler FM, Feng J, Malvin RL (1988) Functional differences of six forms of renin in rats. Am J Physiol 254: F432–F439
3. Rosenthal J, Pfeifle B, Michailov ML, Pschorr J, Jacob ICM, Dahlheim H (1984) Investigations of components of the renin-angiotensin system in rat vascular tissue. Hypertension 6:383–390
4. Rosenthal J, v Lutterotti N, Thurnreiter M, Gomba S, Rothemund J, Reiter W, Kazda S, Garthoff B, Jacob I, Dahlheim H (1987) Suppression of renin-angiotensin system in the heart of spontaneously hypertensive rats. J Hypertension 5 [Suppl 2]:23–31

Regulation of Atrial Natriuretic Peptide in Primary Aldosteronism and in Cushing's Disease

G. Opocher, S. Rocco, G. Carpenè, M. Scarante, and F. Mantero^

Institute of Semeiotica Medica, University of Padua, and Institute of Clinica Medica III, University of Catania, Italy

Key words: ANF – Aldosteronism – Cushing's disease

Supine posture and volume expansion stimulate Atrial Natriuretic Peptide (ANF) secretion by atrial myocytes (Espiner and Nicholls 1987). In primary aldosteronism (PA), a condition of chronic hypervolemia, ANF has been found increased; however, the differences of ANF levels and its regulation in the two main forms of primary aldosteronism, aldosterone producing adenoma (APA) and idiopathic aldosteronism (IHA) are still unknown.

The secretion of ANF seems to be stimulated also by glucocorticoids. This seems to be due to a direct effect on gene expression since and is present in vitro, in cultured atrial myocytes of rats (Matsubara et al. 1987) and in vivo, in rats (Gardner et al. 1986). In normal subjects, cortisol or ACTH long term administration can enhance ANF plasma levels (Connel et al. 1987) but in condition of chronic glucocorticoid hypersecretion, as in Cushing's syndrome, the determinations of ANF levels gave partially contradictory results (Naruse et al. 1987; Sugawara et al. 1988; Yamaji et al. 1988). In order to clarify these points, we have studied 14 patients affected by primary aldosteronism (7 APA and 7 IHA) and 8 patients affected by Cushing's disease of pituitary origin: any therapy had been withdrawn from at least 2 weeks. The patients were overnight fasting and in recumbent position from at least two hours. The study protocol was the following:

Postural test: The patients were fasting from midnight, and placed in supine position from 06.00 a.m. until 08.00 a.m., then they assumed upright posture until 10.00 a.m. and were in supine again for 15 minutes. At the end of each time blood samples for determination of aldosterone, PRA and ANF were drawn.

Saline load test: At 08.00 a.m. to the patients sitting in easy comfortable position, a saline isotonic solution was infused at rate of 8.4 ml/min for 240 minutes. Plasma aldosterone, PRA and ANF were determined before and after saline load (NaCl 0.9% 2 l in 4 hours).

Spironolactone therapy were aso studied in three patients (2 with APA and one with IHA) after treatment with spironolactone 200 mg per os daily for 30 days.

Surgery: The effect of adrenalectomy on ANF postural and saline load response was also evaluated in patients with APA. Plasma and urinary aldosterone (Aldoctk and Aldok, Sorin, Italy), PRA (Renctk, Sorin, Italy), plasma cortisol (Kit DPC, USA) were measured by RIA; ACTH was assayed by a specific IRMA (Euro-Diagnostic, BV, Holland). Plasma ANF was measured by radioimmunoassay after Sep Pak C_{18} cartridges purification using the following procedure: venous blood was collected in iced polypropilene tubes containing Na-Eparine and stored at $-20°C$ after centrifugation at 4°C; plasma samples were applied to previously activated cartridges, washed with Buffer and eluted with 2 ml of Methanol/Trifluoroacetic acid 0.1% solution. The recovery of ^{125}I alpha human ANF was 79.1 ± 13.9, $n = 48$. The radioimmunoassay was performed using ^{125}I alpha human ANF from Amersham (UK) and a specific anti alpha human ANF from Peninsula Lab. (USA). The sensitivity (ED 80) was 9.0 ± 1.2 pg, the intraassay C.V. was $8.8 \pm 4.6\%$, $n = 38$ and the interassay was $14.4 \pm 3.0\%$, $n = 38$. Normal values: supine 25 ± 12, upright 16 ± 7 pg/ml $n = 16$.

The results were expressed as mean ± S.E. Statistical analysis was performed using one-way analysis of variance and Student t test.

Similarly to other reports, (Tunny et al. 1986) even in our patients with primary aldosteronism the basal ANF values were higher than normals (Fig. 1, top). In APA the mean values of ANF are much elevated, whereas in IHA they are only slightly. This could be correlated to the degree of volume expansion, that has been reported more pronounced in APA than in IHA (Lasaridis et al. 1984): in this view ANF could be considered an interesting marker of hypervolemia in primary aldosteronism. The difference of ANF values between APA and IHA could be an additional tool for the differential diagnosis of APA and IHA.

Moreover, in our patients, a direct, significant correlation between basal aldosterone and ANF values is present. Since several reports indicate that glucocorticoids but also DOCA (Weidmann et al. 1988), can directly act on miocytes to stimulate ANF release, a direct relationship between aldosterone and ANF cannot be ruled out. However, after spironolactone, in spite of increased aldosterone values, a decrease of ANF levels was observed; spironolactone increased also PRA, lowered blood pressure, and decreased body weight, suggesting decrease of plasma volume.

As expected, in IHA patients a significant increase of aldosterone with upright posture was observed, while ANF only slightly decreases; in APA, the decrease of ANF in upright posture was evident even if aldosterone did not change; furthermore in both conditions ANF increased shortly after reassuming supine position while aldosterone did not change.

This indicates that the two hormones are independently regulated, in this syndrome. Similarly, a different pattern of the two hormones was observed also after saline load (Fig. 1, bottom). Aldosterone levels were only slightly reduced, whereas ANF increased markedly in both groups, more significantly in IHA than in APA. This could be due to the fact that in APA, ANF secretion is closer to its maximal stimulatory tone; alternatively, chronic ANF hypersecretion which has been involved in the genesis of the "escape phenomenon" would promote a faster sodium excretion after sodium loading, thus blunting further volume expansion. It has been suggested that in normal and essential hypertensive subjects, ANF has a role in the inhibition of aldosterone secretion after saline load. In primary aldosteronism this mechanism does not seem to operate: this could be due to im-

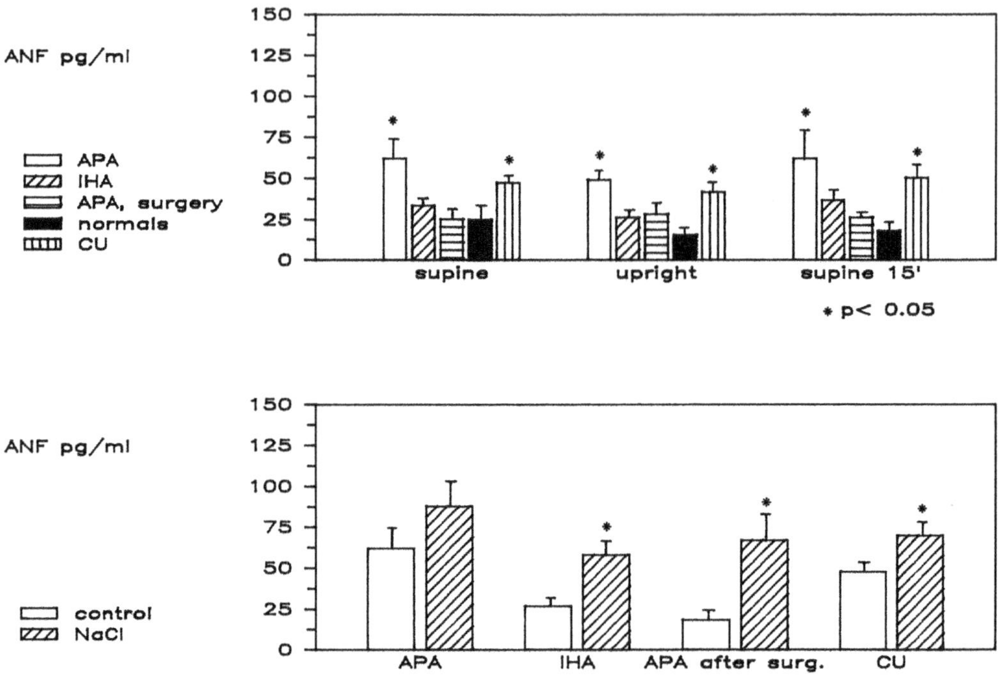

Fig. 1. *Top:* ANF values in patients affected by APA (n = 7), IHA (n = 7), APA after surgery (APA, surgery), Cushing's disease (CU, n = 8) and normal subjects (n = 16). Effect of posture. *Bottom:* Effect of saline infusion on ANF values in patients affected by APA (n = 7), IHA (n = 7) APA after surgery (surg.) (n = 5) and Cushing's disease (CU, n = 8)

paired action of ANF at adrenal level or to suppresion of RAS system as discussed below.

Adrenalectomy was able to decrease blood pressure and normalize aldosterone secretion, PRA and potassium levels: ANF values became normal. Aldosterone and PRA showed a normal regulation after posture and saline load while ANF showed a hyperreactivity to volume expansion (increased sensitivity of atria previously exposed to prolonged stimulation?).

We demonstrated that, in humans, chronic glucocorticoid hypersecretion due to Cushing's disease is associated with elevated ANF values: both in supine and in upright position (47 ± 3.2 and 41.7 ± 5.1 pg/ml, respectively): they are significantly higher than in normal subjects and similar to the levels we found in patients with primary aldosteronism. Saline load significantly stimulated ANF secretion from 47.8 ± 5.1 to 69.9 ± 7.0 pg/ml, $p < 0.05$; no correlation was found between ANF and plasma or urinary cortisol. Our results are in agreement with the results of Yamaji et al. who demonstrated, in a substantial number of patients with Cushing's syndrome, increased plasma levels of Atrial Natriuretic Peptide.

The high levels of ANF in Cushing's disease can be correlated to the hypersecretion of adrenal steroids with sodium retaining action: but recently, it has been observed that chronic administration of prednisone (Weidmann et al. 1988) is associated with a significant elevation of ANF levels without any significant sodium and fluid retention. Volume expansion is not usually present in Cushing's disease (Saruta et al. 1986); moreover, in our patients, plasma renin activity was never suppressed and mineralocorticoid hormones (aldosterone, DOC, B, 18-OH-DOC and 18 OH-B) were in most cases within the normal range. Thus, a lack of a significant mineralocorticoid activity can be hypothesized. Moreover, ANF has been reported to be high or slightly elevated in some forms of hypertension (Sugawara et al. 1988) as a consequence of increased central volume and atrial distention. However, in 3 cases ANF was elevated despite the presence of normal blood pressure and no correlation was found between ANF and blood pressure levels. The postural response of ANF was less evident than in primary aldosteronism, while volume expansion still significantly increased ANF: this can be related to a decreased storage of ANF during chronic stimulation or, in alternative, to a partial insensibility to volume manipulation in Cushing's disease. Our results indicate that the regulation of ANF in these patients is somewhat different to what already reported in normal sujects, in hypertensive and in volume expanded patients.

Since dexamethasone directly stimulates ANF as well as ANF gene expression in rats, in Cushing's syndrome, the chronic glucocorticoid hypersecretion could have a direct effect on ANF secretion; the possibility of a direct action on ANF is supported also by the presence of cardiac glucocorticoid receptors, isolated several years ago (Funder et al. 1973) and whose role is still largely unknown. In conclusion, chronic GC as well as MC excess are associated with increased ANF levels. Basal supine ANF is higher in APA than in IHA and in Cushing's disease. Postural responses are better detectable in PA than in Cushing's disease; saline load increases ANF in each group, but the relative increments are inversely proportional to basal levels. Differences in ANF regulation in adrenal hyperfunctioning states could be related to different haemodynamic patterns and/or to the superimposition of the direct GC effect.

References

Connel JMC, Whitworth JA, Davies DL, Lever AF, Richards AM, Fraser R (1987) Effects of ACTH and cortisol administration on blood pressure, electrolyte metabolism, atrial natriuretic peptide and renal function in normal man. J Hypertension 5:425–433

Espiner EA, Nicholls MG (1987) Human atrial natriuretic peptide. Clin Endocrinol 26: 637–650

Funder JW, Duval D, Meyar F (1973) Cardiac glucocorticoid receptors: the binding of tritiated dexamethasone in rat and dog heart. Endocrinology 93:1300–1307

Gardner DG, Hane S, Trachewsky D, Schenk D, Baxter JD (1986) Atrial natriuretic peptide mRNA is regulated by glucocorticoids in vivo. Biochem Biophys Res Commun 139: 1047–1054

Lasaridis A, Brown JJ, Davies DL, Fraser R, Robertson JIS, Lever AR (1984) Arterial blood pressure and plasma and body electrolytes in idiopathic hyperaldosteronism: a comparison with primary hyperaldosteronism (Conn's syndrome) and essential hypertension. J Hypertens 2:329–336

Matsubara H, Hirata Y, Yoshimi H, Takata S, Takagi Y, Iida T, Yamane Y, Umeda Y, Nishikawa M, Inada M (1987) Effects of steroid and thyroid hormones on synthesis of atrial natriuretic peptide by cultured atrial myocytes of rat. Biochem Biophys Res Commun 145:336–343

Naruse M, Obana K, Naruse K, Yamaguchi H, Demura H, Tadashi I, Shizume K (1987) Atrial natriuretic polypeptide inhibits cortisol secretion as well as aldosterone secretion in vitro from human adrenal tissue. J Clin Endocrinol Metab 654:10–16

Saruta T, Suzuki H, Handa M, Igarashi Y, Kondo K, Senba J (1986) Multiple factors contribute to the pathogenesis of hypertension in Cushing's syndrome. J Clin Endocrinol Metab 62:275–279

Sugawara A, Nakao K, Kono T, Morii N, Yamada T, Itoh H, Shiono S, Saito Y, Mukoyama M, Arai H, Imura H (1988) Atrial natriuretic factor in essential hypertension and adrenal disorders. Hypertension 11 [Suppl I]:I-212–I-216

Tunny TG, Higgins BA, Gordon RD (1986) Plasma levels of atrial natriuretic peptide in primary aldosteronism, Gordon's syndrome and Bartter's syndrome. Clin Exp Pharmacol Physiol 13:341–385

Weidmann P, Matter DR, Matter EE, Gnadinger MP, Uehlinger DE, Shaw S, Hess C (1988) Glucocorticoid and Mineralocorticoid stimulation of atrial natriuretic peptide release in man. J Clin Endocrinol Metab 66:1233–1239

Yamaji T, Ishibashig M, Sekihara H, Takaku F, Nakaoka H, Fujii J (1986) Plasma levels of atrial natriuretic peptice in primary aldosteronism and essential hypertension. J Clin Endocrinol Metab 63:815–818

Yamaji T, Ishibashi M, Yamada A, Takaku F, Itabashi A, Katayama S, Ishii J, Takami M, Fukushima T (1988) Plasma levels of atrial natriuretic hormone in Cushing's syndrome. J Clin Endocrinol Metab 67:348–352

Subject Index

GPSR Compliance

The European Union's (EU) General Product Safety Regulation (GPSR) is a set of rules that requires consumer products to be safe and our obligations to ensure this.

If you have any concerns about our products, you can contact us on ProductSafety@springernature.com

In case Publisher is established outside the EU, the EU authorized representative is:

Springer Nature Customer Service Center GmbH
Europaplatz 3
69115 Heidelberg, Germany

Batch number: 10704771

Printed by Printforce, the Netherlands